Veterinary Techniques in Llamas and Alpacas

Veterinary Techniques in Llamas and Alpacas

Edited by

David E. Anderson, DVM, MS, DACVS
Professor and Associate Dean for Research and Graduate Studies
College of Veterinary Medicine
University of Tennessee Knoxville, Tennessee

Matt Miesner, DVM, MS, DACVIM
Clinical Professor and Section Head Livestock Services
College of Veterinary Medicine
Kansas State University Manhattan, Kansas

Meredyth Jones, DVM, MS, DACVIM
Associate Professor, Farm Animal Medicine and Surgery
College of Veterinary Medicine
Oklahoma State University
Stillwater, Oklahoma

Second Edition

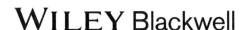

Contents

Preface

Traditional farm animal species are routinely included in veterinary curricula, have immense volumes of published information, and most large animal veterinarians and veterinary technicians possess experience and a general understanding of procedures to be performed on these species. This wealth of resources greatly outweighs that available regarding South American camelids for most veterinarians. South American camelids are increasingly ingrained in modern veterinary culture, but this experience is relatively new—measured in decades versus centuries for that of traditional species. Early on, medical and surgical care was directed toward specialty clinics and veterinarians with special interest. This was largely due to the extreme monetary value of animals and veterinarians' apprehension to treat animals in which they have little to no experience. Also, many practitioners have limited direct practice experience with llamas and alpacas. Many methods for common procedures as well as specialized investigative procedures have been developed through trial and error. The general acceptance of South American camelids as a common component of mixed animal veterinary practice has led to veterinarians finding themselves performing examinations, diagnostic testing, and medical and surgical procedures on llamas and alpacas. Comfort working with the species has grown as graduating veterinarians receive more formal training and experience during their education.

We receive and address many calls from the field and from other academic institutions on how to perform varying procedures. Our goal with this text is to synthesize our combined experience with procedures from routine maintenance to advanced procedures into a single, organized, concise, visually descriptive volume for veterinary reference. This manual is intended to serve as a reference and patient-side guide for veterinarians and veterinary technicians to facilitate performance of these procedures. We gratefully acknowledge the input of our fellow veterinary practitioners who have contributed to the advancement of knowledge about these species and to increasing the standard of care provided to llamas and alpacas.

Section I

Behavior and Capture Techniques

1

Behavior and Capture Techniques

David E. Anderson

Behavior

Llamas and alpacas are intensely herd oriented. Each group of animals has a distinct social structure including a command hierarchy. Interestingly, group hierarchy often changes when the makeup of the group is altered. When herds are moved to a different location, a member of the group is removed, or members of different groups in different pastures are mixed, a period of reorganization occurs.

These dynamics are important when llamas and alpacas are maintained in involuntary groupings based on management decisions (e.g., breeding groups, weaning groups, etc.). Involuntary grouping refers to the fact that small groups are assembled by humans for the purpose of management structure, pasture availability, or other matters of convenience or necessity relative to the working of the farm. Thus, the llamas and alpacas are forced to create stable groups that may not be ideal and, in rare cases, are incompatible. The likelihood of establishing an integrated and stable group can be reduced by limited space. High stocking density creates social stress that is often not perceptible to farm personnel or veterinarians. When regulations are developed for minimum space needs for various species of animals, these guidelines most commonly refer to critical self-care needs to lay down, stand up, turn around, eat, drink, etc. With llamas and alpacas, we have found that these animals seem to have a need for "psychological space." Thus, when herd groups are assembled, space requirements should take into account the need for llamas and alpacas to have the freedom to lay down, eat, move, and so on without disruption of this individual space.

Any assessment of llama and alpaca herds should include an analysis of the herd structure, group compatibility, and space limitations. Occasionally, llamas and alpacas that are losing weight, suffering early embryonic losses, or failing to produce hair or fleece optimally are manifesting these problems as a reflection of herd stress or social stress. This may be present in a herd as a whole or with specific individuals. For example, a herd of 200 alpacas was examined because of a history of weight loss and sudden death. Diagnostic testing suggested deaths were associated with *Clostridium perfringens* Type A overgrowth in the small intestine. Upon inspection of the herd, the 200 alpacas were found to be residing in a rectangular barn of 80 feet by 60 feet square and a 10-acre pasture, and were being fed a daily ration of hay and commercial pelleted supplement. The hay was of good quality (TDN 55%; crude protein 16%) and the grain supplement was appropriate for alpacas and included trace minerals. Observation of hay and supplement feeding revealed that, hay

Veterinary Techniques in Llamas and Alpacas, Second Edition. Edited by David E. Anderson, Matt Miesner, and Meredyth Jones.

was fed based on expected intake with the desire to minimize waste in a feeding trough 60 feet long. The hierarchy of the herd created a dynamic of limited feed access for subordinate members of the herd. Feeding space was inadequate (desired bunk space >18 inches per alpaca; actual bunk space <6 inches per alpaca). Thus, the dominant members of the herd consumed a diet in excess of nutritional requirements, the middle hierarchy alpacas consumed an adequate diet, and the subordinate members of the herd received inadequate nutrition. This problem was resolved by segregating the herd into groups based on body condition score and changing feeding practices such as provision of unlimited grass hay. This achieved the goal of grouping the alpacas based on social compatibility and also matched feeding sources and feeding space to stocking needs more appropriately.

An example of an individual problem occurred in an alpaca herd of 140 alpacas segregated into groups of 20 to 30 alpacas on 5-acre pastures. One alpaca was noted to be progressively losing weight and had a body condition score of 2 out of 10 (1 = emaciated; 10 = obese). Diagnostic investigation revealed evidence of chronic malnutrition despite ample pasture, hay, and a grain-based supplement. Observation of the group dynamics revealed that the alpaca was not integrated with the group and was a "social outcast." The alpaca remained in the areas of the pasture distant from the barn and without interaction with the other alpacas. Thus, the alpaca suffered relative malnutrition because of social limitation rather than because of inadequacy of management or diet. This situation was resolved by removing the female from the pasture and comingling her with other subordinates until a social group could be established.

Capture Techniques

Both herd and individual behaviors should be used to assist veterinary interactions with llamas and alpacas. When performing group activities such as annual vaccination and deworming, these procedures can be easily and readily performed in small groups of animals. Small group settings (e.g., < 10 alpacas; < 5 llamas) lessen the stress of individual handling and may help to prevent stress-induced problems such as peracute ulcers, abortion, and premature births. Ideally, the farm facilities should be used to create a series of enclosures such as pens or corrals so that the entire group or herd can be captured in total, and then smaller groups separated off for procedures and interactions.

When there is a need to capture a single animal within a herd group, the entire group should be captured before attempting to single out the individual. For example, a group of 12 alpacas can be gathered from the pasture into a large pen. A subset of 4 alpacas containing the desired alpaca is separated away from the larger group, then the single alpaca captured, haltered, and taken to the working area. When females have a cria at their side, the cria should be taken to the working area as well. Ideally, the cria would be contained within a small pen adjacent to the female and in full view. This prevents the cria from "wandering off" during the exam resulting in the dam becoming agitated.

Alpacas and llamas have similar "flight zones" as cattle and small ruminants. Cattle, sheep, and goats have different behavioral responses to people. Goats tend to be interactive with people; sheep often respond with fear and run away from humans; cattle tend to be calmer than sheep but less interactive than goats with regard to human interaction. Llamas are most similar to dairy cattle and goats. Llamas are inquisitive but stoic. Human interaction most often is readily achieved, and llamas are less likely to react with sudden or violent maneuvers. Llamas are typically halter trained and can be led easily. This training makes group handling less important for brief activities in llamas. Alpacas are more similar to beef cattle and sheep. Alpacas accept human interaction to a point but will flee if a perceived threat is present. Alpacas are best worked in groups and using pens or stalls to achieve a close confinement area for whatever activity is needed.

When groups of llamas or alpacas need to be brought in from an open pasture, people doing the herding should use behavioral traits and barriers, such as fence lines, to facilitate driving the group into a containment area. The "flight zone" for llamas and alpacas allows for a single person to drive a herd into an enclosure by maintaining a position relative to the point of the shoulder. By stepping in front of the point of the shoulder, the llamas or alpacas are expected to move away and backward. When the person is behind the animal and distant from them, no movement is expected. The animals can be driven forward when movement toward the animal is done from a position well behind the point of the shoulder. The closer the handler is to the animal the more likely the llamas or alpacas are to turn away from the drivers. The further away the driver is, the more likely the animals are to maintain forward progress. Fence lines are useful to limit side-to-side and sudden reverse movements. If the group is uncooperative or resistant to being driven into the working area, a rope may be used to create a moving barrier or fence line (Figure 1.1). The rope can be anchored to a stationary post at the entryway

to the containment area and then a single driver can close this rope around the group to create an ever-decreasing space until the animals move into the capture pen (Figure 1.2). Rope barriers are also useful in open pasture areas if at least two drivers are present. These two people can suspend the rope between them in order create a long barrier to make herding easier until the group is within the capture pen. The rope barrier limits any sudden reversal, or escape movements, by expanding the driving zone and moving the handlers further away from the animals and their pivot point. However, overly aggressive movements, progressing too close to the animals, or making threatening gestures will cause the herd to seek and escape from the situation. In this instance, the herd may charge and break through the barrier. Once the group is in a smaller containment area, each animal can be captured and haltered if needed.

Although many llamas and alpacas are trained to be handled and haltered, uncooperative individuals can easily be captured in a small catch pen (Figure 1.3). The camelid is positioned against a solid barrier or toward a corner of the enclosure and approached from the neutral point of the shoulder. Then the lead rope is swung over the back at the base of

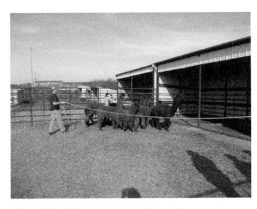

Figure 1.1 A long rope can be used as a movable barrier to herd llamas and alpacas into a containment area.

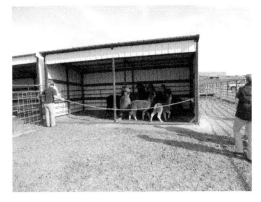

Figure 1.2 The long rope used as a mobile barrier can be suspended between two people or may be attached to a stationary object and used to gradually reduce the area of containment.

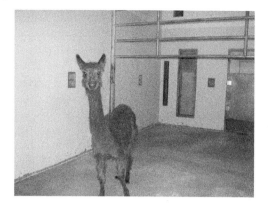

Figure 1.3 Uncooperative patients, such as this alpaca, are most easily captured by initial containment in a stall or pen.

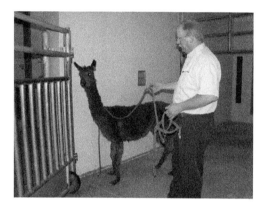

Figure 1.4 A length or rope, such as a lead rope, may be draped across the back while standing behind the point of the shoulder.

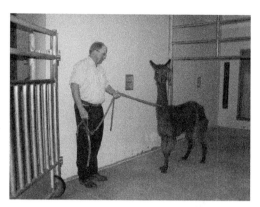

Figure 1.5 After placement of the rope across the shoulders, the handler walks in front of the animal toward the opposite shoulder. This movement encourages the patient to pivot away and expose the free end of the rope. The free end is grasped and the newly formed loop used to control the position of the alpaca.

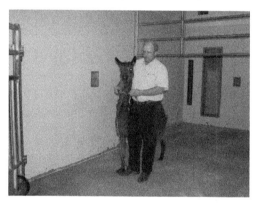

Figure 1.6 The length of rope is shortened until the handler's arms can be encircled around the base of the neck. Then the arms are moved forward along the neck until positioned behind the head.

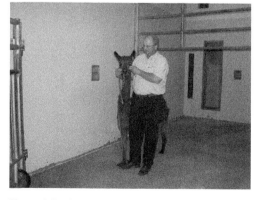

Figure 1.7 An alpaca halter is fitted over the nose by first approaching the head with the halter below the jawline.

the neck (Figure 1.4). Then, the handler slowly walks around the front of the camelid to the neutral point of the opposite shoulder until the animal turns away. The free end of the lead rope is grasped and the rope held firmly to restrain the animal's movement (Figure 1.5). The handler then moves toward the side of the neck closest to the shoulder and wraps the arms around the neck and firmly grasps the neck for restraint (Figure 1.6). A halter is placed on the head (Figure 1.7) and positioned so that the cross strap of the halter is maintained on the bony bridge of the nose (Figure 1.8).

This is important because the rostral end of the nose is cartilaginous and easily collapses under pressure, which can obstruct breathing (Figure 1.9). Llamas and alpacas that are halter trained are most often accustomed to being held and lead from the left hand side of the animal (Figure 1.10).

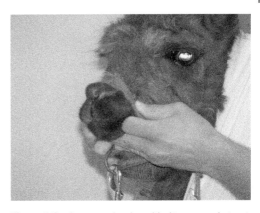

Figure 1.9 Improperly placed halters can obstruct breathing by compressing the cartilaginous bridge of the nose.

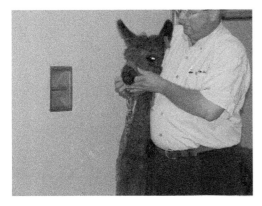

Figure 1.8 The size of the halter is assessed to ensure proper fitting. The nose bridge of the halter should cross immediately in front of the eyes in such a way that the halter is entirely positioned on the bony bridge of the nose.

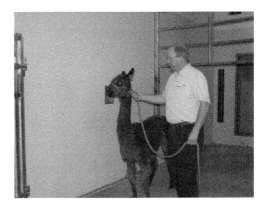

Figure 1.10 Once a halter has been properly fitted, the lead rope should be attached to the halter. Llamas and alpacas are typically led from the left-hand side.

Section II

Physical Restraint and Injection Sites

2

Haltering

Meredyth L. Jones

Purpose or Indication for Procedure

This procedure provides sufficient restraint for physical examination, injection, blood collection, nasal swabbing, and other minor procedures.

Equipment Needed

Alpaca and llama halters (Figure 2.1) are commercially available in various sizes to allow proper fitting and should be used with a lead rope. Additionally, sheep or goat halters and even cattle rope halters (Figure 2.2) may be used if properly adjusted.

Restraint/Position

Standing, sternal recumbency (cushed), or laterally recumbent positions may be used.

Technical Description of Procedure/Method

The handler should place one arm around the animal's neck and gently slide the halter over the bridge of the nose, with the strap placed behind the ears and secured. All types of halters should be checked for proper fit. On a properly fitting halter, the portion over the bridge of the nose should ride over the caudal one-third of the bridge (Figure 2.1). The rostral one-third to one-half of the bridge of the nose is comprised of soft cartilage and is easily compressed by ill-fitting halters. Ill-fit results in occlusion the nasal passages, especially when the animal is resisting leading and is pulling back on the halter. Camelids are nasal breathers and will panic and further resist restraint because of an inability to breathe easily (Figure 2.3). Continued compression can lead to asphyxiation and death. When animals are unattended or out to pasture, halters always be removed; they should never be tied and left unattended. In uncooperative camelids, a surgical huck towel, stocking cap, large sock, or other fabric can be tucked into the halter at the bridge of the nose to keep regurgitate from hitting the handler (Figure 2.4). Lightweight fabric should not be used for this purpose due to the risk of the fabric being pulled to the nostrils with inhalation.

Practice Tip to Facilitate Procedure

Alpacas and llamas are most easily gathered as a group. They can be gathered into a corner using lightweight pipes or a rope (Figures 2.5a and 2.5b) or with a team of people and then individuals restrained.

Veterinary Techniques in Llamas and Alpacas, Second Edition. Edited by David E. Anderson, Matt Miesner, and Meredyth Jones.
© 2023 John Wiley & Sons, Inc. Published 2023 by John Wiley & Sons, Inc.

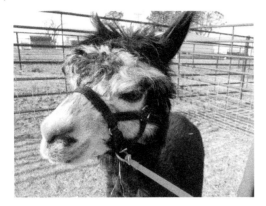

Figure 2.1 A properly fitted alpaca halter. The muzzle portion of the halter encircles the jaws in the caudal third of the nasal passages and fits securely around the head.

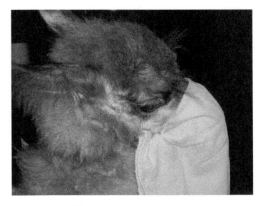

Figure 2.4 The use of a surgical huck towel to manage spitting/regurgitation behavior.

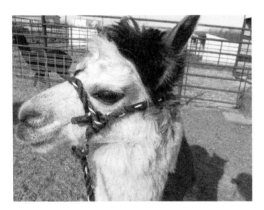

Figure 2.2 A common cattle rope halter is easily adjusted for use with camelids.

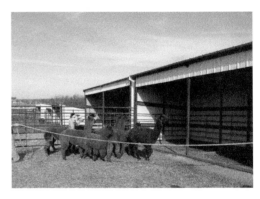

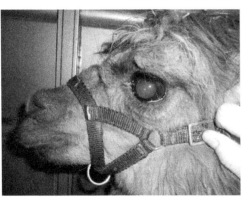

Figure 2.3 This halter is too small for this animal, as evidenced by the muzzle portion, which sits too far rostrally and is compressing the soft nasal cartilage of the nasal passage, restricting airflow.

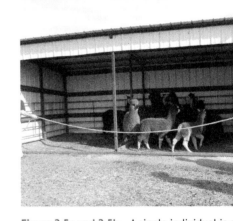

Figure 2.5a and 2.5b A single individual is able to herd a group of alpacas by the use of a rope (or long piece of lightweight conduit), tied at one end at an appropriate height. The rope or conduit is then secured and the animals contained for individual handling.

Potential Complications

Camelids have a soft, cartilaginous rostral end of the nasal passage, and nasal occlusion may occur with ill-fitting halters. Cervical injuries may occur in animals that violently resist haltering and leading.

It is not recommended that camelids be allowed to wear halters except during handling. Friction from the nosepiece can cause fiber loss and reduce the ability of animals to open their mouth and prehend feed. Their curious nature also increases the risk of catching the halter on environmental obstacles.

3

Manual Restraint
David E. Anderson

Purpose or Indication for Procedure

Manual restraint is needed for a wide variety of procedures. Most often, standing restraint is utilized, but either sternal recumbency ("cush"; alternative spelling "kush") or lateral recumbency is desired to facilitate procedures such as ultrasound examination, toenail trimming, and whenever access to the ventral aspect of the body is desired.

Equipment Needed

Halter, lead rope, 2-meter length of cotton rope, or cattle hobbles are needed.

Restraint/Position

Standing, sternal recumbency ("cush"), or lateral recumbency positions may be used.

Technical Description of Procedure/Method

Standing Restraint

Standing restraint can be achieved with or without a halter. In the absence of a halter,

restraint can be achieved by grasping the neck and pulling the head and neck inward against the handler's body (Figure 3.1). Then, one hand is placed behind the head near the base of the ears and the other hand is placed underneath the jaw at a point midway between the mouth and the eyes (Figure 3.2). The grip should be firm but not tight enough to elicit an adverse response. When needed, the hand placed behind the head can easily be moved onto the ears and used to squeeze the ears tightly (Figure 3.3). An ear squeeze is an effective method to gain additional control for short periods of time similar to a nose twitch in horses. The ears should not be twisted, and the squeeze should not be used often or for long periods of time. Oral examination can be performed by moving the hand from behind the head around the opposite side of the head from the handler and up to the mouth. This position places the head into the crook of the handler's elbow, allows the handler to firmly control the head within the arm, and frees up the hand to stimulate opening of the mouth (Figure 3.4). The mouth can be opened by placing the fingers into the commissure of the lips and pulling backward. Extreme care must be observed not to place the fingers or hand into the diastema of the mouth because of the upper and lower canine teeth and the upper incisor teeth present. In adult males, these teeth are well developed and sharp if they have

Veterinary Techniques in Llamas and Alpacas, Second Edition. Edited by David E. Anderson, Matt Miesner, and Meredyth Jones.
© 2023 John Wiley & Sons, Inc. Published 2023 by John Wiley & Sons, Inc.

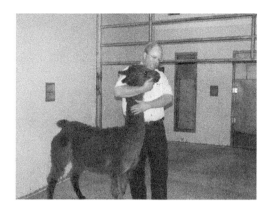

Figure 3.1 The head and neck are grasped and pulled firmly against the handler's body for manual restraint in the absence of a halter.

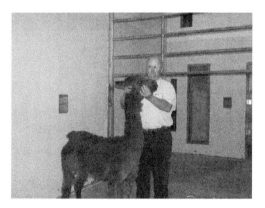

Figure 3.2 Control can be maintained using minimal restraint by grasping the jawbones (mandibles) with one hand and simultaneously placing the other hand behind the poll of the head and the uppermost portion of the neck.

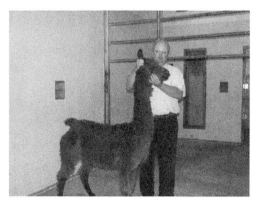

Figure 3.3 An ear squeeze can be used to gain additional control in uncooperative patients.

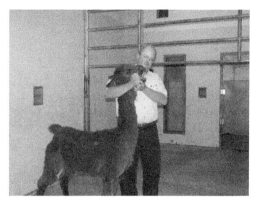

Figure 3.4 Cursory oral examination can be done by placing the poll of the head in the crook of the elbow and then inserting the fingers into the cheek. Care must be exercised so the fingers are not introduced between the teeth.

not been trimmed. The standing restraint position also can be used to obtain blood samples from the jugular vein. For this procedure, the camelid is placed into a submissive posture by tucking the head and neck under the arm and leaning over the animal's back (Figure 3.5). The rostral neck is positioned under the handler's armpit, and that arm is used to restrain the neck and the hand to occlude the jugular vein (Figure 3.6). The free hand is used to palpate the jugular vein and obtain blood samples (Figure 3.7).

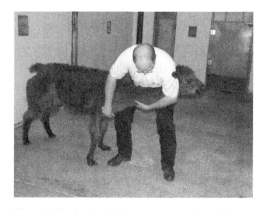

Figure 3.5 A submission posture can be achieved for control during the one-person jugular bleeding method by placing the head and neck beneath the arm and shoulder furthest away from the chest. The handler's knee is braced against the sternum of the animal.

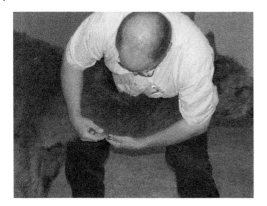

Figure 3.6 The hand of the arm used to apply the head and neck brace is used to occlude the jugular vein.

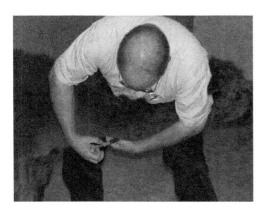

Figure 3.7 The free hand is then used to insert the needle into the jugular vein and the sample obtained.

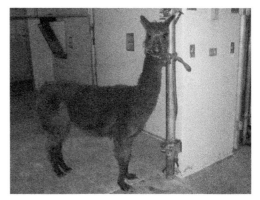

Figure 3.8 A halter and lead rope may be used to tie llamas and alpacas to a stationary post, but these animals should not be left unattended.

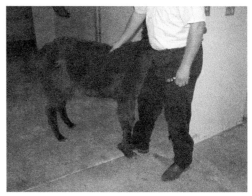

Figure 3.9 The front foot may be raised by inserting the nearside foot in between the patients front feet and bracing the knee against the sternum.

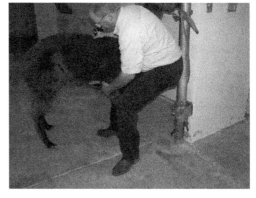

Figure 3.10 The front pastern is firmly grasped and the leg lifted.

Toenail trimming can be done with the animal standing, but it requires coordination to allow the animal to maintain balance. A halter and lead rope are placed on the llama or alpaca and tied to a stationary post (Figure 3.8). Then, the handler approaches the shoulder and places the nearside foot between the front feet of the animal (Figure 3.9). This allows positioning of the handler's knee beneath the sternum and facilitates restraint and encourages the animal to remain standing as well as helping to maintain balance. The handler grasps the metacarpal region firmly and lifts the lower leg (Figure 3.10). The hand is moved down to the pastern region, the toenails trimmed as needed, and the limb released (Figure 3.11).

Next, the handler approaches the hip and places the near-side foot between the rear feet

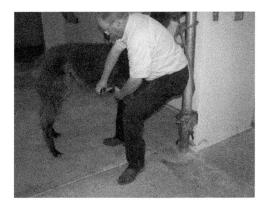

Figure 3.11 The toenails are inspected and trimmed as needed based on growth patterns.

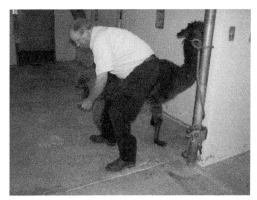

Figure 3.13 The pastern is grasped firmly and the leg lifted.

of the animal (Figure 3.12). This allows positioning of the handler's knee medial to the stifle and facilitates restraint and encourages the animal to remain standing as well as helping to maintain balance. The handler grasps the metatarsal region firmly and lifts the lower leg (Figure 3.13). The hand is moved down to the pastern region, the toenails trimmed as needed, and the limb released (Figure 3.14).

Sternal Recumbency

Sternal recumbency is a natural posture for camelids and is referred to as a "cushed" posture. Alpacas often attain this posture when resisting being handled as a self-protection mechanism. Llamas do this less commonly,

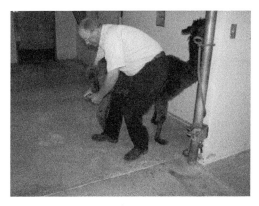

Figure 3.14 The toenails are inspected and trimmed based on growth patterns.

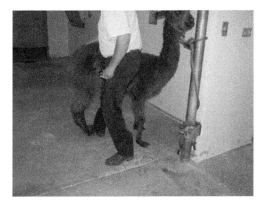

Figure 3.12 The handler places the nearside foot in between the rear feet of the patient and braces the knee against the inner thigh and stifle.

preferring to tuck individual limbs away from the handler but remaining standing. Sternal recumbency can be achieved with manual restraint when needed. First, a halter and lead rope are placed on the head (Figure 3.15). Then, the head is pulled to the ground and the lead rope used to fix the position of the muzzle on the ground (Figure 3.16). The front limb on the same side as the handler is grasped and flexed up off of the ground (Figure 3.17). The position of the head and front limb is maintained until the llama or alpaca lies down in sternal recumbency (Figure 3.18). This can be encouraged by a second handler applying pressure downward on the pelvis and lumbar region. When a sternal posture is attained, the head and neck must be held firmly against the ground to maintain restraint (Figure 3.19).

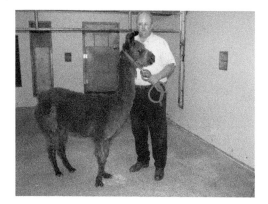

Figure 3.15 The first step in attaining sternal recumbency is to place a halter and lead rope on the animal.

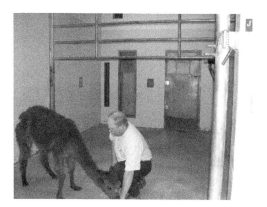

Figure 3.16 Then, the head is pulled tightly against the ground.

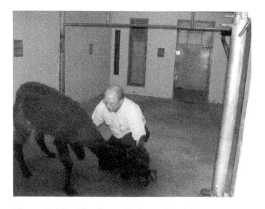

Figure 3.17 The front limb on the side nearest the handler is lifted and held firmly against the body.

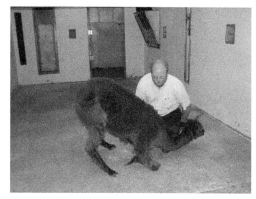

Figure 3.18 The head and neck and the front limb are firmly held in position until the alpaca lies down.

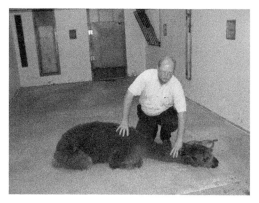

Figure 3.19 The head and neck are held firmly against the ground to ensure that the alpaca remains in a cushed posture.

Lateral Recumbency

Lateral recumbency can be achieved by first placing the camelid in sternal recumbency and then rolling the animal over onto its side (Figure 3.20). This posture can be maintained by having the handler apply firm pressure to the head and neck while simultaneously controlling one front and one rear limb. When longer periods of restraint are desired or additional control is needed, ropes placed on the limbs can be used to stretch the body into a limbs hyperextended posture. These are extremely popular methods of restraint for shearing alpacas and allow for efficient control

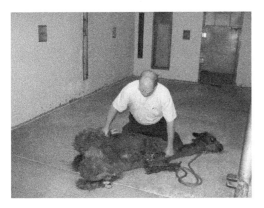

Figure 3.20 With the head and neck held firmly against the ground, the body can be pulled into lateral recumbency.

to optimize the quality of the fleece cut and minimize the risk to the animal. This can be done on the floor or using an elevated platform (Figure 3.21).

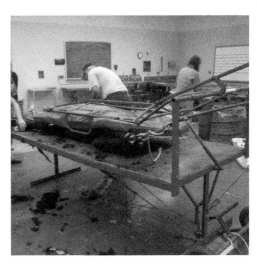

Figure 3.21 Lateral recumbency can be attained using a specially designed camelid restraint chute.

Practice Tip to Facilitate Procedure

During standing restraint and when access to the perineal area is needed (rectal temperature, etc.), relaxation of the animal can be gained by firmly grasping the tail near the base and gently rotating the tail in a circular fashion (Figures 3.22 and 3.23). During restraint in sternal recumbency, a rope may be placed across the dorsum from one hind limb to another to encourage the camelid to remain in sternal posture ("chuckered"). A set of cattle hobbles work well for this purpose. First, the leg strap is firmly applied to one limb at the metatarsal region (cannon bone; Figure 3.24). Then the strap is laid over the back and across the pelvis and attached to the contralateral leg (Figure 3.25). Occasionally, no other restraint is needed to maintain this posture (Figure 3.26).

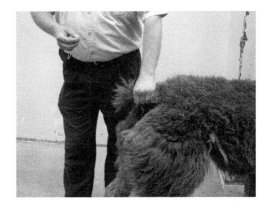

Figure 3.22 During standing restraint, the tail may be grasped at the base to facilitate restraint.

Potential Complications

The handler or animal may be injured during manual restraint if significant resistance to the procedures is encountered.

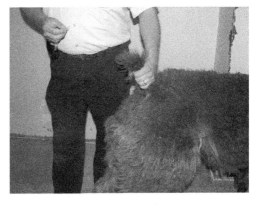

Figure 3.23 Relaxation can often be achieved by gently rotating the tail in a circular motion.

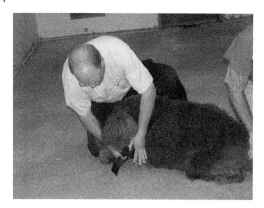

Figure 3.24 Sternal recumbency can be maintained more easily by placement of restraint ropes attached to each of the rear cannon bones and coursing across the back.

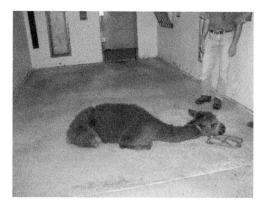

Figure 3.26 Properly fitted back ropes may allow the handler to move about during the procedure, but the patient should not be left unattended while these ropes are in place.

Patient Monitoring/Aftercare

The patient should be monitored for lameness during the 24 hours following restraint.

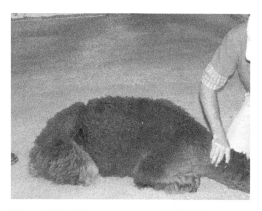

Figure 3.25 These ropes, or cattle hobbles, are tightened to apply gentle pressure against the back so that the alpaca does not attempt to rise.

4

Chute Restraint

Meredyth L. Jones

Purpose or Indication for Procedure

Chute restraint provides restraint sufficient for injections, intravenous catheterization, reproductive examinations, transabdominal and transrectal ultrasonography, radiographs, and minor diagnostic and surgical procedures. Chutes and straps may be used to maintain animals in a standing position and provide access to different areas of the body, while restricting side-to-side movement. Commercial llama and alpaca chutes are available and designed to minimize focal pressure on the neck and head. Ideally, chutes should brace the shoulders while extending the head and neck.

Equipment Needed

A commercially available or manufactured llama or alpaca chute (Figures 4.1 and 4.2), restraint straps (Figure 4.3), halter, and lead rope may be used.

Restraint/Position

Standing/cushed position may be used.

Technical Description of Procedure/Method

Haltered animals may be led or passed into a chute and the shoulder braces locked in alongside the neck. Animals that are reluctant to enter the chute may be pushed in by use of a rump rope (as when loading horses). It may also be helpful to have another camelid in front of the chute to provide companionship. Once restrained in the shoulder brace, the halter or lead rope should be affixed to the chute by use of quick-release hardware or knots (Figure 4.4). Some chutes come with padded straps, which may be placed under the brisket, under the inguinal region, and over the cervico-thoracic spine to limit movement and to keep animals from lying down during procedures or examination (Figure 4.5).

Practice Tip to Facilitate Procedure

Animals restrained in chutes will often cush (sternal recumbency), as a means of self-protection. This is most common with alpacas and less common with llamas. Preparations should be made to perform or complete procedures in a cushed posture if possible

Veterinary Techniques in Llamas and Alpacas, Second Edition. Edited by David E. Anderson, Matt Miesner, and Meredyth Jones.

when working with alpacas. The author finds that it is often easiest to simply work with the animal in this position rather than struggle with the animal. Alternatively, some commercially available chutes have straps that can be used to suspend uncooperative animals in a more suitable stance, but these may result in animals fighting the restraint more. Sedation should be used to facilitate stress-free restraint whenever needed. This is particularly important when performing surgical procedures, obtaining diagnostic specimens, and performing reproductive procedures that involve transrectal or transvaginal ultrasound probes.

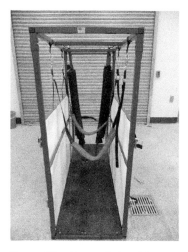

Figure 4.3 Alpaca chute with straps demonstrating means of providing additional restraint.

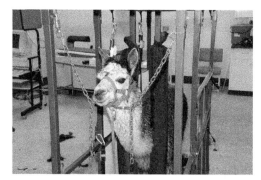

Figure 4.4 An alpaca restrained in the head catch, with the halter held by cross chains with quick release snaps, allowing for immediate release in case of sudden recumbency.

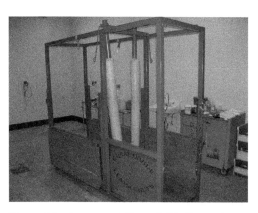

Figure 4.1 A commercially available llama chute.

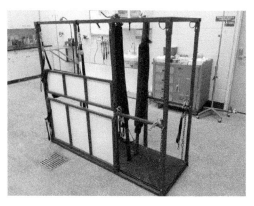

Figure 4.2 A commercially available alpaca chute.

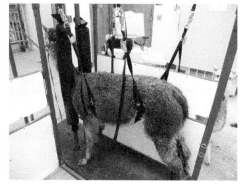

Figure 4.5 Alpaca in a chute with straps applied. These are designed to maintain the animal in the standing position and are affixed to the chute using quick release snaps. The side doors of the chute have been opened for access.

Potential Complications

Animals may suddenly become recumbent in the chute, and accommodations must be made to release the head (quick release hardware and knots). Cervical and thoracolumbar spinal injuries and limb injuries may occur in animals that violently struggle in the chute.

For such animals, sedation is strongly recommended early in the handling process.

Patient Monitoring/Aftercare

Monitor for normal locomotion and behavior postrestraint.

5

Ear Squeeze (Ear Twitch)

Meredyth L. Jones

Purpose or Indication for Procedure

Ear squeeze provides additional standing restraint to fractious animals undergoing halter restraint.

Equipment Needed

A halter and lead rope are recommended.

Restraint/Position

The position for this procedure is standing, with suggested halter restraint.

Technical Description of Procedure/Method

With or without the animal haltered, the operator places the animal's head in the crook of their arm and places one hand at the base of each ear. (See Figures 5.1 and 5.2.) The base of the ear is squeezed firmly, not twisted. Care should be taken that only the base of the ear is squeezed, not the upper cartilage (Figure 5.3). This procedure may also be used in animals to reduce fractious activity while in a chute.

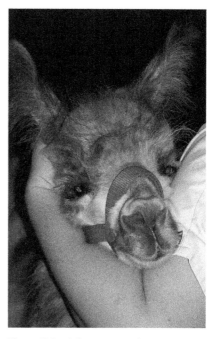

Figure 5.1 A llama correctly restrained with a halter, in the crook of the assistant's arm and with ear squeeze applied.

Practice Tip to Facilitate Procedure

The operator should calmly apply the ear squeeze. Camelids are very head-shy and, while this is quite useful in most animals, others may be very resistant to the method. If the procedure induces extreme resistance, the ear squeeze should not be continued.

Veterinary Techniques in Llamas and Alpacas, Second Edition. Edited by David E. Anderson, Matt Miesner, and Meredyth Jones.

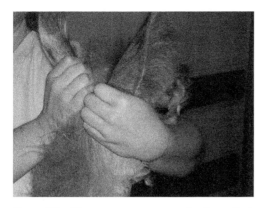

Figure 5.2 The ear squeeze appropriately applied at only the ear base.

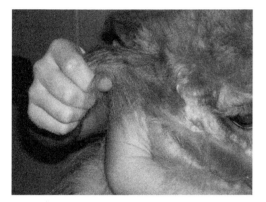

Figure 5.3 Improper handling of camelid ears. This may result in aural cartilage fracture or hematoma.

Potential Complications

Ear cartilage fracture or hematoma may occur when the pressure is not applied at the base of the ear.

6

Injections—Subcutaneous (SC), Intramuscular (IM), Intradermal (ID), Intravenous (IV)

Meredyth L. Jones

Purpose or Indication for Procedure

Injections are administered for deposition of parenteral biologicals and pharmaceuticals. Intradermal injections are utilized for allergen testing and regulatory tuberculosis testing.

Equipment Needed

For injections, a syringe, injection material, and needle are used. For SC or IM injections, a 20 to 18-gauge × 1-inch (2.5-cm) needle is used for adults, and for cria, a 22-gauge by × 1-inch (2.5-cm) needle is used. For IV injections, a 20 to 18-gauge, 1 to 1½-inch (2.5 to 3.8-cm) needle is used. For ID injection, a 27-gauge, ½-inch (1.3-cm) needle is used. New needles should be used for each animal to prevent transmission of blood-borne pathogens, including *Mycoplasma* (*Eperythrozoon*) *haemolamae*.

Restraint/Position

Standing, haltered, and chute restraint positions may be used.

Technical Description of Procedure/Method

Subcutaneous (SC) injections may be made low in the neck, over the caudal cervical epaxial muscles, or over the lateral thoracic wall, behind the elbow. The skin in the selected area is tented, the needle inserted, and the injection made into the subcutaneous tissues (Figure 6.1).

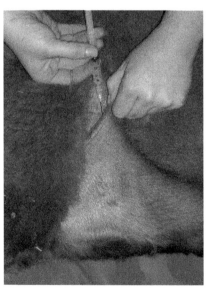

Figure 6.1 Tenting of the fiberless skin behind the left elbow for the injection of a subcutaneous biologic.

Veterinary Techniques in Llamas and Alpacas, Second Edition. Edited by David E. Anderson, Matt Miesner, and Meredyth Jones.

Intramuscular (IM) injections may be made into the caudal cervical epaxial muscles or into the semimembranosus, semitendinosus, or triceps muscles. In the cervical region, the operator should palpate the region to locate the site of greatest muscle mass (Figure 6.2). The needle is inserted perpendicular to the skin and into the center of the muscle mass (approximately 3/4 inch to 1 inch [1.9 to 2.5 cm] in an adult), the plunger pulled back for aspiration, and, if no blood is seen in the hub of the needle, the injection given.

Intradermal (ID) injections are typically given in the fiberless area behind the elbow, on the lateral thoracic wall. A tuberculin needle is superficially inserted to remain within the dermis (Figure 6.3) and the small volume of biologic administered. The skin on the underside of the tail may be used, but camelids do not have a well-defined caudal tail fold, making ID injections in this area less desirable as compared to cattle.

Intravenous (IV) injections are most commonly administered into the jugular vein, although the lateral saphenous and cephalic

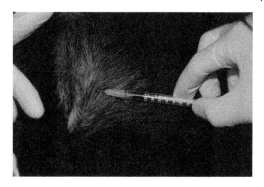

Figure 6.3 Placement of an intradermal injection in the fiberless region behind the elbow. The tuberculin needle is directed at a shallow angle into the dermis and the injection performed.

veins may also be used. The jugular vein is most easily injected in either the upper one-third (high venipuncture) or lower one-third (low venipuncture) of the neck. The mid-portion of the neck is easily accessed, but the carotid artery lies closer to the jugular vein in this region. Thus, caution should be exercised for mid-cervical injections. At the high (proximal) site, the skin is thinner than in the mid-cervical region, and the vein is superficial and somewhat separated from the carotid artery. At the low (distal) site, the carotid is close to the jugular, and there is increased risk of intra-arterial injection. However, the landmarks for puncture of the jugular vein can be easily palpated, and the vein is larger in this location. For both sites, the head and neck should be held upright and the animal well restrained. The operator should palpate the transverse processes of the cervical vertebrae and the trachea medially. The jugular groove lies between these two structures (Figure 6.4), and the vein is rarely visible, particularly when the animal is not clipped. The operator occludes the jugular groove using their thumb, bridging between the transverse process and the trachea, waiting to allow the vein to fill. The vein is then balloted with the opposite hand to confirm position and fill. The needle is inserted at a 45 to 60-degree angle into the skin. After the needle is into the soft tissues of the neck, the plunger is held with negative pressure as the needle is advanced and inserted into the vein (Figure 6.5). It is common to insert the

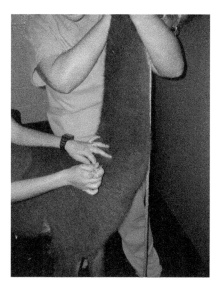

Figure 6.2 Placement of an intramuscular injection into the cervical epaxial musculature. Generally, no more than a 1-inch (2.5-cm) needle is used. The needle is directed perpendicularly to the skin into the muscle followed by aspiration and, if no blood is seen, the injection performed.

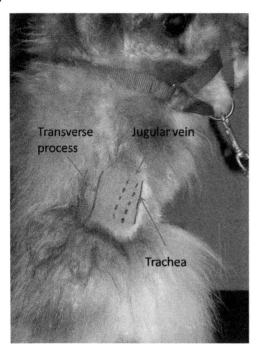

Figure 6.4 Location of the jugular vein within the jugular groove, lying between the transverse processes of the cervical vertebrae laterally and the trachea medially.

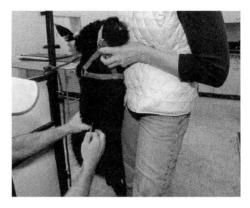

Figure 6.5 Animal receiving an intravenous injection for sedation. Under halter restraint, the neck is extended and the operator has occluded the right jugular vein with his thumb. The needle is directed into the vein at a 45-degree angle, and once confirmed to be in the vein, the injection is completed. After injection, the injection site should be held under slight pressure for a minute to allow for clotting to occur.

needle through and deep to the vein. If this is suspected, negative pressure should be maintained as the needle is withdrawn and re-enters the vein. When blood is easily and consistently aspirated, the injection may be made. For larger volumes of infusion, an intravenous catheter should be used or an extension set attached to the needle to connect the needle to the syringe to prevent dislodging the needle and perivascular extravasation of the drug.

Practice Tip to Facilitate Procedure

When possible, intramuscular injections should be avoided in the cases of large drug volumes, irritating drugs, and in cria because of their small muscle mass. Alternate drugs and biologics that can be administered IV or SC should be considered, where applicable. Lameness has been observed after IM administration of various drugs and vaccines.

Potential Complications

Inadvertent intravascular injection may occur when attempting SC or IM injections and can be prevented by aspiration prior to injection.

Intracarotid injections may occur inadvertently when attempting intravenous injection into the jugular vein. This can cause seizures and loss of consciousness. Immediate medical intervention (IV fluids, NSAIDs, corticosteroids, ventilation, and other supportive care) may be required in these cases.

Anaphylaxis may occur with any exogenous compound and can be treated with 1:1000 epinephrine at 1 mL/50 kg (110#) body weight and other respiratory and cardiovascular support measures.

Significant lameness and tissue damage may occur when irritating solutions are injected into the semimembranosus or semitendinosus muscles or inadvertently injected into or around the sciatic nerve.

Hematoma formation from inadvertent carotid puncture or traumatic jugular puncture may result in esophageal obstruction if formed on the left side of the neck.

Some drugs (for example, sodium iodide) can be extremely irritating when accidentally injected outside the vein. For such injections, the placement of an intravenous catheter is strongly recommended. Treatment of perivascular injection of irritating drugs includes local infusion of Lactated Ringer's solution, lidocaine, and administration of NSAIDs.

Patient Monitoring/Aftercare

Patients should be monitored immediately following the administration of any pharmaceutical or biological for evidence of anaphylaxis. A few days to weeks post-injection with some products, injection-site delayed reactions or abscesses may occur.

Recommended Reading

Jones M, Boileau M. 2009. Camelid Herd Health. *Vet Clin N Am Food Anim Pract*; 25(2):239–263.

Section III

Chemical Restraint and Anesthesia

7

Sedation and Tranquilization

David E. Anderson

Purpose or Indication for Procedure

Sedation or tranquilization may be indicated to complete minor or minimally invasive procedures such as reproductive examination, trimming of teeth, annual shearing in uncooperative patients, etc. Administration of anesthetic agents to camelids is a source of anxiety for many veterinarians and owners. Although specific drug dosages differ between camelids and other livestock and even among llamas and alpacas, all other aspects of the "warm-blooded mammal" apply. Whenever possible, a physical examination should be performed prior to the administration of any sedative to ensure that the patient is not placed at undue risk. The minimum patient assessment before using a sedative is to determine the rectal temperature, heart rate and rhythm, respiratory rate and character, and general demeanor of the patient including body condition score. Heart murmurs, abnormal respiratory sounds, apparent depression or apprehension, or abnormal body temperature may signal conditions that could present risk to the patient for drug administration.

Equipment Needed

The following equipment is needed: 1-mL, 3-mL, 6-mL syringes; 18-gauge × 1.5-inch (3.8-cm) needles; 20-gauge × 1-inch (2.54-cm) needles; hair clippers; alcohol; and desired drugs.

Restraint/Position

Injections may be administered with the llama or alpaca standing or cushed, or in lateral recumbency. The llama or alpaca should be restrained in such a way as to allow access to the area for drug administration with the least risk of an adverse event to the animal or the handler. Intravenous injections usually are administered via the jugular vein, but they may be administered via the ear vein or lateral thoracic vein. Intramuscular drugs are usually administered into the semimembranosus/semitendenosus muscles at a location one hands breadth ventral to the point of the ischium. Alternatively, small volumes of drugs (<5 mL) can be administered in the triceps muscles at a location 5 to 10 cm proximal to the point of the olecranon. Subcutaneous drugs can be administered into the loose tissues at the base of the neck, behind the elbow along the ribcage, or alongside of the sternum cranial to the forelimb.

Technical Description of Procedure/Method

The most commonly used drugs for sedation of llamas and alpacas are butorphanol, xylazine, and acepromazine (Table 7.1). These drugs are relatively safe for use in a field setting for short periods of time and can be administered in combination when synergistic effects are desired.

Veterinary Techniques in Llamas and Alpacas, Second Edition. Edited by David E. Anderson, Matt Miesner, and Meredyth Jones.
© 2023 John Wiley & Sons, Inc. Published 2023 by John Wiley & Sons, Inc.

Table 7.1 Sedation and reversal protocols commonly used in llamas and alpacas.

Use	Drug(s)	Species	Dosage Range	Route
Sedative/Tranquilizer				
Butorphanol		Llama	0.025–0.1 mg/kg body weight	IV, IM, SC
		Alpaca	0.05–0.2 mg/kg body weight	IV, IM, SC
Xylazine				
		Llama	0.05–0.3 mg/kg body weight 0.1–0.4 mg/kg body weight	IV, IM, SC
		Alpaca	0.1–0.4 mg/kg body weight 0.3–0.5 mg/kg body weight	IV,IM, SC
Acepromazine				
		Llama	0.02–0.05 mg/kg body weight	IV, IM, SC
		Alpaca	0.02–0.05 mg/kg body weight	IV, IM, SC
Diazepam				
		Llama or Alpaca	0.05–0.1 mg/kg body weight	IV, IM
Ketamine-Stun				
		Llama	Butorphanol: 0.05 mg/kg; Xylazine: 0.1 mg/kg; Ketamine: 0.2 mg/kg body weight	IV IM
			Butorphanol: 0.1 mg/kg; Xylazine: 0.2 mg/kg; Ketamine: 0.4 mg/kg body weight	
		Alpaca	Butorphanol: 0.05 mg/kg; Xylazine: 0.1 mg/kg; Ketamine: 0.2 mg/kg body weight	IV IM
			Butorphanol: 0.15 mg/kg; Xylazine: 0.3 mg/kg; Ketamine: 0.6 mg/kg body weight	
Xylazine Reversal Agents				
	Yohimbine	Llama or alpaca	0.125 mg/kg body weight	IV or IM
	Tolazoline	Llama or alpaca	1–2 mg/kg body weight	IM recommended; Caution IV: administer slowly
	Atipamezole	Llama or alpaca	0.125 mg/kg body weight	IV or IM
Respiratory Stimulant				
	Doxapram	Llama or alpaca	1 mg/kg body weight	IV or IM
Cardiac Stimulant				
	Epinephrine	Llama or alpaca	1 mL of 1:1000 epinephrine per 100 lb. (50 kg) body weight	IV or IM
	Dobutamine	Llama or alpaca	1–3 µg/kg/minute	IV
	Atropine sulfate	Llama or alpaca	0.01–0.02 mg/kg	IV, IM, or SC

Recently, a Ketamine-Stun protocol has been described for sedation using a combination of butorphanol, xylazine, and ketamine.

Butorphanol (dosage range: 0.025 to 0.2 mg/kg IV, IM, SC) provides safe, reliable, and predictable sedation lasting approximately 20 minutes. Recumbency is not expected. The effect of butorphanol is clinically similar between IV and IM route, but effect is expected to be longer after IM administration.

Diazepam (dosage range: 0.05 to 0.1 mg/kg IV, IM) provides safe but variable sedation lasting approximately 20 minutes. Recumbency is not expected. The effect of diazepam is clinically similar between IV and IM route, but the effect is expected to be longer after IM administration.

Xylazine (dosage range: 0.05 to 0.5 mg/kg IV, IM, SC) provides more profound sedation and analgesia, however, larger dosages are more likely to result in recumbency, bradycardia and bradypnea leading to hypoventilation and hypotension, either of which can be life-threatening. Xylazine has more profound cardiopulmonary effects and can cause significant bradycardia, bradypnea, and bloat. Food and water should be withheld from patients for 12 hours prior to xylazine administration. If fasting is not possible, smaller dosages should be used and titred to effect. Xylazine is most consistent in effect when given IV, but it can be less predictable after IM or SC routes. Clinical effect is expected to last 10 to 20 minutes with maximum sedation and an additional 10 to 20 minutes of mild sedation. Recumbency is not expected at low dosages but will occur more frequently at higher dosages especially when administered IV.

Acepromazine (dosage range: 0.02 to 0.05 mg/kg IV, IM, SC) provides safe, predictable tranquilization lasting approximately 20 minutes. Recumbency is not expected at low dosages, but will occur more frequently at higher dosages, especially when administered IV. Effect of acepromazine is clinically similar between IV and IM route, but the effect is expected to be longer after IM administration.

More recently, a drug combination, referred to as "Ketamine-Stun", utilizes small dosages of butorphanol (0.025 to 0.1 mg/kg), xylazine (0.1 to 0.2 mg/kg), and ketamine (0.2 to 0.4 mg/kg) and can be administered IV or IM depending on the depth of sedation desired.

Practice Tip to Facilitate Procedure

Sedatives or tranquilizers may be administered IV, IM, or SC. Dosages change depending on the route of administration and the desired effect. Drugs administered IV generally cause a more profound effect, have the most rapid onset, can be administered at lower dosages, and are the most consistent in effect from patient to patient. Most IV drugs are administered via the jugular vein to camelids. Drugs administered subcutaneously have the least profound effect, are slowest in onset, and are the least consistent for clinical effect. Clinically, alpacas demonstrate more resistance to anesthetic drugs, and llamas are most susceptible to their effects. In our experience, llamas may require ¼ to 1/3rd less drug on a body-weight basis as compared with alpacas to achieve a similar effect.

Potential Complications

The nature of the hair coat, thickness of the skin, lack of a jugular groove, and proximity of the jugular vein to the esophagus and carotid artery increase the risk of mishaps during drug administration. Puncture of the carotid artery has resulted in extensive hematoma formation. This can cause esophageal obstruction (left carotid artery) or respiratory distress (either carotid artery). If the drug is administered intra-arterially, seizures, hypotension, bradycardia, loss of consciousness, and death may occur. For this reason, many veterinarians prefer to administer sedatives IM or SC unless a venous catheter is in place.

Reversal Agents

Xylazine may cause dangerous cardiopulmonary depression in some patients. In animals that are too heavily sedated or immediate recovery is desired, selective antagonist or general stimulant drugs may be administered. Yohimbine (0.1 mg/kg IV) is the reversal drug of choice for xylazine in llamas and alpacas because this drug is safe and effective. Tolazoline is a selective antagonist for xylazine, but it has been associated with adverse reactions and deaths (possibly caused by cardiac asystole and profound hypotension) when given by IV bolus. This drug is not recommended for use except when it can be administered IM or by slow, controlled IV injection. Atipamezole (0.125 mg/kg IV) also has been used in camelids.

Patient Monitoring/Aftercare

During the period of sedation, the patient's heart rate and respiratory rate should be monitored. If recumbency is achieved, the head should be positioned to facilitate drainage of saliva away from the pharynx and the patient maintained in sternal recumbency. After the conclusion of the procedure, the owner should monitor the animal until it returns to normal mentation and activity. Food and water should not be offered until that time to minimize the risk of aspiration, esophageal choke, or bloat.

Recommended Reading

Abrahamsen EJ. 2009. Chemical restraint, anesthesia, and analgesia for camelids. In Anderson D.E. and Whitehead C., Eds.: *Vet Clin North America*; 25(2):455–494.

Heath RB. 1989 Mar. Llama anesthetic programs. *Vet Clin North Am Food Anim Pract*; 5(1):71–80. doi:10.1016/s0749-0720(15)31004-5. PMID: 2647240.

Larenza MP, Zanolari P, Jäggin-Schmucker N. 2008. Balanced anesthesia and ventilation strategies for an alpaca (Lama pacos) with an increased anesthetic-risk. *Schweizer Archiv für Tierheilkunde*; 150(2):77–81.

Neiger-Aeschbacher G. 1999. Lama–Sedation und Anästhesie (Ubersichtsartikel) [Llamas-sedation and anesthesia (review article)]. *Schweiz Arch Tierheilkd*; 141(7):307–318. German. PMID: 10425887.

Pereira FG, Greene SA, McEwen MM, Keegan R. 2006. Analgesia and anesthesia in camelids. *Small Rumin Res*; 61(2–3):227–233.

Riebold TW, Kaneps AJ, Schmotzer WB. 1989 Sep-Oct. Anesthesia in the llama. *Vet Surg*; 18(5):400–404. doi: 10.1111/j.1532-950x.1989.tb01112.x. PMID: 2683353.

8

Injectable Anesthesia
David E. Anderson

Purpose or Indication for Procedure

General anesthesia may be indicated for a wide variety of procedures, especially surgical procedures such as castration, laceration repair, etc. A physical examination should be performed prior to the administration of any anesthetics to ensure that the patient is not placed at undue risk. The minimum patient assessment before drug administration is to determine the rectal temperature, heart rate and rhythm, respiratory rate and character, and general demeanor of the patient. Heart murmurs, abnormal respiratory sounds, apparent depression or apprehension, abnormal body temperature, or low body condition score consistent with emaciation may signal conditions that could present risk to the patient for drug administration. Prior to general anesthesia, a PCV and TP should be determined. More exhaustive diagnostic tests may be warranted (e.g., hematology, serum biochemistry, etc.) if the patient is geriatric (older than 10 years for llamas and alpacas), has a history of disease, or abnormal physical examination findings are present. An accurate body weight will increase the safety of the procedure, but an estimation of body weight may be obtained by evaluating the body condition score. In general, adult alpacas are expected to weigh between 50 and 70 kg (mean 140 lb.; range 120 to 160 lb.) and adult llamas

between 125 and 204 kg (mean 325 lb.; range 275 to 450 lb.).

Equipment Needed

The following equipment is needed: 1-mL, 3-mL, 6-mL, 12-mL syringes; 18-gauge 1.5-inch (3.8-cm needles); 20-gauge 1-inch (2.54-cm) needles; hair clippers; alcohol; and desired drugs.

Restraint/Position

Adult llamas and alpacas should have all feed withheld for 18 to 24 hours and water withheld for 12 to 18 hours prior to general anesthesia. This will diminish the risks of regurgitation, bloat, respiratory compromise, and post-operative distress.

Injections may be administered with the llama or alpaca standing or cushed, or in lateral recumbency. The llama or alpaca should be restrained in such a way as to allow access to the area for drug administration with the least risk of an adverse event to the animal or the handler. Intravenous injections usually are administered via the jugular vein, but they may be administered via the ear vein or lateral thoracic vein. Intramuscular drugs are usually administered into the semimembranosus/ semitendinosus muscles at a location approximately 10 to 15 cm

Veterinary Techniques in Llamas and Alpacas, Second Edition. Edited by David E. Anderson, Matt Miesner, and Meredyth Jones.
© 2023 John Wiley & Sons, Inc. Published 2023 by John Wiley & Sons, Inc.

ventral to the point of the ischium. Alternatively, small volumes of drugs (<5 mL) can be administered in the triceps muscles at a location 5 to 10 cm proximal to the point of the olecranon. Caution must be exercised when administering drugs IM in the neck because there is relatively little muscle present. The most readily accessible area in the neck is immediately cranial to the shoulder.

Technical Description of Procedure/Method

The most commonly used combination of drugs for general anesthesia of llamas and alpacas are butorphanol, xylazine, and ketamine (Table 8.1).

The combination of diazepam and ketamine also is safe for short procedures, particularly in field settings. These drugs are relatively safe for use in field settings for short periods of time and can be administered in various combinations depending on the desired effect. For procedures requiring > 30 minutes to complete, intravenous access is desirable so that additional anesthetic drugs may be administered during the procedure, IV fluids can be administered, or emergency drugs can be administered if needed. Many veterinarians prefer to administer drug combinations IM rather than IV because of the convenience and minimal risk of adverse events associated with jugular venipuncture. However, the onset, depth, and duration of general anesthesia are more variable after IM administration.

Table 8.1   Injectable general anesthesia protocols commonly used in llamas and alpacas.

Use	Drug(s)	Species	Dosage Range	Route
B:X:K Combination Injectable Anesthesia				
	Butorphanol	Llama	0.05–0.1 mg/kg body weight	IV, IM
		Alpaca	0.05–0.1 mg/kg body weight	IV, IM
	Xylazine	Llama	0.3–0.35 mg/kg body weight	IM
			0.2–0.25 mg/kg body weight	IV
		Alpaca	0.4–0.5 mg/kg body weight	IM
			0.25–0.3 mg/kg body weight	IV
	Ketamine	Llama	3–4 mg/kg body weight	IM
			2–2.5 mg/kg body weight	IV
		Alpaca	4–5 mg/kg body weight	IM
			2.5–3 mg/kg body weight	IV
Ketamine-Diazepam Injectable Anesthesia				
	Diazepam	Llama	0.14 mg/kg body weight	IV, IM
		Alpaca	0.18 mg/kg body weight	IV, IM
	Ketamine	Llama	Ketamine 2.7 mg/kg body weight	IV
		Alpaca	Ketamine 3.6 mg/kg body weight	IV
Respiratory Stimulant				
	Doxapram	Llama or alpaca	1 mg/kg body weight	IV or IM
Cardiac Stimulant				
	Epinephrine	Llama or alpaca	1 mL of 1:1000 epinephrine per100 lb. (50 kg) body weight	IV or IM
	Dobutamine	Llama or alpaca	1–3 µg/kg/minute	IV
	Atropine sulfate	Llama or alpaca	0.01–0.02 mg/kg	IV, IM, or SC

Premedication is not commonly done in llamas and alpacas. The drugs used for general anesthesia are most often given in combination in the same syringe at the same time. Although not commonly recommended, atropine sulfate (0.01 to 0.02 mg/ kg body weight) can be given prior to or during anesthesia to support cardiopulmonary function.

The following anesthetics may be administered as follows:

• BXK (Butorphanol/Xylazine/Ketamine) Anesthesia:
  ○ IM Anesthesia: Combine the butorphanol, xylazine, and ketamine in the same syringe and administer together in one location IM. Butorphanol (dosage range: 0.05 to 0.1 mg/kg) is used to provide sedation and analgesia. Xylazine (dosage range: 0.2 to 0.4 mg/kg) provides profound sedation and analgesia. Xylazine has more profound cardiopulmonary effects and can cause significant bradycardia, bradypnea, and bloat. Clinical effect is expected to last 20 to 30 minutes with maximum sedation and an additional 10 to 20 minutes of mild sedation. Ketamine (dosage range: 2 to 4 mg/kg) provides neuroleptic anesthesia and analgesia lasting 20 to 30 minutes. Given IM, this B:X:K cocktail is expected to provide general anesthesia within 10 minutes following injection and surgical plane analgesia for 20 to 30 minutes. Patients will regain consciousness and the ability to remain sternal within 40 to 60 minutes after injection. If the procedure time is expected to exceed 30 minutes, a supplemental dose of xylazine and ketamine at one-third of the original dosage may be administered at 20 to 30 minutes. A convenient field-ready cocktail can be made by adding butorphanol (1 mL at 10 mg/mL) and xylazine (1 mL at 100 mg/mL) into a vial of ketamine (10 mL at 100 mg/mL). This combination is then administered IM at a dosage rate of 1 mL/18 kg (40 lb.) body weight in alpacas and 1 mL per 23 kg (50 lb.) body weight in llamas.

  ○ IV Anesthesia: Administer the butorphanol and xylazine in the same syringe and administer IV. When sedation is apparent, administer the ketamine dosage. Administer butorphanol (dosage range: 0.05 to 0.1 mg/kg IV) and xylazine (dosage range: 0.2 to 0.3 mg/kg IV). Wait until sedation is apparent and then administer ketamine (dosage range: 2 to 3 mg/kg IV). Given IV, this B:X:K cocktail is expected to provide general anesthesia within 5 minutes following IV injection of ketamine. Surgical plane anesthesia will be sustained for approximately 20 minutes. Patients will regain consciousness and the ability to remain sternal within 30 to 40 minutes after injection. If the procedure time is expected to exceed 20 minutes, a supplemental dose of xylazine and ketamine at one-third of the original dosage may be administered at 15 to 20 minutes.

• Ketamine-Diazepam Anesthesia: The combination of diazepam and ketamine provides a safe method for induction of general anesthesia lasting approximately 15 to 20 minutes. For intravenous induction of llamas, diazepam (0.14 mg/kg) and ketamine (2.7 mg/kg) may be combined and administered simultaneously. For alpacas, diazepam (0.18 mg/kg) and ketamine (3.6 mg/kg) may be combined and administered simultaneously IV. An easy field-ready cocktail is to add equal volumes of ketamine (100 mg/mL) and diazepam (5 mg/mL) into a syringe and administer this combination at a rate of 1 mL/18 kg to llamas or 1 mL/14 kgs to alpacas.

Practice Tip to Facilitate Procedure

Anesthetics may be administered IV or IM. Dosages change depending on the health status and age of the animals, route of administration and the desired effect. Drugs administered IV generally cause a more profound effect, have the most rapid onset, can be administered at lower dosages, and are the most consistent in

(continued)

(continued)

effect from patient to patient. However, IV drugs also present a greater risk for cardiopulmonary instability. IV drugs most often are administered via the jugular vein to camelids. This can present special challenges in these species (see below). Clinically, alpacas demonstrate more resistance to anesthetic drugs as compared with llamas. Thus, llamas are usually dosed at the low-end of the dosage range and alpacas at the middle to upper-end of the dosage ranges.

Potential Complications

The nature of the hair coat, thickness of the skin, lack of a jugular groove, and proximity of the jugular vein to the esophagus and carotid artery increase the risk of mishaps during IV drug administration. Puncture of the carotid artery has resulted in extensive hematoma formation. This can cause esophageal obstruction (left carotid artery) or respiratory distress (either carotid artery). Any drug administered intra-arterially can cause seizures, hypotension, bradycardia, loss of consciousness, and death. For this reason, many veterinarians prefer to administer anesthetic drugs IM unless a venous catheter is in place.

Reversal Agents

Xylazine may cause dangerous cardiopulmonary depression in some patients. In animals that are too heavily sedated or immediate recovery is desired, selective antagonist or general stimulant drugs may be administered. Yohimbine (0.1 mg/kg IV) is the reversal drug of choice for xylazine in llamas and alpacas because this drug has proven to be safe and effective. Tolazoline is a selective antagonist for xylazine but has been associated with adverse

reactions and deaths (possibly caused by cardia asystole and profound hypotension) when given by IV bolus. This drug is not recommended for use except when it can be administered IM or by slow, controlled IV injection. Atapamezole (0.1 mg/kg IV) also has been used in camelids.

Patient Monitoring/Aftercare

During the period of sedation, the patient's heart rate and respiratory rate should be monitored. The head should be positioned to facilitate drainage of saliva away from the pharynx and the animal maintained in sternal recumbency until ready to stand. Consider placement of an orotracheal or nasotracheal tube prior to initiation of the procedure. If available, oxygen may be delivered either via facemask or via an orotracheal or nasotracheal tube. After the conclusion of the procedure, the animal should be closely monitored until it is fully aroused and able to maintain sterna posture. Food and water should not be offered until the patient can stand up and walk around without falling. This will decrease the risk of aspiration, esophageal choke, or bloat.

Recommended Reading

Abrahamsen EJ. 2009. Chemical restraint, anesthesia, and analgesia for camelids. In Anderson D.E. and Whitehead C., Eds.: *Vet Clin North America*; 25(2):455–494.

Larenza MP, Zanolari P, Jäggin-Schmucker N. 2008. Balanced anesthesia and ventilation strategies for an alpaca (Lama pacos) with an increased anesthetic-risk. *Schweizer Archiv für Tierheilkunde*; 150(2):77–81.

Pereira FG, Greene SA, McEwen MM, Keegan R. 2006. Analgesia and anesthesia in camelids. *Small Rumin Res*; 61(2–3):227–233.

9

Orotracheal Intubation

David E. Anderson

Purpose or Indication for Procedure

Orotracheal intubation is indicated whenever ready access to the airway is desired (Abrahamsen, 2009). This is most commonly done to facilitate breathing during anesthesia, but it also may be a lifesaving technique, if the nasopharynx becomes obstructed and percutaneous tracheostomy is not possible. Tracheal intubation is recommended to be used whenever general anesthesia is expected to be maintained for >45 minutes or the procedure being performed necessitates the patient being positioned in dorsal recumbency.

Equipment Needed

The following equipment will be needed: laryngoscope with extended blade (15 cm or longer) and light source; cuffed orotracheal tubes (crias: 15 to 20-cm length, 6 to 10-mm OD; adults: 30 to 50 cm long; 10 to 14-mm OD); semi-rigid stylet 10 to 20 cm longer than the tracheal tube; mouth gag; lidocaine HCl (optional); suction apparatus (optional).

Restraint/Position

Head and neck extended in sternal recumbency (recommended), lateral recumbency, or dorsal recumbency positions may be used.

Technical Description of Procedure/Method

Conscious patients must be induced under general anesthesia or have profound sedation; unconscious patients may or may not require sedation or anesthesia. The llama or alpaca is placed into sternal recumbency, and the head and neck are extended. The mouth is opened by hand or by using a mouth gag, and the tongue is pulled from the mouth and retracted laterally (Figure 9.1). Attention should be paid not to occlude the nostrils prematurely so that breathing is not interrupted before the operator is prepared to introduce the orotracheal tube. A laryngoscope with an extended blade (Figures 9.2 and 9.3) is used to elevate the

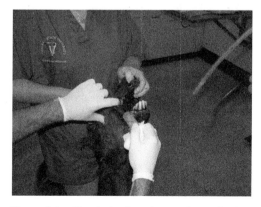

Figure 9.1 After induction of general anesthesia, the head and neck are hyperextended and the tongue pulled from the mouth.

Veterinary Techniques in Llamas and Alpacas, Second Edition. Edited by David E. Anderson, Matt Miesner, and Meredyth Jones.

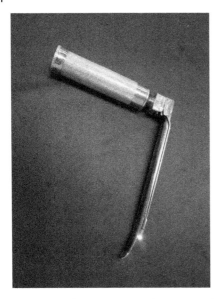

Figure 9.2   A laryngoscope with an extended blade is needed to enable viewing of the larynx.

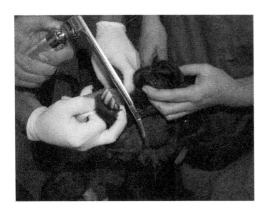

Figure 9.3   The laryngoscope blade must be long enough to extend beyond the base of the tongue.

soft palate and depress the base of the tongue (Figure 9.4) until the epiglottis and arytenoid cartilages can be viewed. Then a semi-rigid stylet (aluminum rod, polyurethane tubing, etc.) is passed through the endotracheal tube and mouth and into the trachea (Figures 9.5 and 9.6). The orotracheal tube is placed over the stylet and advanced into the trachea (Figure 9.7). If the larynx hinders advancement of the endotracheal tube, the tube should be retracted, rotated 90 degrees and advanced again. This procedure is continued until entry into the trachea is successful (Figures 9.8 and

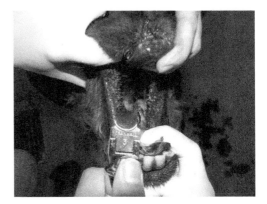

Figure 9.4   The laryngoscope light source must be sufficiently bright so it illuminates the pharynx.

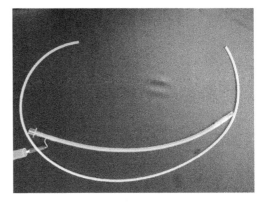

Figure 9.5   A long, thin stylette is used as a guide for the endotracheal tube.

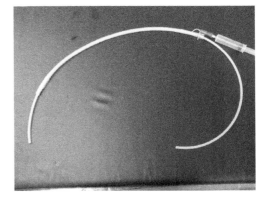

Figure 9.6   The stylette must be long enough to be able to pass into the trachea as well as extend beyond the length of the endotracheal tube.

9.9). The stylet is removed (Figure 9.10) and the cuff inflated to ensure adequate seal in the trachea and the tube tied in place to prevent dislodgement. Manual ventilation assistance devices should be available to provide breaths in the event that the patient develops apnea (Figures 9.11 and 9.12).

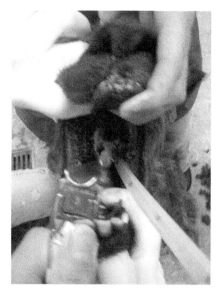

Figure 9.7 The endotracheal tube is passed over the stylette and pushed forward into the trachea.

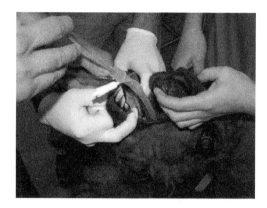

Figure 9.10 Multiple attempts may be required for successful endotracheal intubation.

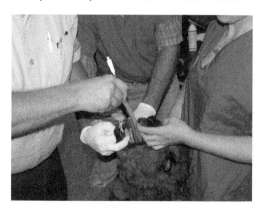

Figure 9.8 Correct placement of the endotracheal tube can be assured by laryngoscope examination.

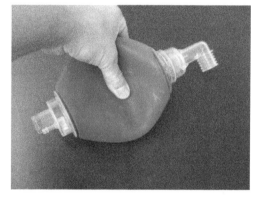

Figure 9.11 An artificial device should be on hand to provide mechanical or manual ventilation if needed.

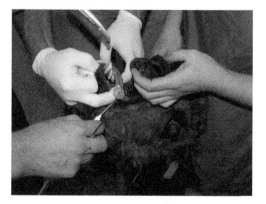

Figure 9.9 If resistance to advancement of the endotracheal tube is felt, the tube can be withdrawn a short distance, rotated, and advanced again.

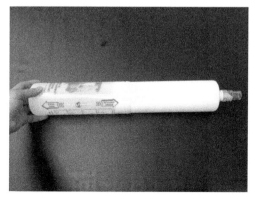

Figure 9.12 Volume-regulated ventilation assistance devices are useful to ensure consistent delivery of air.

Practice Tip to Facilitate Procedure

The laryngoscope blade should be long enough to reach the epiglottis to facilitate viewing of the larynx. A small spray bottle containing 2% lidocaine HCl is useful for management of laryngospasm. If the arytenoids are abducted closed, spray-coat the pharynx and larynx with lidocaine to desensitize the area. A long narrow stylet aids in placement of a tracheal tube without loss of view. This tubing subsequently serves as a guide over which the tube is passed.

Potential Complications

Camelids are semi-obligate nasal breathers. Obstruction of the airway is the primary concern and may occur during intubation or immediately after extubation. Swallowing motions and the ability to lift the head should be present prior to extubation to prevent obstruction associated with dorsal displacement of the soft palate.

Patient Monitoring/Aftercare

Patients should be monitored until they are able to stand to ensure no interruption of airflow.

Recommended Reading

Abrahamsen EJ. 2009. Chemical restraint, anesthesia, and analgesia for camelids. In Anderson D.E. and Whitehead C., Eds.: *Vet Clin North America*; 25(2):455–494.

10

Nasotracheal Intubation

David E. Anderson

Purpose or Indication for Procedure

Nasotracheal intubation is indicated whenever ready access to the airway is desired in conscious patients or when unfettered access to the mouth or oral cavity is needed (Abrahamsen, 2009). This is most commonly done to facilitate breathing during anesthesia, but it also may be a lifesaving technique to provide assisted ventilation in newborn crias or snake-bite victims. Tracheal intubation is recommended to be used whenever general anesthesia is expected to be maintained for >45 minutes or the procedure being performed necessitates the patient being positioned in dorsal recumbency. Ventilation via nasotracheal tubes requires greater care because these tubes are considerably smaller than orotracheal tubes and can become more easily obstructed during the procedure.

Equipment Needed

The following equipment is needed: cuffed orotracheal tubes (crias: 15 to 20-cm length, 4 to 6-mm OD; adults: 30 to 50-cm long, 6 to 12-mm OD); semi-rigid stylet slightly longer than the tracheal tube; sterile lubricant; lidocaine HCl (optional); suction apparatus (optional).

Restraint/Position

Head and neck extended in sternal recumbency (recommended), lateral recumbency, or dorsal recumbency positions may be used.

Technical Description of Procedure/Method

Nasotracheal intubation can be performed in conscious patients but may require sedation if the animal is uncooperative. The llama or alpaca is placed into sternal recumbency, and the head and neck are extended (Figure 10.1). The nasotracheal tube is coated with small amount of sterile lubricant and introduced

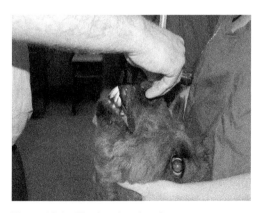

Figure 10.1 The head and neck are hyperextended for nasotracheal intubation.

Veterinary Techniques in Llamas and Alpacas, Second Edition. Edited by David E. Anderson, Matt Miesner, and Meredyth Jones.

through the nares (Figure 10.2). The tube is directed ventrally so that passage occurs along the ventral meatus (Figure 10.3). Deviation of the tube into the middle or dorsal meatus is more likely to cause bleeding because of

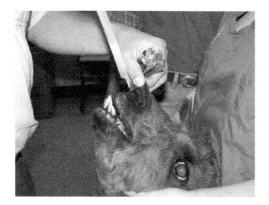

Figure 10.2 The nasotracheal tube is guided into the ventral nasal meatus through the nares.

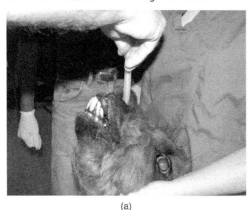

(a)

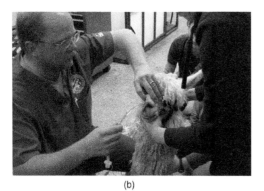

(b)

Figure 10.3 Ventral placement of the tube is crucial to ensure passage without causing trauma. This can be done in the anesthetized (**3a**) or sedated (**3b**) patient.

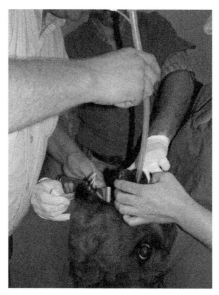

Figure 10.4 The nasotracheal tube is advanced if no resistance is felt. If resistance is felt, the tube is retracted and the placement reassessed.

trauma to the mucosa or ethmoid turbinate. Also, advancement of dorsally directed tubes is not likely to be successful because of entrapment in the caudal dorsal pharyngeal recess. If advancement of the endotracheal tube is hindered, the tube should be partially or completely withdrawn and redirected into the ventral meatus. The ventral meatus merges with the common meatus at the termination of the nasal septum ventrally approximately 6- to 8-cm caudal to the nares (Figure 10.4). If the larynx hinders advancement of the tube, the tube should be retracted, rotated 90 degrees, and advanced again. This procedure is continued until entry into the trachea is successful (Figure 10.5) or an alternative strategy is elected. Entry into the trachea is evident by free movement of air through the endotracheal tube. Palpation of the proximal esophagus during placement can help ensure that accidental intubation of the esophagus does not occur. If a stylet was used within the tube to add rigidity to aid in guidance, it is removed and the cuff inflated to ensure adequate seal in the trachea (Figure 10.6). The tube is tied in place to prevent dislodgement. Manual ventilation assistance devices should be available to provide

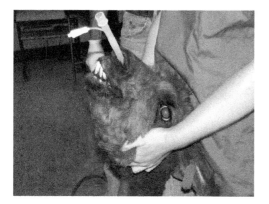

Figure 10.5 Successful intubation is assured by assessment of air movement.

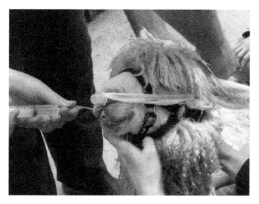

Figure 10.6 The tube is secured in place and the cuff of the tube inflated.

breaths in the event that the patient develops apnea (Figure 10.7).

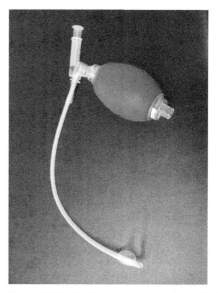

Figure 10.7 Mechanical or manual ventilation should be available if needed.

Potential Complications

Nasal bleeding and excessive hemorrhage are the most common complications. These are self-limiting in most cases. If bleeding seems inappropriate, a coagulation profile is indicated. Failure to successfully intubate the trachea is another common concern. This technique requires patience and practice. The novice initially should attempt this method on llamas or alpacas that have been anesthetized to improve the chances for success.

Patient Monitoring/Aftercare

Patients should be monitored until they are able to stand to ensure no interruption of airflow and stoppage or any bleeding.

Recommended Reading

Abrahamsen EJ. 2009. Chemical restraint, anesthesia, and analgesia for camelids. In Anderson D.E. and Whitehead C., Eds.: *Vet Clin North America*; 25(2):455–494.

Practice Tip to Facilitate Procedure

A small spray bottle containing 2% lidocaine HCl is useful for management of laryngospasm. If the endotracheal tube cannot be passed beyond the larynx, spray lidocaine down the lumen of the tube to coat the nasopharynx and larynx with lidocaine to desensitize the area. In some cases, a stylet aids in placement of a nasotracheal tube by providing rigidity to the tube. These must be used carefully so as not to cause bleeding from trauma to the mucosa.

11

Percutaneous Tracheal Intubation (Also Referred to as Retrograde Tracheal Intubation)

Matt D. Miesner

Purpose or Indication for Procedure

Percutaneous tracheal intubation can imply either direct or indirect endotracheal intubation. Direct tracheal intubation through a tracheotomy is indicated when oropharyngeal procedures require that an endotracheal not obstruct the procedure. Examples may include lesions of the soft palate, arytenoids, intra-oral, or intranasal pathology. In addition to initial case management, a tracheotomy may need to be maintained postoperatively (see tracheostomy procedure in this text).

Alternatively, percutaneous tracheal intubation may imply first passing a guide stylette retrograde from the trachea and out the mouth or nose to provide accurate physical guidance of the endotracheal tube. This method of endotracheal intubation is extensively described in humans. Routine (normograde) orotracheal intubation may be difficult to perform in some camelids with challenging anatomical and pathological reasons. The primary obstacle of orotracheal intubation is poor visualization of the larynx and epiglottis, which can delay intubation, trigger regurgitation, or result in pharyngeal and laryngeal trauma. When difficult intubation is encountered or anticipated, retrograde/cutaneous intubation can be considered. This method may also be used as

an alternative to tracheotomy for acquiring a patent airway during emergency situations in difficult patients. Retrograde or normograde nasotracheal intubation should be considered if the airway is to be maintained in the semi-conscious patient.

Equipment Needed

Sedation and/or preanesthetic induction drugs as well as 2% lidocaine for local anesthesia will be needed. Endotracheal tubes of various sizes, cuff inflation syringe, 14-gauge nested trocar set, stiff polypropylene urinary catheter or guide wire, #10 scalpel blade, and an oral speculum are also needed. The stylette chosen needs to be approximately 2 to 3 feet long (60 to 90 cm). Large animal transtracheal wash kits provide nearly all of the necessary materials for the procedure. It is also advised to have emergency tracheotomy equipment available if needed.

Restraint/Position

Support patient in a cushed or sternal position with the head and neck extended dorsally after administering the sedation. One to two assistants will be needed to help complete the procedure.

Veterinary Techniques in Llamas and Alpacas, Second Edition. Edited by David E. Anderson, Matt Miesner, and Meredyth Jones.
© 2023 John Wiley & Sons, Inc. Published 2023 by John Wiley & Sons, Inc.

Technical Description of Procedure/Method

Aseptically clip and scrub an area at the junction of the proximal and middle third of the neck. Infuse 1 to 2 mL of 2% lidocaine subcutaneously for a small skin incision. Make a midline stab incision (0.5 to 1 cm) with the #10 scalpel blade in the skin overlying the trachea. Insert the nested trocar through the incision, into the lumen of the trachea between cartilaginous rings, and remove the inner trocar, leaving the cannula sleeve in place. (See Figures 11.1 and 11.2.) A fair amount of

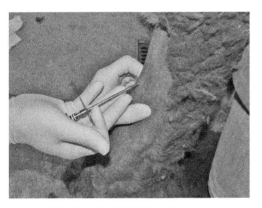

Figure 11.1 A stab skin incision has been made on midline over the trachea, and the nested trocar is positioned for insertion between the cartilaginous rings of the trachea.

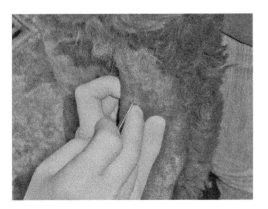

Figure 11.2 The trocar is pushed through the cartilaginous rings. The novice will recognize the unexpected amount of pressure needed to penetrate the lumen of the trachea.

resistance will be encountered when puncturing the trachea. Direct the cannula orally so the guide wire will course toward the larynx (Figure 11.3). Attach a syringe and aspirate to determine correct lumen positioning, which is indicated by no evidence of air resistance. Insert the oral speculum, which can be as simple as a partial roll of bandage tape placed between the lower incisors and dental pad to prevent patient from chewing on the stylette and eventually the tracheal tube (Figure 11.4).

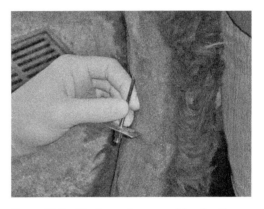

Figure 11.3 The trocar is removed, leaving the cannula sleeve. A syringe can be connected, and if no air resistance is noted when the plunger is withdrawn, correct placement has been achieved into the lumen. This author prefers to just attempt passage of the stylette, which should not meet any resistance.

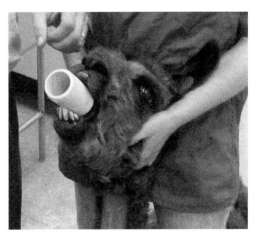

Figure 11.4 An oral speculum has been inserted between the incisors and dental pad to prevent stylette or tube damage from the molars if the animal bites down.

Next, insert the chosen stylette through the cannula directed toward the oropharynx (Figure 11.5). Depending on the method of intubation intended, the guide wire/stylette will exit that orifice (Figure 11.6). The soft palate may need to be directed dorsally to achieve oral intubation; a laryngoscope with a long blade is helpful (Figure 11.7). Thread the stylette through the lumen of the endotracheal tube, and then advance it through the larynx and into the trachea following the stylette. Remove the stylette and the trocar cannula, advance the endotracheal tube to the desired

position, and inflate the cuff (Figures 11.8 and 11.9). Close the skin incision with tissue glue or suture, and bandage with gauze.

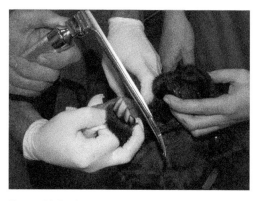

Figure 11.7 A laryngoscope with a long blade is helpful to displace the soft palate dorsally for guided orotracheal intubation.

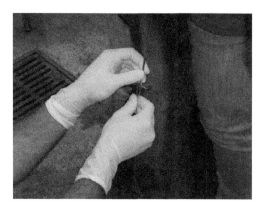

Figure 11.5 A stiff guide wire or catheter is being placed through the cannula and directed toward the oropharynx.

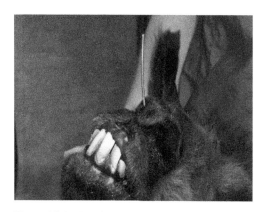

Figure 11.6 In this photograph, the guide wire has passed out the right naris. If orotracheal intubation was preferred, the wire would be withdrawn into the trachea and the head would be repositioned or a laryngoscope would be used to displace the soft palate dorsally to guide the wire orally.

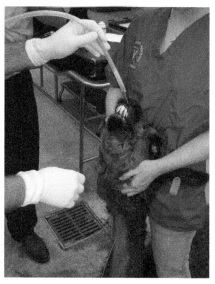

Figure 11.8 The guide wire is passed through the lumen of the endotracheal tube, to guide the tube through the nasal passage and pharynx, and into the trachea.

Practice Tip to Facilitate Procedure

Extend the head as far vertically as possible when passing the stylette to help avoid entrance into the nasal passage when not desired. This helps to displace the soft palate dorsally, which can also be facilitated by using a laryngoscope.

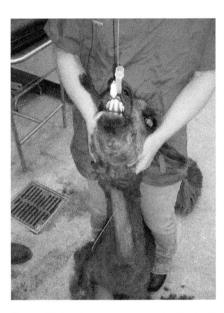

Figure 11.9 Once the endotracheal tube is placed, the guide wire is removed, and the tube is passed distal to the tracheal puncture of the trocar before inflating the cuff.

Potential Complications

The potential for localized infection and tracheal inflammation exists. This procedure is not routinely performed and has not been extensively reviewed regarding potential acute or long-term problem development in camelids. However, only mild epistaxis due to misguided stylette advancement into the nasal cavity was noted in a review of the procedure in llamas (Byers et al. 2009). Difficulty displacing the soft palate dorsally for oral placement of the stylette can be addressed by using a laryngoscope or the endotracheal tube to be placed. It should also be recognized that the cuff of the endotracheal tube should be distal to the area of the trachea that was punctured by the trocar to avoid development of subcutaneous emphysema.

Patient Monitoring/Aftercare

Monitor patient for signs of coughing, dyspnea, and localized infection at the tracheal insertion site.

Recommended Reading

Byers SR, Cary JA, Farnsworth KD. 2009. Comparison of endotracheal intubation techniques in llamas. *Can Vet J*; 50:745–749.
Riebold TW, Engel HN, Grubb TL, et al. 1994. Orotracheal and nasotracheal intubation in llamas. *J Am Vet Med Assoc*; 204(5):779–783.

Section IV

Catheterization

12

Vascular Catheterization—Jugular Vein

Meredyth L. Jones

Purpose or Indication for Procedure

This procedure allows administration of pharmaceuticals or fluids and collection of serial blood samples.

Equipment Needed

The following equipment is needed: clippers with #40 blade; gauze; iodine or chlorhexidine preparatory solutions; isopropyl alcohol; 2% lidocaine; #10, #11, or #15 scalpel blade; exam gloves; catheter or catheter set; 4 U/mL heparin flush solution; extension set; Elastikon or other neck wrap material; nonabsorbable suture.

Use the following guidelines for catheter selection:

- Adult jugular: 14 gauge × 5.5 inch (14 cm) or 16 gauge × 5.25 inch (13 cm)
- Cria jugular: 16 gauge to 20 gauge × 2 inch (50 mm) or 3.5 inches (8.9 cm)

These size recommendations are for over-the-needle catheters. Similar sizes are available for J-wire and camelid "peel away" catheters (MILA Int., Florence, KY), which are very useful in camelids, particularly for long-term usage.

Restraint/Position

Standing, recumbent, haltered, or chute restraint may be used.

Technical Description of Procedure/Method

For jugular catheterization, jugular catheters can be placed at any point along the length of the neck. However, these catheters are most easily placed without trauma to the carotid artery or esophagus when placed in the upper third or lower third of the neck. The jugular groove is easily located by palpation of the transverse processes of the cervical vertebrae and the trachea. (See Figure 12.1.) The fiber over the selected area is clipped and the area aseptically prepared. An amount of 0.5 cc of 2% lidocaine is instilled subcutaneously at the site of catheter insertion (Figure 12.2). The skin of the neck is quite thick in camelids, and over-the-needle catheters are easily damaged during insertion. A stab incision or tunnel into the skin (Figure 12.3) serves to minimize drag of the catheter in the skin. The jugular vein should be occluded with the thumb of one hand and the stylette/catheter unit flushed with dilute heparin. An effective

Veterinary Techniques in Llamas and Alpacas, Second Edition. Edited by David E. Anderson, Matt Miesner, and Meredyth Jones.

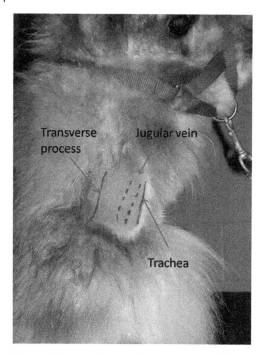

Figure 12.1 Location of the jugular vein within the jugular groove, lying between the transverse processes of the cervical vertebrae laterally and the trachea medially.

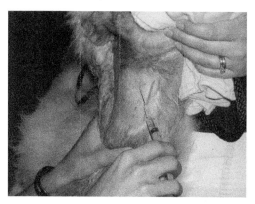

Figure 12.2 Injection of 2% lidocaine for local anesthesia subcutaneously over the jugular vein prior to catheterization.

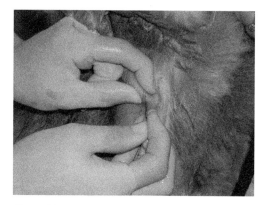

Figure 12.3 Stab incision made with a scalpel blade through the skin overlying the jugular vein. This can be helpful in minimizing catheter drag.

and thrust into the vein (Figure 12.4). Once there is blood flash, the angle of the stylette/catheter unit should be reduced toward the neck and the catheter fed off into the lumen of the vein (Figure 12.5). Pressure should be maintained on the jugular vein throughout the procedure to minimize the risk of dislodgement from the vein. The stylette should be removed and an extension set or injection port attached to the catheter (Figure 12.6). The catheter should be aspirated and flushed

blocking technique is to grasp the nuchal ligament with the tips of the fingers and roll the thumb over the transverse process of the cervical vertebra to compress the jugular groove. The trachea is positioned off the tip of the thumb. Then, the catheter is inserted through the skin at an approximately 45-degree angle

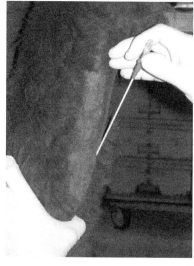

Figure 12.4 Occlusion of the jugular vein with the veterinarian's left hand with placement of the catheter/stylette unit into the jugular vein.

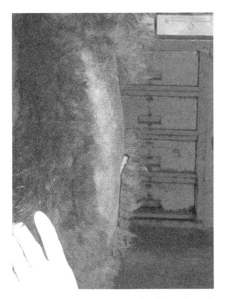

Figure 12.5 The catheter has been introduced fully into the jugular vein and the stylette removed. The vein is occluded to confirm placement.

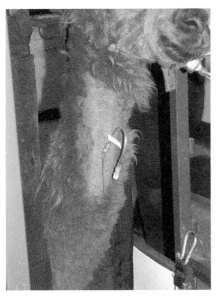

Figure 12.6 Attachment of an extension set to the catheter for ease of bandaging and fluid administration.

to ensure patency and location within the lumen. The catheter may then be secured with either adhesive elastic bandaging material, or with nonabsorbable suture (Figure 12.7).

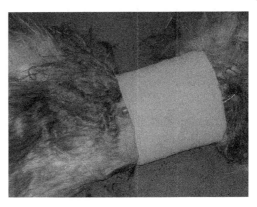

Figure 12.7 A neck wrap placed over a jugular catheter. The injection port is left outside the wrap for easy access.

Care must be taken, particularly in crias, to "lay" adhesive bandaging onto the neck, rather than wrapping the material to prevent neck and head edema. The adhesive tape is first placed around the neck and then over the catheter in such a way that the catheter hub is encased within the adhesive tape. This technique minimizes movement of the catheter.

Camelid "peel away" catheters (Figures 12.8–12.13) and J-wire catheters (Figures 12.14–12.22) require additional steps for placement as compared to over-the-needle catheters, and step-by-step photos are provided for these.

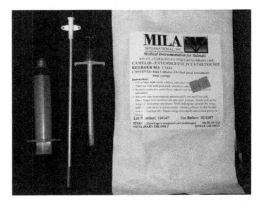

Figure 12.8 This package contents of the camelid "peel away" catheters, which includes a syringe, catheter, and insertion catheter and stylette.

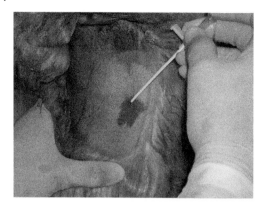

Figure 12.9   Insertion of the stylette and tabbed insertion catheter into the jugular vein.

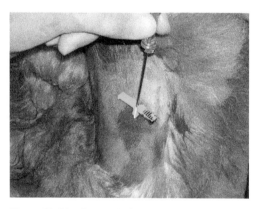

Figure 12.10   Removal of the stylette once blood flash has occurred and the insertion catheter is passed into the vein.

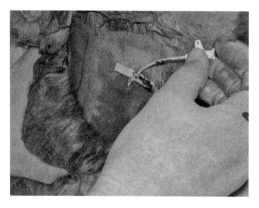

Figure 12.11   Passage of the actual catheter into the vein via the tabbed insertion catheter, which is acting as a conduit.

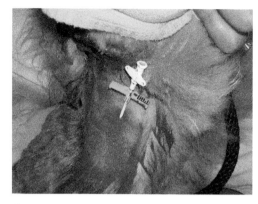

Figure 12.12   The insertion and actual catheters within the jugular vein.

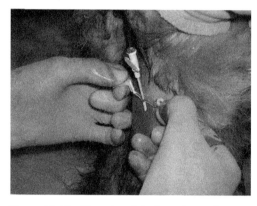

Figure 12.13   The tabs of the insertion catheter are grasped and peeled apart and away from the actual catheter and then removed. The remaining catheter is then advanced if necessary and secured.

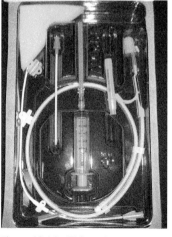

Figure 12.14   This package contents of a J-wire catheter set, which includes a syringe and needle, insertion needle, tissue separator, J-wire, and catheter.

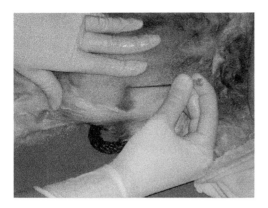

Figure 12.15 The insertion needle is placed within the lumen of the jugular vein.

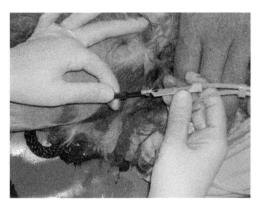

Figure 12.16 The J-wire is fed down through the insertion needle into the jugular vein, taking care to keep a grip on the end of the wire.

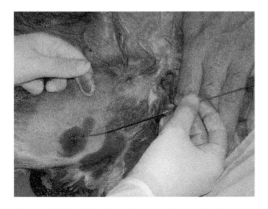

Figure 12.17 The insertion needle is withdrawn from the jugular, leaving the wire in place. Care must be taken to maintain a firm hold on the J-wire.

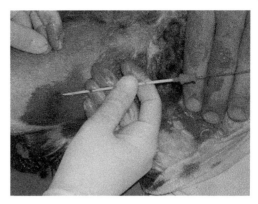

Figure 12.18 The tissue spreader is passed over the wire and pushed through the skin and soft tissues to make a wide passage for the catheter.

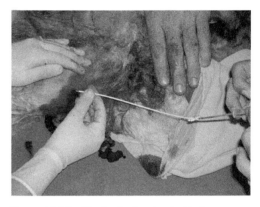

Figure 12.19 The J-wire is retracted to longer than the length of the catheter, and the catheter is fed over the wire. An assistant watches for the wire to emerge from the external catheter port and grasps the wire.

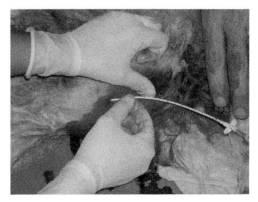

Figure 12.20 The catheter is fed along the wire and into the jugular vein.

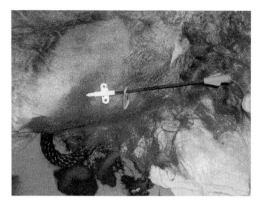

Figure 12.21 Once the catheter is in the vein, the J-wire is removed.

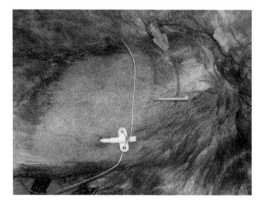

Figure 12.22 The built-in extension port on the catheter is sutured to the skin.

Practice Tip to Facilitate Procedure

In the author's experience, camelid owners are generally not concerned with fiber removal in ill animals for medical procedures, particularly of the neck. Clipping a wide area for catheterization is useful for visualization and hygiene. If the clip area is to be minimized, the fiber around that area can be taped away from the catheterization site to minimize interference. Part the fiber longitudinally overlying the vein, fold the fiber laterally on both sides flat against the neck, and use adhesive tape to secure the fiber in place.

Venous catheters should be flushed every 4 to 6 hours with 4 U/mL heparin flush.

Potential Complications

The esophagus or carotid artery may be inadvertently punctured when attempting to place jugular catheters. Hematoma formation, which is of little consequence in most cases, may become large enough to cause esophageal obstruction if it occurs on the left side of the neck from inadvertent puncture of the carotid artery. Thrombophlebitis may also occur.

Patient Monitoring/Aftercare

Catheters without a constant flow of fluids should be flushed every 4 to 6 hours to ensure patency and placement. The head and neck should be monitored for swelling secondary to a tight catheter wrap or thrombus formation.

13

Vascular Catheterization—Cephalic Vein

Meredyth L. Jones

Purpose or Indication for Procedure

This procedure allows administration of pharmaceuticals or fluids and serial blood collection.

Equipment Needed

Clippers with #40 blade; gauze; iodine or chlorhexidine preparatory solutions; isopropyl alcohol; 2% lidocaine; #10, #11, or #15 scalpel blade; exam gloves; catheter or catheter set; 4 U/mL heparin flush solution; extension set; Elastikon or other neck wrap material; and nonabsorbable sutures are needed.

Use the following guidelines for catheter selection: 18 gauge to 22 gauge × 1.5 to 2 inch (3.8 cm to 5.1 cm).

Restraint/Position

Standing, recumbent, haltered, or chute restraint positions may be used.

Technical Description of Procedure/Method

For cephalic catheterization, the cephalic vein may be catheterized in camelids as in small animals through the use of an assistant or tourniquet occluding the vein at the level of the elbow. The region over the antebrachium is clipped and aseptically prepared (Figure 13.1) and an over-the-needle catheter placed (Figure 13.2), an extension set attached (Figure 13.3), and the catheter is secured with adhesive tape or suture material.

Practice Tip to Facilitate Procedure

In the author's experience, camelid owners are generally not concerned with fiber removal in ill animals for medical procedures, particularly the fiber of the distal limbs. Clipping a wide area for catheterization is useful for visualization and hygiene. If the clip area is to be minimized, the fiber around that area can be taped away from the catheterization site to minimize interference. Part the fiber longitudinally overlying the vein, fold the fiber away on both sides flat against the leg, and use adhesive tape to secure the fiber in place.

Venous catheters should be flushed every 4 to 6 hours with heparin flush solution.

Potential Complications

Hematoma formation and thrombophlebitis are potential complications.

Veterinary Techniques in Llamas and Alpacas, Second Edition. Edited by David E. Anderson, Matt Miesner, and Meredyth Jones.

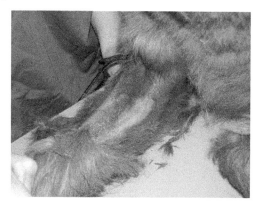

Figure 13.1 Preparation of the forelimb for cephalic vein catheterization. A rubber tourniquet has been placed proximal to the elbow, and the dorsal surface of the antebrachium has been clipped and prepared.

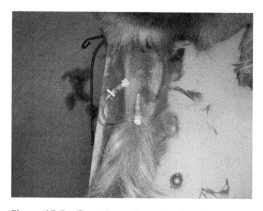

Figure 13.3 Once the catheter is placed, an extension set is attached and the catheter is bandaged to the limb.

Patient Monitoring/Aftercare

Catheters without a constant flow of fluids should be flushed every 4 to 6 hours to ensure patency and placement. The limb containing the catheter should be monitored for swelling secondary to a tight catheter wrap or thrombus formation.

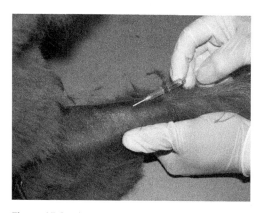

Figure 13.2 An over-the-needle catheter is placed into the cephalic vein.

14

Vascular Catheterization—Saphenous Vein

Meredyth L. Jones

Purpose or Indication for Procedure

This procedure is used for the administration of pharmaceuticals or fluids and serial blood collection.

Equipment Needed

The following equipment is needed: clippers with #40 blade; gauze; iodine or chlorhexidine preparatory solutions; isopropyl alcohol; 2% lidocaine; #10, #11, or #15 scalpel blade; exam gloves; catheter or catheter set; 4 U/mL heparin flush solution; extension set; Elastikon or other neck wrap material; and nonabsorbable suture.

Use the following guidelines for catheter selection, 18 gauge to 22 gauge × 1.5 to 2 inch (3.8 cm to 5.1 cm).

Restraint/Position

Standing, recumbent, haltered, or chute restraint positions may be used.

Technical Description of Procedure/Method

For saphenous catheterization, the lateral saphenous vein is catheterized proximal to the hock, on the lateral aspect of the tibia (Figure 14.1). The area is clipped and aseptically prepared, and an assistant wraps a hand around the distal muscle belly of the gastrocnemius muscle, occluding the vein. An over-the-needle catheter is used and secured using adhesive tape.

Practice Tip to Facilitate Procedure

In the author's experience, camelid owners are generally not concerned with fiber removal in ill animals for medical procedures, particularly on the limbs. Clipping a wide area for catheterization is useful for visualization and hygiene. If the clip area is to be minimized, the fiber around that area can be taped away from the catheterization site to minimize interference. Part the fiber longitudinally overlying the vein, fold the fiber away on both sides flat against the leg, and use adhesive tape to secure the fiber in place.

Venous catheters should be flushed every 4 to 6 hours with 4 U/mL heparin flush.

Veterinary Techniques in Llamas and Alpacas, Second Edition. Edited by David E. Anderson, Matt Miesner, and Meredyth Jones.
© 2023 John Wiley & Sons, Inc. Published 2023 by John Wiley & Sons, Inc.

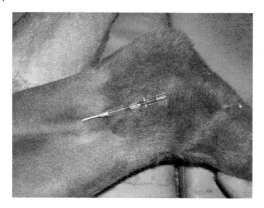

Figure 14.1 Catheterization of the lateral saphenous vein of a llama. An assistant has occluded the vein at the level of the gastrocnemius muscle at the proximal tibia.

Potential Complications

Hematoma formation and thrombophlebitis may occur.

Patient Monitoring/Aftercare

Catheters without a constant flow of fluids should be flushed every 4 to 6 hours to ensure patency and placement. The limb containing the catheter should be monitored for swelling secondary to a tight catheter wrap or thrombus formation.

15

Vascular Catheterization—Lateral Thoracic Vein

Meredyth L. Jones

Purpose or Indication for Procedure

This procedure is for administration of pharmaceuticals or fluids and serial blood collection.

Equipment Needed

The following equipment is needed: clippers with #40 blade; gauze; iodine or chlorhexidine preparatory solutions; isopropyl alcohol; 2% lidocaine; #10, #11, or #15 scalpel blade; exam gloves; catheter or catheter set; 4 U/mL heparin flush solution; extension set; Elastikon or other neck wrap material; and nonabsorbable suture.

Use the following guidelines for catheter selection: 18 gauge to 22 gauge × 1.5 to 2 inch (3.8 to 5.1 cm).

Restraint/Position

Standing, recumbent, haltered, and chute restraint positions may be used, but lateral recumbency is preferred.

Technical Description of Procedure/Method

For lateral thoracic vein catheterization, the lateral thoracic vein lies superficially on the ventrolateral body wall, just ventral to the costochondral junctions. The vessel is most easily identified in the standing animal. When the vessel is located, the animal is restrained in lateral recumbency and the area is clipped, prepared, and occluded just caudal to the elbow (Figures 15.1a and 15.1b). The vein may be viewed after soaking of the skin with alcohol, particularly in light-colored animals or it can be palpated. An over-the-needle catheter is directed cranially into the vessel (Figure 15.2) and secured using suture and/or butterfly tabs of bandaging tape.

Practice Tip to Facilitate Procedure

In the author's experience, camelid owners are generally not concerned with fiber removal in ill animals for medical procedures, however, the location of the lateral thoracic vein is near the prime fiber. Clipping a wide area for catheterization is useful for visualization and hygiene. If the clip area is to be minimized, the fiber around that area can be taped away from the catheterization site to minimize interference. Part the fiber overlying the vein, fold the fiber flat against the body, and use adhesive tape to secure the fiber in place. Venous catheters should be flushed every 4 to 6 hours with 4 U/mL heparin flush.

Veterinary Techniques in Llamas and Alpacas, Second Edition. Edited by David E. Anderson, Matt Miesner, and Meredyth Jones.
© 2023 John Wiley & Sons, Inc. Published 2023 by John Wiley & Sons, Inc.

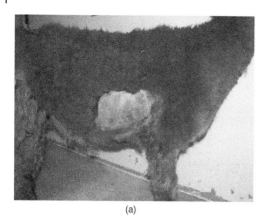

(a)

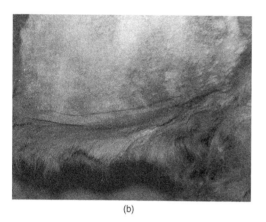

(b)

Figure 15.1 Location of the lateral thoracic vein in a standing alpaca. The vein is located between the blue lines in Figure 15.1b.

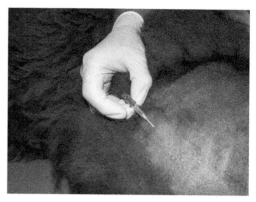

Figure 15.2 Placement of an over-the-needle catheter into the lateral thoracic vein of a laterally recumbent alpaca.

Potential Complications

Hematoma formation and thrombophlebitis are possible.

Patient Monitoring/Aftercare

Catheters without a constant flow of fluids should be flushed every 4 to 6 hours to ensure patency and placement.

16

Vascular Catheterization—Auricular Artery and Vein

Meredyth L. Jones

Purpose or Indication for Procedure

This procedure is used for administration of pharmaceuticals or fluids, serial blood collection, or arterial blood gas determination.

Equipment Needed

The following equipment is needed: clippers with #40 blade; gauze; iodine or chlorhexidine preparatory solutions; isopropyl alcohol; 2% lidocaine; #10, #11, or #15 scalpel blade; exam gloves; catheter or catheter set; 4 U/mL heparin flush solution; extension set; Elastikon or other neck wrap material; and nonabsorbable suture or skin stapler.

Use the following guidelines for catheter selection:

- Auricular artery: 20 gauge to 22 gauge × 1 inch (2.5 cm)
- Auricular vein: 18 gauge to 20 gauge × 1 to 1.5 inch (2.5 to 3.8 cm)

Restraint/Position

Standing, recumbent, haltered, and chute restraint positions may be used.

Technical Description of Procedure/Method

Auricular Vein Catheterization

Auricular veins are located on the dorsum of the ear. The ear is clipped and prepared, and a rubber band is placed around the base of the ear to occlude the vein (Figure 16.1). An over-the-needle catheter is placed and the rubber band cut off. The catheter is secured using an adhesive tape butterfly, with the tape wings sutured or stapled to the ear (Figure 16.2). Alternately, a gauze roll may be placed in the ear and the catheter secured using bandaging material around the ear.

Auricular Artery Catheterization

The auricular arteries are located on the dorsum of the ear and are most easily palpated on the upper one-third of the ear. Using digital palpation, each vessel on the ear is palpated for a pulse and the artery identified. Good head restraint is used and an over-the-needle catheter is placed and taped into place. A pulsing flow of bright red blood confirms arterial placement. Hematoma formation is common from arterial catheterization and after a failed attempt at catheterization or after removal of a catheter, firm pressure should be applied to the insertion site for several minutes.

Veterinary Techniques in Llamas and Alpacas, Second Edition. Edited by David E. Anderson, Matt Miesner, and Meredyth Jones.
© 2023 John Wiley & Sons, Inc. Published 2023 by John Wiley & Sons, Inc.

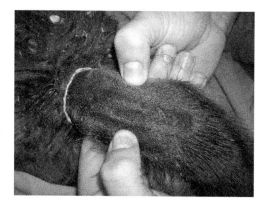

Figure 16.1 Locating the auricular vein after placement of a rubber band tourniquet around the base of the ear.

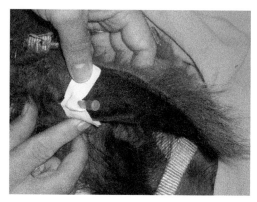

Figure 16.2 Butterfly taping of an auricular vein catheter, which may be sutured/stapled into place, or the ear may be bandaged for catheter security.

Practice Tip to Facilitate Procedure

Arterial catheters should be flushed with a 4 U/mL heparin solution every 2 hours, and venous catheters should be flushed every 4 to 6 hours.

Potential Complications

Hematoma formation, thrombophlebitis, and thromboarteritis are potential complications.

Patient Monitoring/Aftercare

Venous catheters without a constant flow of fluids should be flushed every 4 to 6 hours to ensure patency and placement. Arterial catheters should be flushed every 2 hours. The ear should be monitored for signs of an excessively tight catheter wrap.

17

Vascular Catheterization—Femoral Artery

Meredyth L. Jones

Purpose or Indication for Procedure

This procedure is for arterial blood gas analysis or blood pressure monitoring under anesthesia.

Equipment Needed

The following equipment is needed: clippers with #40 blade; gauze; iodine or chlorhexidine preparatory solutions; isopropyl alcohol; 2% lidocaine; #10, #11, or #15 scalpel blade; exam gloves, catheter or catheter set; 4 U/mL heparin flush solution; extension set; Elastikon or other neck wrap material; and nonabsorbable suture.

Guidelines for catheter selection follow: 20 gauge to 22 gauge × 1.5 to 2 inch (3.8 to 5.1 cm).

Restraint/Position

Standing, recumbent, haltered, and chute-restraint positions may be used.

Technical Description of Procedure/Method

For femoral artery catheterization, the femoral artery is located on the medial aspect of the upper hind limb, running alongside the femoral vein (Figure 17.1). This artery is more often single sampled (Figure 17.2), but it may be catheterized using an over-the needle catheter.

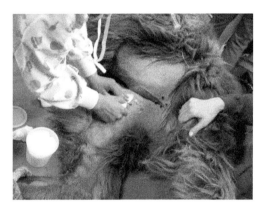

Figure 17.1 A femoral artery catheter placed in a llama undergoing general anesthesia. This catheter may be maintained for systemic blood pressure monitoring or arterial blood gas determination.

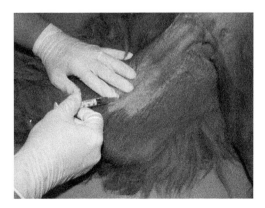

Figure 17.2 An arterial blood sample being drawn from the femoral artery on the medial aspect of the femur. This location may also be used for catheter placement for continuous arterial sampling.

Veterinary Techniques in Llamas and Alpacas, Second Edition. Edited by David E. Anderson, Matt Miesner, and Meredyth Jones.

Potential Complications

Hematoma formation and thromboarteritis are possible.

Patient Monitoring/Aftercare

Arterial catheters should be flushed with heparin every 2 hours to ensure patency and placement. The limb should be monitored for swelling around the catheter placement site.

18

Intramedullary Cannulation of the Femur for Administration of Parenteral Fluids

David E. Anderson

Purpose or Indication for Procedure

Intramedullary cannulation provides access to the medullary cavity and bone marrow for administration of IV drugs intended to be rapidly absorbed and distributed systemically through the blood stream of neonates (<3 months old). This technique is useful for emergency resuscitation of patients where intravenous access is not possible. Examples of these patients include extreme or life-threatening dehydration, hypothermia, and/or hypotension. This method of fluid therapy is less efficient in older patients because of fatty infiltration of the bone marrow and diminished trabecular bone network.

Equipment Needed

The following equipment is needed: clippers; povidone-iodine scrub; alcohol; 4 × 4 gauze sponges; 1 × 14-gauge; 3.5-inch intraosseous needle (bone marrow aspiration and biopsy needle); sterile gloves; IV fluid administration set (used for administration of crystalloids or colloids) or whole blood administration set (used for plasma or whole blood transfusion); and bandage material (sterile 4 × 4 gauze pads, skin adhesive tape, triple antibiotic ointment).

Restraint/Position

This procedure is normally performed in young, moribund patients, therefore, the llama or alpaca should be placed into lateral recumbency. The patient may be placed in right or left lateral recumbency to allow ease of insertion of the intraosseous needle. Right-handed individuals may prefer right lateral recumbency so that the left hand may grasp the stifle while standing behind the dorsal midline of the patient and the right hand used to drive the needle into the bone. Sedation may be required but should be used cautiously depending on the medical condition of the animal. When needed, butorphanol (0.1 mg/kg IM or IV) is most often sufficient. When needed, xylazine HCl (0.2–0.3 mg/kg for llamas; 0.3–0.4 mg/kg for alpacas IV or IM) will provide profound sedation.

Technical Description of Procedure/Method

A 10-cm × 10-cm area, centered over the dorsal aspect of the greater trochanter of the femur, is clipped using a No. 40 clipper blade (Figure 18.1). Aseptic preparation of the skin is done by using 4 × 4 gauze sponges in three consecutive cycles of povidone-iodine scrub followed by alcohol over a

Veterinary Techniques in Llamas and Alpacas, Second Edition. Edited by David E. Anderson, Matt Miesner, and Meredyth Jones.
© 2023 John Wiley & Sons, Inc. Published 2023 by John Wiley & Sons, Inc.

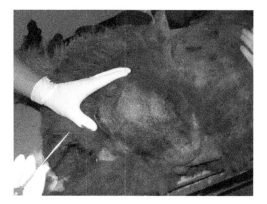

Figure 18.1 A large area centered around the greater trochanter of the femur is clipped and aseptically prepared.

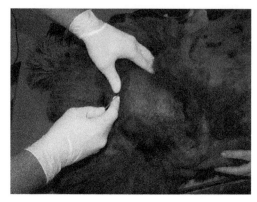

Figure 18.3 The greater trochanter is palpated and the muscle mass overlying the trochanteric fossae identified.

5-minute period. In extremely urgent situations, an abbreviated preparation may be done. Proper technique for aseptic preparation should be followed. Gauze sponges are touched to the skin at the center of the intended procedure area and moved in concentric circles of increasing diameter extending out toward the periphery of the prepared area, and then the gauze is discarded. The intraosseous needle (Figure 18.2) is inserted into the intramedullary space of the femur by palpating the greater trochanter and inserting the needle 1- to 2-cm medial (Figure 18.3). Then the needle is probed along the proximal aspect of the femur, medial to the greater trochanter so that the needle may be inserted through the center of the trochanteric fossa (Figure 18.4). The direction of the needle is parallel and central in the femur in such a way that the needle may be threaded down the femur in a manner similar to an intramedullary pin (Figure 18.5). The direction of the needle is best estimated by grasping the stifle with the free hand and palpating the femoral condyles and patella. The angle of the pin should be toward the midpoint

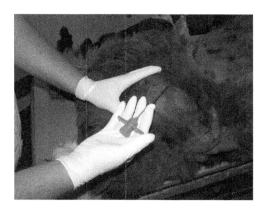

Figure 18.2 A bone biopsy and aspiration needle is grasped firmly and readied for percutaneous insertion into the intramedullary canal of the femur.

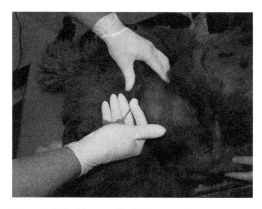

Figure 18.4 The needle is inserted through the skin and inserted into the trochanteric fossae. This may require "walking" the needle off of the medial aspect of the greater trochanter.

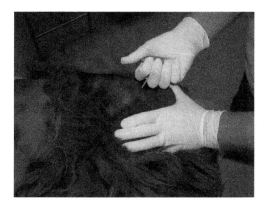

Figure 18.5 The position of the diaphysis of the femur should be assessed during insertion to ensure that the needle is threaded into the medullary canal and not placed trans-cortically.

between these two landmarks. Resistance is felt as the needle penetrates the proximal bone; this is followed by marked decrease in resistance to advancement of the needle while traversing the trabecular bone of the medullary cavity. The needle should be fully inserted (Figure 18.6). If resistance is felt again, this may indicate that the needle is being directed into cortical bone and the position of the needle reassessed. The desired location of the end of the needle is for the length of the needle to be fully engaged and the tip positioned within the center of the medullary canal. Urgency and expediency require that the location

of the needle be estimated, but radiographs may be obtained to verify correct placement prior to institution of therapy in stable patients. The trocar is removed and the fluid administration set attached to the hub of the intraosseous needle (Figure 18.7). With correct needle placement, fluids should flow easily but may not flow rapidly. A pressure bag or other means of increasing fluid administration pressure will increase fluid flow rate, and this rate may approach high volumes in neonates.

Practice Tip to Facilitate Procedure

This procedure can be readily performed under field conditions, but the operator is advised to practice the insertion technique on a cadaver to gain experience prior to clinical use. This technique may be used to improve circulating blood volume and pressure sufficiently to allow intravenous catheterization.

Potential Complications

The most common complication is failure to establish adequate fluid flow and accidental insertion of the needle through the bone into

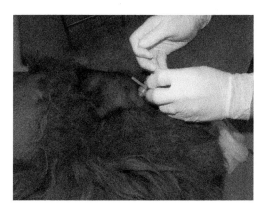

Figure 18.6 The needle is fully inserted to ensure that no displacement is encountered.

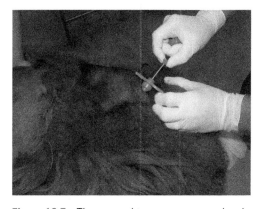

Figure 18.7 The cap and trocar are removed and the fluid line or a syringe attached to the proximal portion of the cannula.

the soft tissue compartment. This method can be used for fluid administration for up to 24 hours after needle placement, but the risk of ascending infection into the bone increases with the duration of use.

Patient Monitoring/Aftercare

Patients should be monitored for lameness or infection at the needle insertion site.

19

Intraperitoneal Cannula for Plasma or Fluid Administration

David E. Anderson

Purpose or Indication for Procedure

Intraperitoneal (IP) administration of plasma is popular among veterinarians working with neonatal llamas and alpacas. This technique offers a time efficient method for administration of plasma without the need to catheterize the jugular vein. Many people find catheterization of veins in llamas and alpacas to be challenging and prefer to use other techniques to achieve therapy goals. IP cannulas can be useful in crias < 30 days old for administration of predetermined volumes of fluids. These cannulas are not intended for continuous use. One rationale often used to justify IP administration of plasma is the expectation of lower complication rates as compared to plasma administered intravenously. This is based on anecdotal evidence. In fact, similar complication rates have been observed for both methods.

Equipment Needed

The following equipment is needed: clippers, aseptic preparation kit including povidone-iodine or chlorhexidine and alcohol, metal teat cannula, sterile gloves, IV administration set, lidocaine 2% HCl, No. 15 scalpel blade, and 6-mL syringe.

Restraint/Position

Lateral recumbency with or without sedation depending on the condition of the patient is recommended. Sedation may be required but should be used cautiously depending on the medical condition of the animal. When needed, butorphanol (0.05 to 0.1 mg/kg IM or IV) is most often sufficient. When needed, xylazine HCl (0.1 to 0.3 mg/kg for llamas; 0.2 to 0.4 mg/kg for alpacas IV or IM) will provide sufficient sedation.

Technical Description of Procedure/Method

Sedation is indicated in uncooperative patients to minimize the risks of untoward events during placement of the intraperitoneal cannula. Although intravenous catheters and needles may be used for IP administration, these are discouraged because of the increased risk of perforation of the intestines and abdominal viscera. In young crias (<30 days old), the left flank is the preferred site for IP cannula placement because the C1 compartment is small. The spleen is positioned in the left lateral abdominal space; care must be exercised to avoid puncture of the spleen. The right side of the abdomen is occupied by the C3 and intestinal mass. Care must be taken not to place the cannula in the dorsal aspect of the abdomen because this

Veterinary Techniques in Llamas and Alpacas, Second Edition. Edited by David E. Anderson, Matt Miesner, and Meredyth Jones.
© 2023 John Wiley & Sons, Inc. Published 2023 by John Wiley & Sons, Inc.

increases the risk of retroperitoneal placement or perforating the kidney or liver on the right side and the kidney or spleen on the left side.

A 10- × 10-cm area of hair is clipped from the skin of the left flank at a point adjacent to the costochondral arch of the last rib and at the junction of the ventral and middle third of the abdominal wall (Figure 19.1). The area is aseptically prepared using povidone-iodine- and alcohol-soaked gauze pads. The intended site for placement of the cannula is locally anesthetized using 1 mL of 2% lidocaine HCl. Sterile gloves should be used to ensure aseptic placement of the cannula. A small stab incision is made in the skin using a No. 15 scalpel blade (Figures 19.2 and 19.3). A teat cannula (Figure 19.4) is inserted through the skin defect and advanced through the abdominal muscular using continuous but gentle force (Figure 19.5). The cannula is directed into the abdomen at a 60-degree angle to the skin and advanced until the peritoneum is penetrated. This is usually evident by a sudden release of resistance. The intraperitoneal placement of the cannula is confirmed by gently rotating the cannula to ensure that the end is freely movable. The syringe is attached to the cannula and suction applied to verify that viscera have not been penetrated. Finally, the IV administration set is attached and fluid flow established (Figure 19.6). If the cannula is correctly positioned, the fluids should flow without resistance.

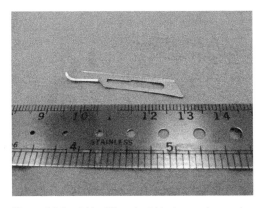

Figure 19.2 A No. 15 scalpel blade may be used to create a small skin incision to facilitate passage of the cannula.

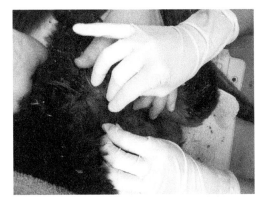

Figure 19.3 The skin incision may be made using a skin tenting technique to ensure that the abdomen is not inadvertently penetrated.

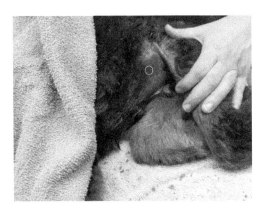

Figure 19.1 The site for cannulation of the left lateral abdominal wall is selected.

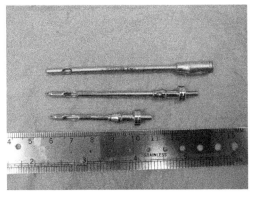

Figure 19.4 A variety of lengths of teat cannulas are available for use.

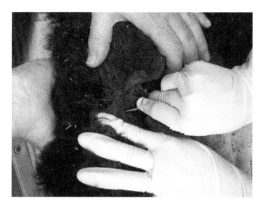

Figure 19.5 Placement of the teat cannula into the peritoneal cavity is achieved by steady pressure.

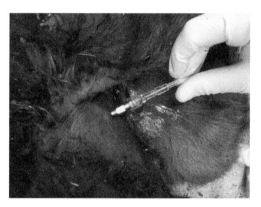

Figure 19.6 Intraperitoneal position of the cannula should be ensured prior to infusion of any fluid or plasma.

Practice Tip to Facilitate Procedure

Sedation improves the efficiency and safety of the procedure. Use of a short teat cannula diminishes the risk of incorrect placement of the cannula. Attachment of a syringe containing sterile saline to the cannula during placement allows infusion of a small amount of saline during introduction of the cannula. The saline will be freely and rapidly injected immediately upon penetration of the peritoneum and will decrease the risk of visceral puncture. Administration of flunixin meglumine (1 mg/kg IV) up to 30 minutes prior to administration of plasma may decrease the risk or severity of adverse reactions.

Potential Complications

Visceral perforation is the most significant concern, and this can be life threatening. Understanding of abdominal anatomy of the camelid will minimize the risk. Adverse reactions have been noted following IP administration of plasma and is recognized by vocalization, restlessness, increased heart rate, increased respiratory rate, recumbency, colic, and fever. Colic has also been noted after administration of sterile crystalloid fluids. Septic peritonitis has also been observed following IP fluid administration.

Patient Monitoring/Aftercare

The llama or alpaca should be monitored for 24 hours for evidence of adverse events including colic, lethargy, fever, anorexia, and recumbency.

Recommended Reading

Whitehead, Claire E., and Christopher Cebra. *"Neonatology and Neonatal Disorders."* Llama and Alpaca Care: Medicine, Surgery, Reproduction, Nutrition, and Herd Health: First Edition. N.p., 2013. 552–575. Web.

20

Caudal (Sacro-coccygeal) Epidural Anesthesia

Matt D. Miesner

Purpose or Indication for Procedure

This procedure provides regional anesthesia of the perineum for facilitating procedures and pain management. Caudal epidural anesthesia is most commonly performed during reproductive and rectal surgery as well as manipulating fetuses during dystocia but can also be used as an effective pain management technique. Lumbosacral epidural catheterization is recommended for long-term management of pain. See lumbosacral anesthesia and catheterization elsewhere in this text.

Equipment Needed

The following equipment is needed: 20-gauge × 1 inch (25-mm) to 18-gauge × 1.5-inch (38-mm) hypodermic needle, syringe, and 2% lidocaine.

Restraint/Position

Standing or cushed (sternal) positions may be used.

Technical Description of Procedure/Method

Palpate the movable sacro-coccygeal space by manipulating the tail head in dorsal and ventral motion. (See Figure 20.1.) Clip and aseptically prepare the area. Insert the needle through the skin with the bevel facing forward just caudal to the sacral vertebra and cranial to the first coccygeal vertebra. (See Figure 20.2.) Angle the needle approximately 60 degrees off the skin, directed so that it will travel ventral to the body of the sacrum into the vertebral column. In camelids, the epidural space has limited relative vacuum, rendering the hanging drop technique for verifying appropriate location of the needle unreliable. Therefore, the user is encouraged to attach the syringe with the anesthetic solution to the needle and apply gentle pressure to the plunger while advancing the needle. Inject solution into the epidural

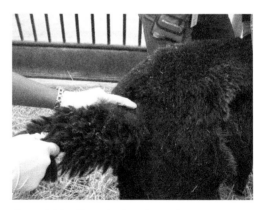

Figure 20.1 The clinician's index finger is placed over the moveable space between the last sacral and first caudal vertebrae. Moving the tail dorsal and ventral will allow palpation of this space for injection.

Veterinary Techniques in Llamas and Alpacas, Second Edition. Edited by David E. Anderson, Matt Miesner, and Meredyth Jones.

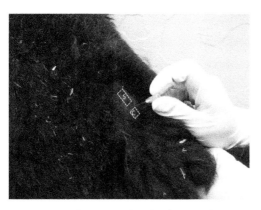

Figure 20.2 The needle is being inserted just caudal to the sacral vertebrae (**S**) and cranial to the first coccygeal vertebrae (**C**). Note that the clinician will have to decrease the angle of the needle to advance ventral to the sacral vertebrae into the epidural space.

Potential Complications

The volume of anesthetic injected may be sufficient to travel cranial to the nerve root branches of the sciatic and femoral nerves, causing recumbency with some drugs. The volume of 2% lidocaine injection should not exceed 1 mL per 50 kg (110 lb.) of body weight for standing procedures. The total dose of lidocaine administered to a llama or alpaca should not exceed 5 mg/kg body weight to prevent lidocaine toxicity. Neurologic and systemic complications from localized and ascending infection are possible, therefore an aseptic preparation of the area is required.

space. The epidural space is recognized when little to no resistance is encountered while injecting. The anatomical angles and narrow epidural space of the caudal region of camelids causes difficulty locating the epidural space by first observing free flow of anesthetic from the needle hub before attaching the syringe. Correct positioning can be confirmed by relaxation of the tail within 30 to 60 seconds after injection. Finish the injection and remove the needle.

Patient Monitoring/Aftercare

The duration of the lidocaine epidural lasts 1 to 2 hours. If the patient becomes recumbent due to the volume of lidocaine used, assure that they have solid traction during recovery and possibly consider hobbles to prevent pelvic limb splaying trauma.

Recommended Reading

Padula AM. 2005. Clinical evaluation of caudal epidural anaesthesia for the neutering of alpacas. *Vet Rec May*; 156:616–617.

Saltet J, Dart AJ, Dart CM, et al. 2000. Ventral midline caesarean section for dystocia secondary to failure to dilate the cervix in three alpacas. *Aust Vet J*; 78(5):326–328.

Shoemaker RW, Wilson DG. 2007. Surgical repair of femoral fractures in New World Camelids: five cases (1996–2003). *Aust Vet J*; 85(4):148–152.

Tibary A, Rodriguez J, Sandoval S. 2008. Reproductive emergencies in camelids. *Therio*; 70(3):515–534.

Practice Tip to Facilitate Procedure

Retain a small air pocket in the syringe with the anesthetic. Note the compression or displacement of air during injection. Lack of resistance during injection is observed when the air pocket does not compress during injection. This indicates that the needle is most likely in the epidural space.

21

Epidural Catheterization
Matt D. Miesner

Purpose or Indication for Procedure

This procedure is primarily indicated for situations needing prolonged analgesia or anesthesia. It can be used as adjunctive therapy for acute situations or as pre-emptive pain management. It is useful for preoperative and postoperative management of pain associated with surgical procedures of the pelvic limbs, abdomen, rectum, and reproductive disorders, as examples. This allows for provision of repetitive doses of analgesics to combat severe, persistent, or pathologic pain by way of repetitive epidural punctures. Repeat epidural becomes difficult after only a few repetitions due to localized inflammation and trauma. In addition, analgesics can lose potency resulting in shortened and escalating cycles of pain relapse with repetitive doses in some situations. For example, in severe cases of rectal prolapse, repeat lidocaine epidurals to alleviate discomfort after replacement or repair is met with shorter action and exponential relapse in severity of exhibited discomfort. Epidural catheterization provides a portal for repetitive dosing or constant rate infusion of anesthetics/analgesics tailored to pain response.

Equipment Needed

The following equipment is needed: clippers, scrub, sterile surgical gloves, epidural catheter setup, Tuohy needle, 2% lidocaine, white tape, and adhesive flexible bandage material. (See Figure 21.1.)

Restraint/Position

The procedure can be completed with the patient standing or in sternal recumbency. Sternal positioning has the benefit of widening the epidural space for catheter placement. Sedation may be necessary in some cases.

Technical Description of Procedure/Method

The area of catheterization must be clean and sterile techniques used. Clip and surgically prep the lumbar sacral area for catheter placement. (See Figure 21.2.) Inject 1 to 2 mL of 2% lidocaine in the subcutaneous tissues, but avoid puncture of the ligamentum flavum and dura, then surgically prepare the area again. (See Figure 21.3.) Place the materials needed for catheter placement in a sterile field. (See Figure 21.4.)

Insert the Tuohy needle through the skin to the epidural space. (See Figure 21.5.) Advance the needle toward the epidural space slowly so that you do not puncture the dura into the subarachnoid space. When you feel the epidural space has been reached, remove the stylette

Veterinary Techniques in Llamas and Alpacas, Second Edition. Edited by David E. Anderson, Matt Miesner, and Meredyth Jones.

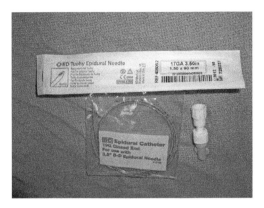

Figure 21.1 Epidural catheter setup including a Tuohy needle, epidural catheter, and injection port. The catheter and injection port are included in a package, but the needle will need to be purchased separately.

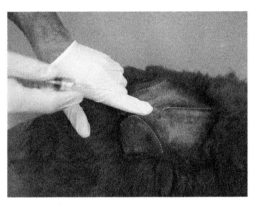

Figure 21.2 The clinician's index finger is placed on the location of the lumbar-sacral space approach. The tuber coxae of the pelvis and the dorsal spinous processes of the sacral vertebrae are marked with dashed white lines.

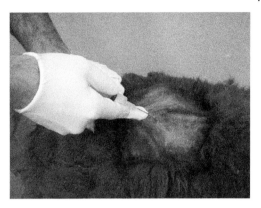

Figure 21.3 One to two milliliters of 2% lidocaine are injected into the subcutaneous tissues en route to the epidural space.

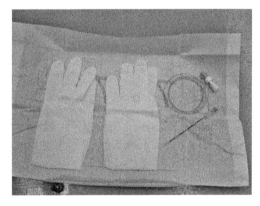

Figure 21.4 The materials needed for epidural catheterization are placed in a sterile field for efficient use. It is very important to be sterile in placement of the catheter.

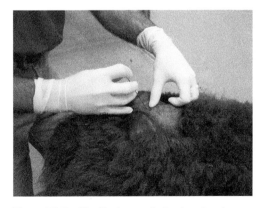

Figure 21.5 The Tuohy needle is placed and advanced toward the epidural space. Be sure the curve of the needle faces forward. Do not insert the needle too deep (refer to text for discussion).

and test for proper placement. If spinal fluid is observed in the hub of the needle, the needle is positioned too deep and should be retracted. Methods to test for epidural placement include the following: (1) saline solution freely flows from the hub of the needle into the space, or (2) the epidural catheter is easily advanced. (See Figure 21.6.) The epidural catheter placement will be met with some resistance even when correctly entering the epidural space. Resistance to advancement must be interpreted carefully so as to minimize repositioning of a correctly placed needle.

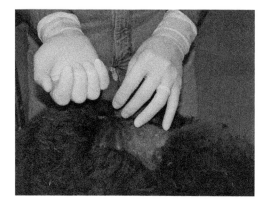

Figure 21.6 Saline is being placed in the hub of the needle to test for correct placement. The fluid should flow freely into the epidural space.

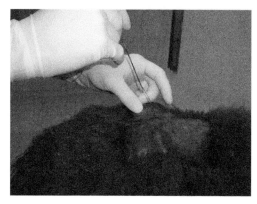

Figure 21.8 After the catheter is placed, the Tuohy needle is removed while the catheter remains in place.

When the epidural space is identified, insert the catheter through the needle into the epidural space, taking note of the length of catheter being inserted. (See Figure 21.7.) After placing the catheter, remove the Tuohy needle leaving the catheter in place. (See Figure 21.8.) Cut off the unnecessary length of catheter and assemble the injection port. (See Figure 21.9.) Affix one to two sections of tape to the catheter to serve as fixation points and attach them to the skin. The author prefers a tissue stapler to anchor the catheter. (See Figure 21.10.) Finally, place flexible adhesive bandaging tape over the

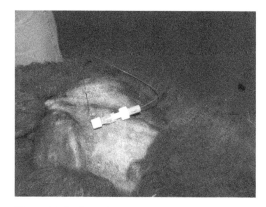

Figure 21.9 Extra length of catheter has been cut off and the injection port setup has been assembled to the catheter.

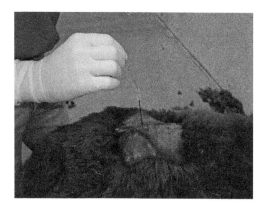

Figure 21.7 The epidural catheter is being placed through the Tuohy needle. Note: Some resistance will be encountered when the catheter is turning at the tip of the Tuohy needle as well as being advanced in the epidural space. The patient may show mild discomfort while advancing the catheter.

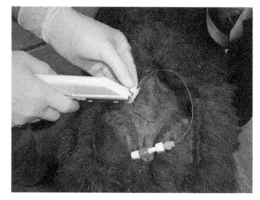

Figure 21.10 A section of white tape has been fixed to the catheter and is being stapled to the skin.

catheter and attach to skin in a manner to protect the catheter and site from contamination during use. (See Figures 21.11–21.13.)

Practice Tip to Facilitate Procedure

Local lidocaine anesthesia in the skin and soft tissue dorsal to the epidural space provides more cooperation from the patient while advancing the spinal needle.

Potential Complications

Infection is a serious concern. Use meticulous techniques to ensure sterile preparation and catheter management. Potential side effects of drugs being administered should be considered (Kalchofner et al. 2007; Martin-Bouyer et al. 2010).

Patient Monitoring/Aftercare

While the catheter is in place and for several days after removal, monitor for signs of lethargy, neurologic deficits, and body temperature.

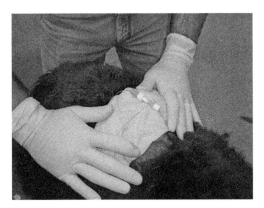

Figure 21.11 An adhesive flexible bandage material is being placed over the catheter insertion site to protect it from environmental contamination or damage.

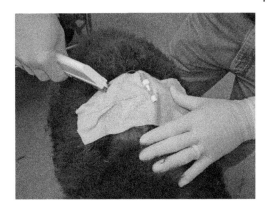

Figure 21.12 Additional support is being applied by stapling the bandage to the skin. Be careful not to staple the catheter directly.

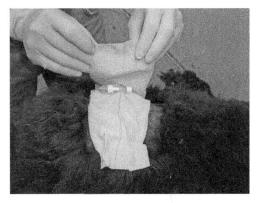

Figure 21.13 A second strip of bandage material is being applied for protection and easy access to the injection port.

Recommended Reading

Hansen BD. 2011. Epidural catheter analgesia in dogs and cats: technique and review of 182 cases (1991–1999). *J Vet Emerg Critical Care*; 11(2):95–103.

Kalchofner KS, Kummer M, Price J. 2007. Pruritis in two horses following epidurally administered morphine. *Equine Vet Educ*; 19(11):590–594.

Martin-Bouyer V, Schauvliege S, Duchanteau L, et al. 2010. Cardiovascular effects following epidural injection of romifidine in isoflurane-anesthetized dogs. *Vet Anes and Analgesia*; 37(2):87–96.

Smith JS, Schleining J, Plummer P. 2021. Pain management in small ruminants and camelids. *VCNA Food An Pract*; 37:17–31.

Sysel AM, Pleasant RS, Jacobson JD, et al. 1997. Systemic and local effects associated with long-term epidural catheterization and morphine-detomidine administration in horses. *Vet Surg*; 26(2):141–149.

22

Lumbo-Sacral Epidural Anesthesia

Matt D. Miesner

Purpose or Indication for Procedure

This procedure provides regional anesthesia of the abdomen, perineum, and rear limbs to facilitate restraint and pain management. Lumbosacral epidural anesthesia is most commonly performed for facilitating abdominal surgery and orthopedic procedures of the pelvic limbs. Lumbosacral epidural catheterization is recommended for long-term management of pain.

Equipment Needed

The following equipment is needed: 18- to 20-gauge × 3-inch-long (25-mm) spinal needle, syringes, 2% lidocaine, and sterile gloves.

Restraint/Position

Standing or cushed in sternal recumbency positions may be used.

Technical Description of Procedure/Method

Clip and aseptically prepare a generous area along the dorsal midline centered on the lumbar-sacral junction between the palpable tuber-coxae. Palpate the evident depression about 2 centimeters caudal to the last palpable dorsal spinous process of the lumbar vertebra. (See Figure 22.1.) Inject approximately 2 mL of 2% lidocaine subcutaneously and into the soft tissues en route to the epidural space, but avoid puncture of the ligamentum flavum and dura. (See Figure 22.2.) Aseptically prepare the area again before inserting the spinal needle.

Insert the needle through the skin and approximately 1 cm into the soft tissues just caudal to the last palpable dorsal spinous process of the lumbar vertebrae (Figure 22.3). Fill the hub of the needle with anesthetic solution but do not secure the syringe to the hub yet (Figure 22.4). Advance the spinal needle toward the epidural space slowly. Watch for disappearance of the anesthetic solution from the hub of the needle. If spinal fluid is noted to flow from the needle, it is positioned too deeply, and should be withdrawn slightly into the epidural space. (See Figure 22.5.) Attach the syringe with the anesthetic solution and inject the solution into the epidural space. The epidural space is recognized when little to no resistance is encountered while injecting. Finally, remove the needle. If spinal fluid was seen during the procedure, the volume of injection should be reduced by 50% so that untoward effects of the anesthetic do not occur.

Veterinary Techniques in Llamas and Alpacas, Second Edition. Edited by David E. Anderson, Matt Miesner, and Meredyth Jones.

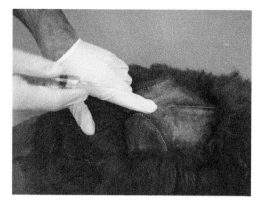

Figure 22.1 The clinician's index finger is placed on the location of the lumbar-sacral space approach. The tuber coxae of the pelvis and the dorsal spinous processes of the sacral vertebrae are marked with dashed white lines.

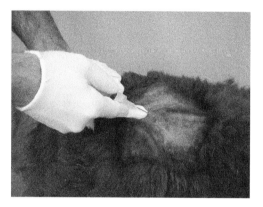

Figure 22.2 One to two milliliters of 2% lidocaine are injected into the subcutaneous tissues en route to the epidural space.

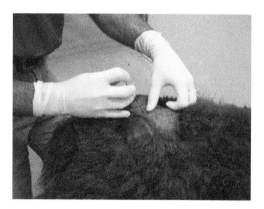

Figure 22.3 The spinal needle is placed through the skin prepared to be advanced toward the epidural space. Be sure the bevel of the needle faces forward. Do not insert the needle too deep. (See the text for further discussion).

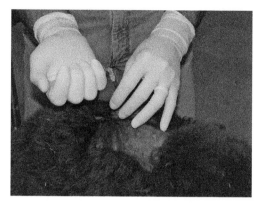

Figure 22.4 Saline is being placed in the hub of the needle to test for correct placement when advanced. The fluid should flow freely when the epidural space is entered.

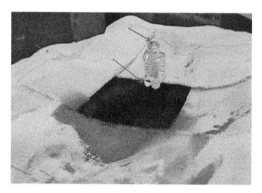

Figure 22.5 Spinal fluid is seen flowing out of the hub of the needle (*arrows*). Anesthetic volume should be reconsidered.

Practice Tip to Facilitate Procedure

Local lidocaine anesthesia in the skin and soft tissue dorsal to the epidural space provides more cooperation from the patient while advancing the spinal needle.

Potential Complications

The volume of anesthetic injected may be sufficient to travel cranial to the nerve root branches supporting cardio-respiratory function or brain and brainstem function. Be sure to keep the head and neck elevated to avoid undue cranial migration of the drug. Neurologic and systemic complications from localized and ascending infection are possible; therefore, an aseptic or sterile prep of the area is required.

Patient Monitoring/Aftercare

The duration of the lidocaine epidural lasts 1 to 2 hours. The patient will become recumbent, and residual effects will be apparent for a variable duration, therefore, assure that they have solid traction during recovery and possibly consider hobbles to prevent pelvic limb trauma.

Recommended Reading

Garcia Pereira FL, Greene SA, McEwen MM, et al. 2006. Analgesia and anesthesia in camelids. *Sm Rum Res*; 61(2–3):227–233.

Grubb TL, Riebold TW, Crisman RO, et al. 2002. Comparison of lidocaine, xylazine, and lidocaine-xylazine for caudal epidural analgesia in cattle. *Vet Anes and Analgesia*; 29(2):64–68.

Martinez M, Murison PJ, Murrell J. 2014. Possible delayed respiratory depression following intrathecal injection of morphine and bupivacaine in and alpaca. *J Vet Emer and Crit Care*; 29(4):450–454.

Scott PR, Sargison ND, Penny CD, et al. 1994. Application of lumbosacral spinal anesthesia for ovine caesarian surgery and for vasectomy under field conditions. *Therio*; 42(5):891–893.

Smith JS, Schleining J, Plummer P. 2021. Pain management in small ruminants and camelids. *VCNA Food An Pract*; 37:17–31.

Section V

Head and Neck

23

Anatomical Features of the Head and Neck

David E. Anderson

Purpose or Indication for Procedure

The head and neck region of llamas and alpacas is unique among ruminants (Figure 23.1).

The neck is long and has a wide range of motion in multiple orientations: dorsal-to-ventral, side-to-side, and rotationally. The vertebrae of the neck (C1 through C7) are prominent and form the majority of the bulk of the neck. Laterally and dorsally, muscle coverage in the neck is sparse, but camelids do have a well-developed nuchal ligament (Figure 23.2). Ventrally, the space between the transverse processes of the cervical vertebrae contains the trachea, esophagus, vagosympathetic trunk, jugular veins, and carotid artery. Camelids lack a jugular groove because of the absence of prominent musculature (Figure 23.3). Thus, venipuncture is more challenging and has a greater risk of complication, such as carotid artery or esophageal puncture, as compared with horses and other livestock species. Cervical subluxation and fracture seems to be more common in camelids than other livestock and may be associated with the combination of range of motion without significant supportive muscle mass (Figure 23.4).

The head of camelids features large eyes having a wide field of view, split upper lips that possess some tactile and prehensile ability, and a soft, cartilaginous nose (Figure 23.5). Llamas and alpacas are semi-obligate nasal breathers and cannot mouth breath effectively or for prolonged periods of time. Camelids are the only domesticated ruminant to have upper incisor and canine teeth. The upper incisor and canine teeth and the lower canine teeth are referred to as the "fighting teeth" because males use these teeth for defense and when fighting for hierarchy within a group. Camelids have a limited range of motion in their temporomandibular joint and therefore cannot open the mouth widely. Although this poses no difficulty for the animal, oral examination by handlers is limited in view.

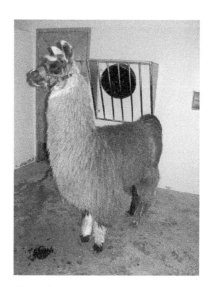

Figure 23.1   Llamas and alpacas have long, dense hair or fiber that covers the neck and shoulders.

Veterinary Techniques in Llamas and Alpacas, Second Edition. Edited by David E. Anderson, Matt Miesner, and Meredyth Jones.
© 2023 John Wiley & Sons, Inc. Published 2023 by John Wiley & Sons, Inc.

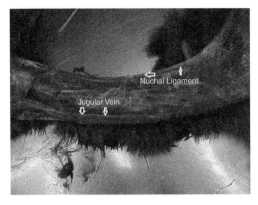

Figure 23.2   Relatively little muscle mass is present in the neck of llamas and alpacas, but a prominent nuchal ligament and jugular vein are present.

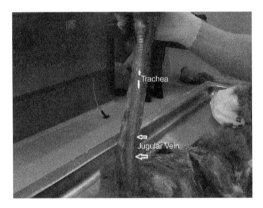

Figure 23.3   The ventral aspect of the neck includes the trachea on midline and the paired jugular veins, carotid arteries, vagosympathetic trunks, and the single esophagus (to the left side of the trachea).

Restraint/Position

Standing restraint is used. The head and neck are most easily examined with the animal restrained in a standing chute so as to minimize the side-to-side and evasive movements.

Technical Description of Procedure/Method

The neck is easily palpated, but hair or fiber coverage may interfere with visual examination. A

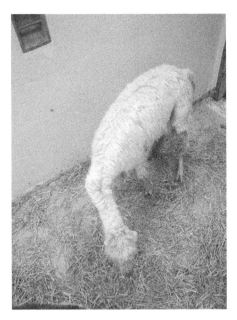

Figure 23.4   Cervical injuries such as subluxation of the C4-5 and C5-6 vertebra seem to be more common among llamas and alpacas as compared with other livestock.

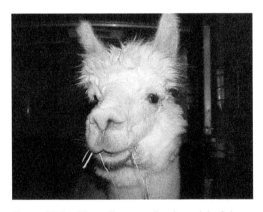

Figure 23.5   The split upper lips (muzzle) of the camelids serve to improve foraging capability.

mouth gag is useful to facilitate oral examination. Mouth gags designed for swine and small ruminants are effective in llamas and alpacas. Alternatively, homemade mouth gags can be readily constructed from PVC pipe, wood dowels, or similar materials (Figure 23.6). The gums of llamas and alpacas are easily traumatized, and the use of mouth gags frequently results in bleeding. This complication is self-limiting but

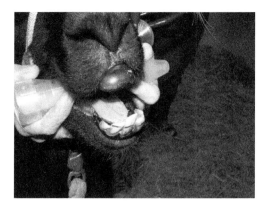

Figure 23.6 An oral speculum can be constructed from a variety of materials such as this 60-cc syringe case.

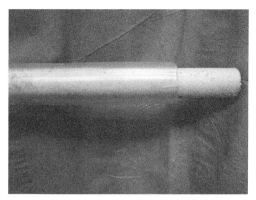

Figure 23.7 A PCV pipe with a rubber tube placed over top provides a firm but soft speculum for oral examination.

unsightly. Mouth gags should be covered with a soft material to minimize oral trauma (e.g., rubber coating, adhesive tape layering as shown in Figures 23.7 and 23.8). The lower incisor teeth of camelids should line up with the rostral edge of the dental pad when the mouth is closed (Figure 23.9). The cheek teeth normally have multiple points that interdigitate for grinding of forages (Figure 23.10). Flattened occlusal surfaces of the crowns of the cheek teeth are not desirable and may contribute to weight loss because of diminished grinding efficiency.

Practice Tip to Facilitate Procedure

Camelids resist oral examination, and sedation is recommended to facilitate complete inspection of the mouth (e.g., butorphanol at 0.1 mg/kg IV or xylazine at 0.2 mg/kg IV). A powerful light source should be available, and a head-mounted light allows for easy illumination.

Potential Complications

The most common complications during handling of the head and neck are bleeding of the gums during oral examination and obstruction of breathing under halter or manual restraint if the rostral nose is compressed. The

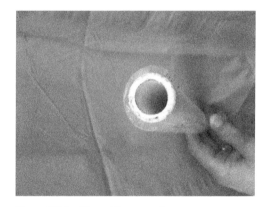

Figure 23.8 The rubber covering prevents bleeding from the sensitive gumline during use.

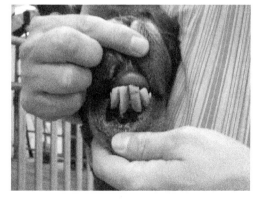

Figure 23.9 Camelids have a lower mandibular row of incisors that should meet the dental pad but not extend beyond its rostral margin.

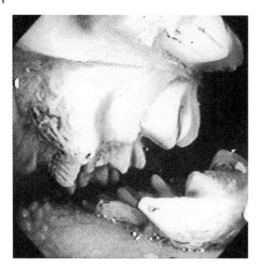

Figure 23.10 The premolars and molars (cheek teeth) are normally pointed and should not be filed down (floated) unless a specific problem has been identified.

handler should be aware of the risk of cervical vertebral injury and not leave the camelid unattended while restrained in a chute or tied at halter, or engage in uncontrolled, forced restraint.

Recommended Reading

Fowler, M. E. "Clinical Anatomy of the Head and Neck of the Llama, Lama Glama." *One Medicine*. Berlin, Heidelberg: Springer Berlin Heidelberg. 141–149. Web.

24

Dental Examination and Trimming

Meredyth L. Jones

Purpose or Indication for Procedure

This procedure is used for estimation of age, diagnosis of diseases including malocclusion, retained deciduous incisors, tooth root abscesses, wave-mouth, and tooth loss, and determination of causes of weight loss. The lower incisors and fighting teeth are routinely trimmed in most animals, especially males, until the teeth no longer actively grow (at approximately 7 years of age).

Equipment Needed

The following equipment will be needed: mouth speculum (1-inch [2.2-cm] polyvinyl chloride (PVC) pipe, bandage roll, swine oral speculum), exam gloves, light source, flush and dosing syringe, and rotary cutting tool with diamond cutting blade. Miniature horse floats or rasps may be needed in rare cases.

Restraint/Position

Chute restraint and sedation may be necessary for a full oral examination. Animals may be restrained by halter, but this limits opening the mouth for full exam.

Technical Description of Procedure/Method

The animal is restrained, preferably without a halter, in the standing position, and the operator's hand is placed in the commissure of the mouth. This action will cause the animal to open its mouth for incisor examination (Figure 24.1). The cheek teeth may be palpated with the mouth closed through the cheek walls for initial evaluation of the occlusal surfaces before the mouth is opened. Missing teeth may also be identified in this way. For oral examination, the mouth is opened using a swine oral speculum or PVC pipe and a light source used to visualize the tooth crowns, tongue, and oral mucosa.

Normal Anatomy and Examination Findings

The dental formula for llamas and alpacas follows:

- Deciduous: I 1/3, C 1/1, PM 2–3/1–2
- Permanent: I 1/3, C 1/1, PM 1–2/1–2, M 3/3

Camelids have a unique dentition. Unlike ruminants, the diastema contains incisor and canine teeth. The examiner should use caution, especially when examining adult males, not to injure their hand or fingers during dental examination. There are no incisors contained

Veterinary Techniques in Llamas and Alpacas, Second Edition. Edited by David E. Anderson, Matt Miesner, and Meredyth Jones.
© 2023 John Wiley & Sons, Inc. Published 2023 by John Wiley & Sons, Inc.

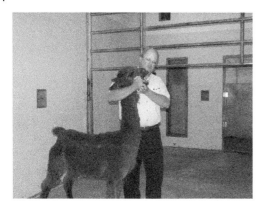

Figure 24.1 The operator restrains the animal in the standing position without a halter to allow full oral evaluation. The operator's hand is introduced into the oral commissure in order to open the mouth for initial examination.

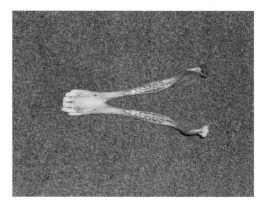

Figure 24.3 Alpaca mandibles showing the lower incisors and cheek teeth. The alveolar sulci are present with the mandibular canines unerupted.

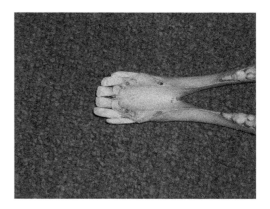

Figure 24.4 The mandibular incisors, demonstrating the initiation of eruption of the two permanent, central incisors behind the deciduous teeth.

within the upper dental pad. The single upper incisor is caudal to the dental pad and is shaped identically to a canine tooth. Caudal to it, there is a canine tooth, followed by the premolars and molars (Figure 24.2). On the mandible, there are three incisors, followed by a single canine, premolars, and molars (Figure 24.3).

Crias born at full term will have all three lower incisors erupted. The permanent incisors will come in at 2–2.5 years for I1, 3–3.25 years for I2, and 3–6 years for I3 (Figure 24.4). The canines and upper incisor (fighting teeth) are commonly erupted at 2.5–3.5 years. In males, these teeth grow to be long, curved, and extremely sharp.

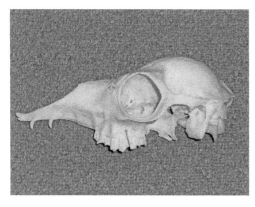

Figure 24.2 Alpaca skull demonstrating the single upper incisor, canine, and cheek teeth.

Alpacas have long, narrow incisors that continue to grow into adulthood, and enamel is only present on the labial side of the teeth. Llamas have broader incisors, which do not continuously grow, and have enamel surrounding the tooth (Figure 24.5).

The cheek teeth of camelids do not continuously grow, and the mandibular cheek teeth extend 3- to 4-mm medial (lingually) to the maxillary teeth, resulting in normal points on the crowns lingually on the mandibular teeth and buccally on the maxillary teeth. These points develop normally and should *not* be floated unless there is evidence of oral laceration, ulceration, or stomatitis adjacent to the

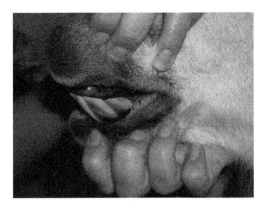

Figure 24.5 Normal incisor conformation in an alpaca, with the teeth just meeting the dental pad.

point. Additionally, the occlusal surface of camelid cheek teeth normally has sharp ridges for grinding coarse feeds (Figure 24.6). Came lids rarely get abnormal sharp enamel points, as horses do, except in cases of significant malocclusion due to congenital malformations, trauma, or tooth loss. Routine "floating" of camelid cheek teeth is strongly discouraged.

Externally, the maxilla and mandible, along with the lymph nodes of the head and neck, should be palpated, due to the high incidence of tooth root abscesses (mandibular abscesses are most common) in camelids.

Teeth Trimming

There are two main methods that are used to trim lower incisors. The first is a commercially available guarded power saw, which is available at many llama and alpaca supply houses. This author uses a diamond rotary tool bit (Figure 24.7). A PVC speculum, swine oral speculum, or bandage roll (Figure 24.8) is placed to lower the incisors away from the dental pad, and the rotary tool is used to cut the incisors off so that they just meet the dental pad when the mouth is closed (Figure 24.9). Some animals have incisors that have significantly overgrown and have begun to move horizontally away from the dental pad. These

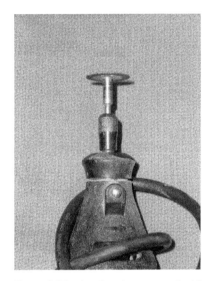

Figure 24.7 An electric rotary tool with a diamond blade, ideal for trimming the incisor and fighting teeth of camelids.

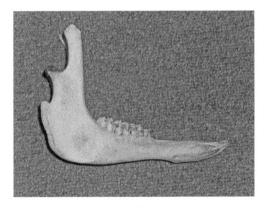

Figure 24.6 Alpaca mandible showing the normal sharp, rough surface of camelid cheek teeth.

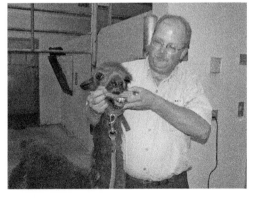

Figure 24.8 A 60-mL syringe barrel used as an oral speculum for incisor examination and trimming.

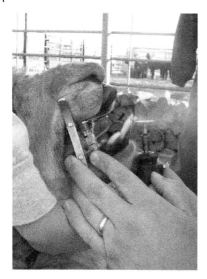

Figure 24.9 Severely overgrown mandibular incisors being trimmed with a rotary tool with the use of a swine oral speculum.

should be trimmed in such a way to maximize occlusion with the dental pad (Figure 24.10). Annual incisor exam is suggested, especially in older camelids, as well as teeth trimming of individuals as indicated.

Fighting teeth (upper incisor 3, upper and lower canines) should be trimmed in all intact males over 2 to 3 years of age and may also require trimming in aggressive females or geldings. These teeth can be trimmed by using a rotary tool with a diamond blade or obstetric wire. Obstetric wire can be difficult to seat on

the tooth. The sharp point should be trimmed off of these teeth, leaving 2 to 4 mm of the tooth above the gumline (Figure 24.11). Cutting them off lower can result in gum swelling, fossa formation, and feed material packing into the space. Fighting teeth should never be cut using side cutters or similar devices.

Practice Tip to Facilitate Procedure

Halters that fit well will often impede opening of the mouth, and it is useful to have a chute or standing sedation available to provide restraint for detailed oral exams. Standing sedation is strongly encouraged for a thorough oral exam. Most camelids are head shy and are resistant to manipulation of the jaws and oral speculum placement.

External palpation of the cheek teeth is easily performed due to the thin skin of the cheeks in camelids and can provide valuable information about the cheek teeth contour or loss prior to significant head restraint.

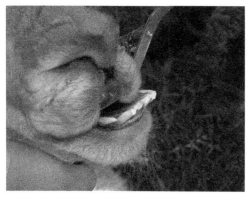

Figure 24.10 After trimming of severely overgrown incisors, the conformation remains abnormal but allows for improved function.

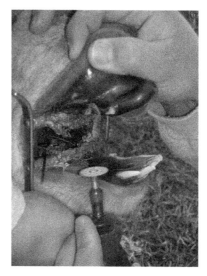

Figure 24.11 Use of a rotary tool for trimming fighting teeth. The upper fighting teeth have been trimmed to an acceptable level to remove the sharp point, while leaving sufficient exposure beyond the gumline.

Potential Complications

Teeth may become fractured by improper speculum use.

Fighting teeth may become fractured if cut with tools such as side cutters, resulting in root fracture and tooth root abscess. The use of such tools is strongly discouraged.

Patient Monitoring/Aftercare

The patient should be monitored as indicated by examination and treatments. No aftercare is generally necessary after fighting teeth or incisor trimming.

Recommended Reading

Cebra ML, Cebra CK, Garry FB. 1996. Tooth root abscesses in New World camelids: 23 cases (1972–1994). *J Am Vet Med Assoc*; 209(4):819–822.

Niehaus A. 2009. Dental disease in llamas and alpacas. *Vet Clin N Am Food Anim Pract*; 25(2):281–293.

25

Tooth Extraction – Oral Approach
David E. Anderson

Purpose or Indication for Procedure

Dental disease is increasingly diagnosed in llamas and alpacas. Although tooth root abscesses may be seen in llamas and alpacas of any age, most affected alpacas are aged 4 to 8 years. The most commonly affected teeth are the premolars and molars of the mandible, but infections of the incisor and canine teeth are seen as well. In the case of premolars and molars, the onset of tooth root abscess occurs during or immediately following the period of eruption of the permanent teeth (Table 25.1). Clinical experience suggests that infection of the incisors is more common among juveniles and may be associated with septicemia. When incisor tooth infection is seen in adults, these infections often are associated with trauma or as a consequence of retained deciduous incisors in young adults (3 to 5 years old). Infections of the canine teeth are most commonly associated with trauma or following excessive teeth trimming. Tooth root abscess involving the canine teeth are unique in that trimming of the crown of the tooth is a routine procedure, especially in males, to reduce animal–to–animal and/or handler trauma. Trimming of the fighting teeth (upper incisor and canine; lower canine) is done annually and is done most often in males during the period of prominent tooth growth (3 to 8 years old). Trauma to the tooth is most likely to occur when side-cutting tools are used or when trimming is done without sedation. Exposure of the pulp cavity or splitting of the tooth during trimming may result in bacterial infection of the tooth root or dental alveolus.

Equipment Needed

Chute, mouth gag, periodontal elevator, pliers, dental forceps (molar forceps), and sedation or injectable general anesthesia will be needed.

Restraint/Position

Standing, sternal recumbency (cushed), lateral recumbency position may be used.

Technical Description Of Procedure/Method

Incisor and canine teeth may be removed orally (Video 25.1: PM4 oral extraction). The third premolar tooth is also easily accessed and removed orally. When palpably loose, the fourth premolar or first molar teeth also may be removed transorally (Video 25.2: Removal of Deciduous Incisors). In many cases, sedation is adequate, in combination with a mouth

Veterinary Techniques in Llamas and Alpacas, Second Edition. Edited by David E. Anderson, Matt Miesner, and Meredyth Jones.

Table 25.1   Dental Anatomy and Eruption Times.

Tooth	Deciduous (1/3,1/1,2−3/1−2,0/0)	Adult (1/3,1/1,1−2/1−2,3/3)
I1	birth	2 years
I2	birth	3 years
I3	birth	3 to 6 years
C1	±, usually −	2 to 7 years
PM3	birth	3.5 to 5 years
PM4	birth	3.5 to 5 years
M1	—	6 to 9 months
M2	—	1.5 to 2 years
M3	—	2.75 to 3.75 years

gag, to gain access to the oral cavity for removal of these teeth.

When prolonged procedure times are expected, general anesthesia with orotracheal or nasotracheal intubation is advisable. When the procedure is done under sedation, infiltration of local anesthesia or blockade of the mental nerve diminishes adverse stimuli during the procedure and improves postoperative pain management. The rostral opening of the mental foramen can be palpated in the lateral aspect of the rostral mandible immediately caudal to the lower canine tooth (Figure 25.1). Retrograde infusion of 5 mL of lidocaine HCl 5% is done by inserting a 20-gauge needle into the foramen under palpation guidance. Anesthetic blockade of the mental nerve is more effective when done at the point of insertion of the nerve into the origin of the mental canal. The caudal foramen is located on the medial aspect of the mandible along the rostral aspect of the vertical ramus (Figure 25.2).

After sedation or induction of anesthesia, a mouth gag is placed so that the mouth can be held open throughout the procedure (Figure 25.3). Then, a periodontal elevator or small periosteal elevator is used to disrupt the periodontal ligament surrounding the tooth (Figure 25.4). A periodontal elevator may be sufficient

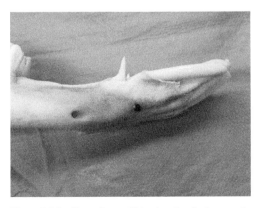

Figure 25.1   Rostral mandible showing incisor teeth, canine tooth, and rostral opening of the mental foramen on the lateral aspect of the rostral mandible immediately caudal to the lower canine tooth.

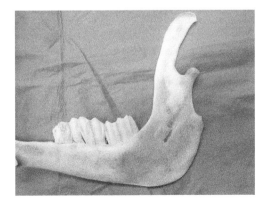

Figure 25.2   Anesthetic blockade of the mental nerve is done at the point of insertion of the nerve at the caudal opening of the mental canal, which is located on the medial aspect of the mandible along the rostral aspect of the vertical ramus.

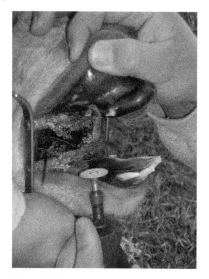

Figure 25.3 A mouth speculum, or "gag," is used to separate the maxillary and mandibular arcades for dental work. The mouth speculum pictured is a swine mouth gag.

to loosen the tooth until it can be extracted. The tooth should be extracted intact. In the event that the tooth root fractures in the process of being extracted, thorough debridement of the alveolus should be done to ensure that all remaining enamel and debris are removed.

If the tooth cannot be loosened sufficiently with a periodontal elevator, an osteotome or curette may be used to remove the lateral alveolar bone shelf and expose the tooth root. The infected tooth is removed, the cavity debrided thoroughly, and the mucosal flap sutured closed if possible. In cases with extensive bone involvement or when the mucosal flap cannot be closed over the defect, a drainage port is created ventrally through the skin and a passive drain (e.g., Penrose drain) placed to facilitate drainage. This is not necessary for maxillary incisor or canine teeth. When the third or fourth premolar is being removed, a molar extractor is useful to grasp the tooth and facilitate elevation out of the alveolus (Figure 25.5). When premolars and molars cannot be loosened, surgical removal may require a lateral approach through the skin or a buccotomy incision.

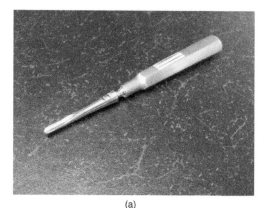

(a)

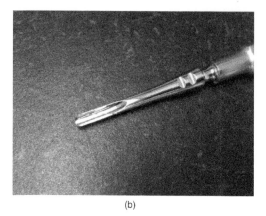

(b)

Figure 25.4 A dental elevator (25.4a), also referred to as a wolf tooth extractor, can be used to loosen incisor and canine teeth for extraction. The beveled edge of the extractor (25.4b) assists in disruption of the periodontal ligament.

Practice Tip to Facilitate Procedure

Commercial mouth gags are not available for llamas and alpacas. Sheep and goat mouth gags or a swine oral speculum may be used. These devices may include cheek teeth wedges or transverse U-bar inserts. When the transverse U-bar mouth gags are used, these bars should be padded because the oral mucosa of camelids is more delicate than that of other livestock, and bleeding and ulceration of tissues may result from use of the mouth gag. Retained mandibular incisor teeth are common findings in llamas and alpacas (Figure 25.6). If these teeth have

(Continued)

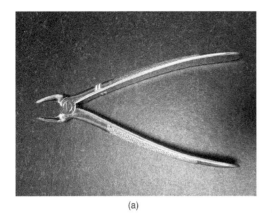

(a)

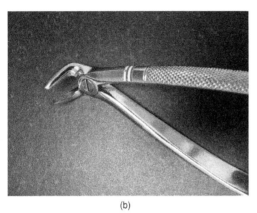

(b)

Figure 25.5 Angled molar, or cheek tooth, extractors are useful for loosening the tooth until extraction is possible (25.5a). The beveled edge of the grasping surface facilitates engagement of the edges of the tooth.

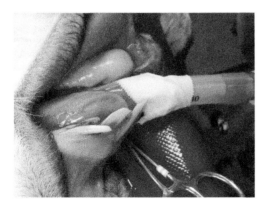

Figure 25.6 Retained deciduous third mandibular incisor in an alpaca.

(Continued)

not been expulsed by 36 months of age, they should be removed to prevent infection or damage to the permanent incisors. The deciduous incisors are lost by being extruded through the rostral gumline. The permanent incisors erupt caudal to the deciduous teeth and, therefore, the most cranial row of teeth is easily identified as the retained deciduous teeth.

Potential Complications

Fracture of the maxilla or mandible has been seen when extensive osteomyelitis is present and is more common with maxillary teeth extraction. Orocutaneous fistulas can occur and may be more common with mandibular cheek teeth extraction and when multiple teeth are removed simultaneously. Bone sequestra may occur at the surgery site if infection is not controlled. Long-term complications of tooth root infection are not well documented. Continued weight loss, anorexia, difficult mastication, septicemia, endocarditis, osteomyelitis, bone sequestra, damage to adjacent tooth roots or teeth, fracture of the mandible or maxilla, aspiration pneumonia, and bacterial embolization of internal organs have been diagnosed. Dysphagia or malocclusion may occur but are not as commonly seen because llamas and alpacas do not erupt their teeth throughout life.

Patient Monitoring/Aftercare

The ventral drainage wound is flushed twice daily until covered with granulation tissue. For incisors and canine teeth, this usually occurs over a period of 7 to 10 days. If draining tracts persistent beyond

30 days after surgery, radiographs should be obtained to evaluate the healing of the surgical

site. Antibiotics are continued for 10 to 14 days after surgery.

Recommended Reading

Cebra ML, Cebra CK, Garry FB. 1996. Tooth root abscesses in New World camelids: 27 cases (1972–1994). *J Am Vet Med Assoc*; 209:819–822.

Coyne BE, Frey RE. 1995. Tooth root abscess in llamas: 22 cases (1986–1995). *Vet Surg*; 24(5):423.

Fowler ME. 1998a. Ed., Digestive system. In: *Medicine and Surgery of South American Camelids*. Iowa State University Press, Ames, pp. 306–319.

Fowler ME. 1998b. Ed., Surgery. In: *Medicine and Surgery of South American Camelids*. Ames, Iowa State University Press, pp. 112–120.

Koch MD. 1984. Canine tooth extraction and pulpotomy in the adult male llama. *J Am Vet Med Assoc*; 185(11):1304–1306.

Niehaus A. 2009. Dental disease in llamas and alpacas. In Anderson DE and Whitehead CE, Eds.: *Vet Clin N Amer Food Animal Pract*; 25(2):281–294.

Niehaus AJ, Anderson DE. 2007 Jul 15. Tooth root abscesses in llamas and alpacas: 123 cases (1994–2005). *J Am Vet Med Assoc*; 231(2):284–289. doi: 10.2460/javma.231.2.284. PMID: 17630900.

Wheeler JC. 1982. Aging llamas and alpacas by their teeth. *Llama World*; Summer:12–17.

26

Tooth Extraction—Lateral Approach to Premolars and Molars
David E. Anderson

Purpose or Indication for Procedure

Mandibular and maxillary bone infections may be caused by trauma (e.g., resulting in bone sequestra), infection of a tooth, or hematogenous spread of bacteria (e.g., mandibular osteomyelitis). Although tooth root abscesses may be seen in llamas and alpacas of any age, most affected alpacas are aged 4 to 8 years. The most commonly infected teeth are the mandibular molars (M1, M2, M3) and premolar (PM4), and the onset of tooth root abscess often occurs during or immediately following the period of eruption of the permanent molars and loss of the deciduous cap. Treatment options for tooth root infections include no treatment, antibiotic therapy, drainage and debridement of the tooth, and extraction of the affected tooth. Tooth extraction is most often performed after failure to resolve the infection by means of antibiotics and drainage (Table 26.1).

Equipment Needed

The following equipment is needed: general anesthesia, soft tissue surgery pack, sterile gloves, face mask, rotating burr (osteotome or Dremel tool), periosteal elevators, self-retaining retractors (Gelpi, Weitlaner), and No. 0 PG-910 or other absorbable suture material.

Restraint/Position

Lateral recumbency with the affected side uppermost and under general anesthesia with cuffed endotracheal tube in place may be used.

Technical Description of Procedure/Method

Although the canine, incisor, and first cheek teeth (premolar 3, ± PM4) can be removed orally, the caudal cheek teeth, premolar-4 and molars 1, 2, and 3, are most easily removed via a ventral lateral surgical approach to the mouth. In most cases, only a single root of a single tooth is compromised, but both roots may be diseased (Figure 26.1). Occasionally, extensive mandibular osteomyelitis is present, and computed tomography scans can be helpful to delineate the extent of the disease and determine what teeth, if any, may be involved (Figure 26.2). When only one tooth root is involved, the remaining root is most often securely attached in the bone and considerable effort must be afforded to loosen or remove the tooth. A lateral approach to the mandible is made by a semi-curved incision along the ventral aspect of the mandible (Figure 26.3). The skin incision is centered over the draining tract (if present), bone enlargement, or diseased tooth root. The skin incision should

Veterinary Techniques in Llamas and Alpacas, Second Edition. Edited by David E. Anderson, Matt Miesner, and Meredyth Jones.
© 2023 John Wiley & Sons, Inc. Published 2023 by John Wiley & Sons, Inc.

Table 26.1 Dental Anatomy and Eruption Times.

Tooth	Deciduous (1/3,1/1,2–3/1–2,0/0)	Adult (1/3,1/1,1–2/1–2,3/3)
I1	birth	2 years
I2	birth	3 years
I3	birth	3 to 6 years
C1	±, usually −	2 to 7 years
PM3	birth	3.5 to 5 years
PM4	birth	3.5 to 5 years
M1	—	6 to 9 months
M2	—	1.5 to 2 years
M3	—	2.75 to 3.75 years

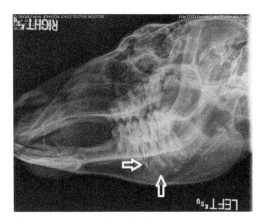

Figure 26.1 Lateral oblique radiographic image of an adult alpaca. The second molar tooth of the left mandible has extensive periodontal disease with widening of the alveolar space and lucency consistent with periapical tooth root abscess of the caudal root of M2.

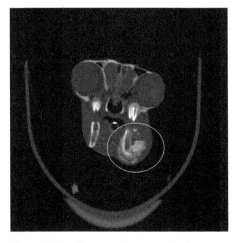

Figure 26.2 Computed tomography image of an alpaca with extensive bony proliferation surrounding the second molar tooth of the right mandible, loss of alveolar bone, evidence of osteomyelitis, and disruption of the tooth.

be located ventral and lateral on the mandible and should be no longer than that needed to access the tooth so as to minimize the risk of damage to adjacent structures of importance (e.g., parotid salivary duct, facial artery, facial nerve). Risk of damage to the salivary ducts or facial artery can be reduced by continuing the ventral aspect of the incision through the periosteum and onto the mandible bone. Then, the skin, subcutaneous tissues, muscle masses, parotid salivary duct, facial artery, vein and nerve, and the periosteum are all reflected dorsally as one unit (myoperiosteal elevation flap; Figure 26.4). If a draining tract

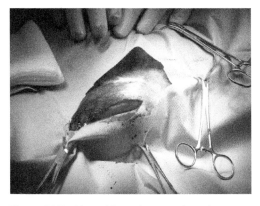

Figure 26.3 Ventral lateral approach to the mandibular arcade in a llama.

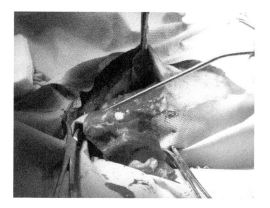

Figure 26.4 Myoperiosteal elevation flap reflected dorsally to expose the underlying bone to provide access to surgically approach the lateral alveolar plate and entry into the oral cavity to exposure the crown of the effected tooth.

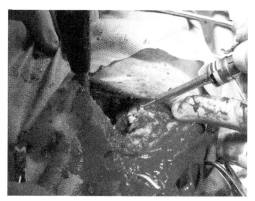

Figure 26.5 The lateral alveolar plate of bone overlying the effected tooth is most easily removed using a rotating burr such as this pneumatic osteotome.

is present, curettes, an osteotome (e.g., a compressed air-driven burr), and rongeurs can be used to enlarge the tract and search for the affected tooth root. After the compromised tooth root has been identified, the bone overlying the tooth is removed until both roots have been exposed. A periodontal elevator is used to disrupt the periodontal ligament and elevate the tooth. When a draining tract is not present, the myoperiosteal flap is elevated to the level of the oral cavity and the buccal mucosae overlying the affected tooth is incised and elevated from the gingiva to expose the crown of the cheek teeth. The affected tooth is confirmed either by anatomical comparison to preoperative radiographs or by intraoperative radiographs. After confirmation, an osteotome (e.g., a compressed air-driven burr) is used to remove the lateral alveolar plate of the mandible overlying the infected tooth (Figure 26.5). The tooth is removed using a periodontal elevator. Tooth repulsion by dental punches and mallet, such as that used in horses, is not recommended for use in llamas because the thin mandible is prone to fracture. Maxillary teeth are somewhat more challenging to remove. Intraoperative radiographs are useful to guide dissection. The maxilla is easier to fracture than the mandible, but these teeth can be equally as difficult to repulse. The parotid

duct, externally, and the nasolacrimal duct, internally, should be avoided during dissection and repulsion. After removal of the affected tooth, the alveolus is debrided and thoroughly lavaged. The ventral most part of the incision may be left open to facilitate drainage and daily care. Dental plugs, such as polymethylmethacrylate, are not used in most cases because of the complications encountered with their use in llamas and alpacas. Instead, cotton packing, such as tampons, is placed in the draining tract to partially fill the alveolus and prevent excessive salivary losses (Figure 26.6).

Practice Tip to Facilitate Procedure

Wolf tooth extractors are useful to disrupt the periodontal ligament and elevate teeth being extracted (Figure 26.7).

Potential Complications

Fracture of the mandible has been seen when extensive osteomyelitis is present and when dental punches have been used to perform retropulsion of the tooth. Salivary loss acidosis has been seen when ventral drainage wounds are left unattended. Orocutaneous fistulas and salivary fistulas can occur and

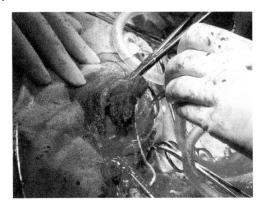

Figure 26.6 After tooth extraction, a temporary plug may be inserted using silicone dental putty, polymethylmethacrylate, or gauze sponges (depicted here).

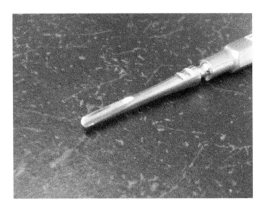

Figure 26.7 Dental elevators (Wolf tooth) extractors are useful to disrupt the periodontal ligament and elevate teeth being extracted.

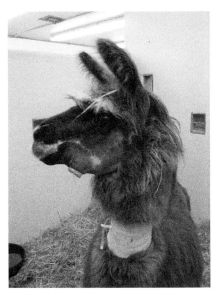

Figure 26.8 A cotton plug made from gauze sponges may be used to occlude drainage of food and saliva from the empty dental space between wound treatments.

may be more common when multiple teeth are removed simultaneously. Bone sequestra may occur at the surgery site if infection is not controlled.

Long-term complications of tooth root infection can include weight loss, anorexia, difficult mastication, septicemia, endocarditis, osteomyelitis, bone sequestra, damage to adjacent tooth roots or teeth, fracture of the mandible or maxilla, aspiration pneumonia, and internal abscesses affecting the liver or lung. Dysphagia or malocclusion does occur in some cases, but these are not seen as commonly as in horses because llamas and alpacas do not erupt teeth throughout

life. Over time, molar drift occurs to partially close the gap remaining after tooth extraction.

Patient Monitoring/Aftercare

The ventral drainage wound is flushed daily until covered with granulation tissue. This is expected to occur over a period of 14 to 21 days. A cotton plug may be used to occlude drainage of food and saliva between wound flushing (Figure 26.8). Plugs are no longer needed when sufficient granulation tissue is present to prevent excessive salivary loss and food contamination of the wound. The use of intra-oral plugs (e.g., silicone rubber, PMMA, etc.) has been discontinued because of complications (prolonged retention of the plug, infection associated with the plug, dysphagia, etc.) associated with the presence of the dental plug. If draining tracts persistent beyond 30 days after surgery, radiographs should be obtained to evaluate the healing of the surgical site. Antibiotics are continued for 14 to 21 days after surgery and nonsteroidal anti-inflammatory drugs are used as needed.

Recommended Reading

Cebra ML, Cebra CK, Garry FB. 1996. Tooth root abscesses in New World camelids: 27 cases (1972–1994). *J Am Vet Med Assoc*; 209:819–822.

Coyne BE, Frey RE. 1995. Tooth root abscess in llamas: 22 cases (1986–1995). *Vet Surg*; 24(5):423.

Fowler ME. 1998. Ed., Digestive system. In: *Medicine and Surgery of South American Camelids*. Ames, Iowa State University Press, pp. 306–319.

Fowler ME. 1998. Ed., Surgery. In: *Medicine and Surgery of South American Camelids*. Ames, Iowa State University Press, pp. 112–120.

Koch MD. 1984. Canine tooth extraction and pulpotomy in the adult male llama. *J Am Vet Med Assoc*; 185(11):1304–1306.

Niehaus A. 2009. Dental disease in llamas and alpacas. In Anderson DE and Whitehead CE, Eds.: *Vet Clin N Amer Food Animal Pract*; 25(2):281–294.

Niehaus AJ, Anderson DE. 2007 Jul 15. Tooth root abscesses in llamas and alpacas: 123 cases (1994–2005). *J Am Vet Med Assoc*; 231(2): 284–289. doi: 10.2460/javma.231.2.284. PMID: 17630900.

Wheeler JC. 1982. Aging llamas and alpacas by their teeth. *Llama World*; Summer:12–17.

27

Examination of the Ear
Matt D. Miesner

Purpose or Indication for Procedure

Llamas and alpacas show a variation in shape and size of the pinna of the ears. Llamas have longer ears that vary in shape from straight to curved, whereas alpaca ears are short and spear shaped. Hair length is also variable. The cartilage of the pinna may be abnormally weak or misshapen from environmental insults (e.g., hypothermia "frost bite"), infection, trauma, premature births, and congenital birth defects (Fowler 1998).

The clinician is occasionally called upon to examine an animal with a droopy ear or evaluate a foul discharge noted by the owner (Figure 27.1). Clinical examination may indicate irritation from a foreign body (grass awn), infestation (spinose ear ticks), or infection (otitis externa) possibly triggered by trauma such as fighting. Clinical signs may be more dramatic, having originally appeared localized to the ear but now apparently affecting cranial nerves and vestibular system indicating otitis media/ interna (Fowler and Gillespie 1985; Koenig et al. 2001; Van Metre et al. 1991).

However, moderate to severe destruction of the tympanic bullae, as seen on CT scans, has been diagnosed with little to no outward clinical signs in the patient. Otitis media/interna in llamas and alpacas is thought to develop after ascending infection from the external auditory canal. However, these infections may also arise from the nasopharynx by ascension through the Eustachian tubes. Herd outbreaks of otitis externa have been observed when alpacas were randomly misted with water to keep them cool during the heat of summer. Herd outbreaks of otitis interna/media have been diagnosed after infestation with spinose ear ticks.

Difficulty arises when examining the ear and ear canal in camelids. Llamas and alpacas resist handling of the ear especially if there is a history of frequent use of the ear during manual restraint. This procedure may require sedation. Otoscopic examination is very limited due to the anatomical shape and size of the ear canal (Fowler and Gillespie 1985) (Figure 27.2). Flexible endoscopes, radiographs, and computed tomography are often required to evaluate problems involving the ear canal, internal ear, and tympanic bullae.

Equipment Needed

An otoscope with a long slender cone will be needed. Optional equipment may include a flexible pediatric endoscope (<6 mm diameter), radiographic equipment, and computed tomography. In llamas or alpacas suspected of having congenital ear defects, otic biopsy may be performed for histopathologic examination. A 2-mm to 4-mm diameter skin biopsy punch

Veterinary Techniques in Llamas and Alpacas, Second Edition. Edited by David E. Anderson, Matt Miesner, and Meredyth Jones.
© 2023 John Wiley & Sons, Inc. Published 2023 by John Wiley & Sons, Inc.

or a swine ear-notching tool is an efficient method for specimen collection.

Restraint/Position

Camelids resist examination and handling of the ear for examination, especially when the ears are painful or inflamed. Sedation is usually necessary. Butorphanol (0.1 mg/kg IV) and/or xylazine (0.2 mg/kg IV) are sufficient to facilitate most otic examinations.

Technical Description of Procedure/Method

First, view the external pinna of the ear for clinical signs of trauma (laceration, aural hematoma), alopecia, infection, or parasite infestation. The integrity of the cartilage should be evaluated in neonates in conjunction with physical exam and signalment parameters to attempt to differentiate weak cartilage from congenital defects (Fowler 1998) (Figure 27.3).

The external vertical ear canal lies adjacent to the lateral portion of the annular cartilage of the pinna. There is a conchal eminence medial to the vertical canal, which can lead to

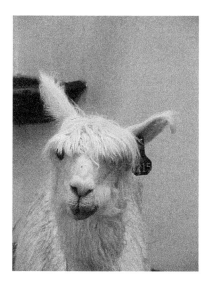

Figure 27.1 Photograph of an alpaca with otitis media/interna. Note the deviated nasal septum indicating nerve paralysis.

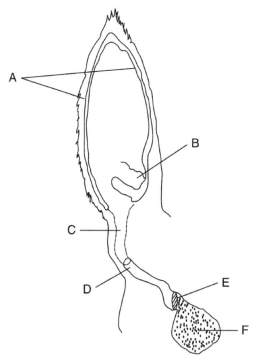

Figure 27.2 Sketch diagram (cutaway anterior view) of the structures of the external, middle, and inner right ear: (**A**) the cartilage of the external pinna, (**B**) the area of the conchal eminence, (**C**) the lateral vertical canal, (**D**) the beginning of the bony horizontal canal, (**E**) the tympanic membrane, and (**F**) the tympanic bulla.

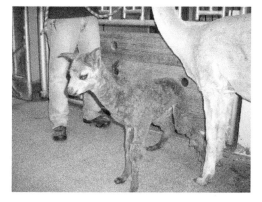

Figure 27.3 Photograph of a newborn cria that was showing signs of prematurity. Note the lax cartilage of the external pinna, which resolved within a few days of birth. Congenital cartilage laxity is more pronounced and does not resolve.

confusion when attempting to insert the otoscope (Figure 27.4). A marked medial curvature is noted when entering the horizontal or external osseous ear canal, which tapers to only a few millimeters in diameter. Then, the ear canal courses ventral and medial making viewing of this portion of the ear and tympanic membrane extremely difficult with routine otoscopic equipment (Figure 27.2). Flexible image-generating otoscopy of pediatric sizes (4-mm bronchoscope) can be used if available. However, plain and contrast radiography and/or computed tomography (CT) are recommended to best evaluate the deeper structures of the ear (Figures 27.5 to 27.7). Computed tomography has proven to be the most

effective tool for assessment of the inner ear and tympanic bullae because interpretation of radiographic images is often inconclusive.

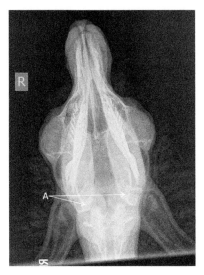

Figure 27.6 Skull radiograph of a young alpaca with acute external otitis. Tympanic bulla (**A**) are radiographically normal. The level of interpretation of skull radiographs regarding otic pathology can be difficult in some patients depending on age and the degree and duration of inflammation.

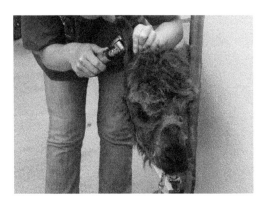

Figure 27.4 Otoscopic exam of the external canal of camelids is limited due to anatomy and natural patient resistance. A narrow cone should be used and placed lateral to the conchal eminence of the external pinna. The angle of the otoscope in this picture is directed toward the conchal eminence and needs to be directed more lateral and vertically to visualize the ear canal.

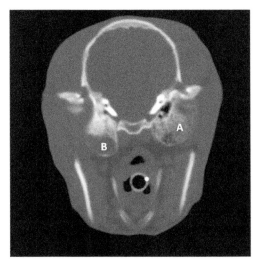

Figure 27.7 CT image of a patient with severe right-sided otitis interna. The abnormal tympanic bulla (**B**) can be compared to the normal left bulla (**A**). Interestingly, this patient did not have any obvious neurologic deficits. Foul discharge from the right ear was the only presenting complaint.

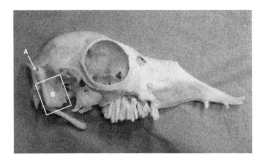

Figure 27.5 Picture of an alpaca skull showing the bony ear canal (**A**), and right tympanic bulla (**B**).

Recommended Reading

Fowler ME. 1998. *Medicine and Surgery of South American Camelids*, 2nd Edition. Blackwell Publishing, Ames, IA, pp. 441–444.

Fowler ME, Gillespie D. 1985. Middle and inner ear infection in llamas. *J Zoo Anim Med*; 16:9–15.

Gauly M, Vaughan J, Hogreve SK, et al. 2008. Brainstem auditory evoked potential assessment of auditory function and congenital deafness in llamas (Lama glama) and alpacas (L pacos). *J Vet Intern Med*; 19(5):756–760.

Koenig JB, Watrous BJ, Kaneps AJ, et al. 2001. Otitis media in a llama. *J Am Vet Med Assoc*; 218(1):1619–1623.

Mazulis CA, Erb HN, Thachil A, et al. 2019. External ear cytological results and resident flora of clinically normal alpacas (Vicugna pacos). *Vet Derm*; 30:337–341.

Van Metre DC, Barrington GM, Parish SM, et al. 1991, July 15. Otitis media/interna and suppurative meningoencephalomyelitis associated with Listeria monocytogenes infection in a llama. *J Am Vet Med Assoc*; 199(2):236–240.

Section VI

Skin

28

Anatomical Comments on the Skin

Matt D. Miesner

Purpose or Indication for Procedure

Dermatologic diseases in camelids may be infectious, parasitic, and metabolic in origin. Comments on normal anatomy of the skin are warranted to better identify actual problems or recognize normal variation from more commonly encountered species. Gross anatomical distinctiveness should be recognized, and histological aspects have been classified in the llama (Atlee et al. 1997).

Restraint/Position

The standing restraint position is used. For evaluation of the skin, a "hands on" approach is needed, where the entire animal can be examined.

Technical Description of Procedure/Method

Hair or fiber character and quality of camelids vary dependent upon species as well as genetic selection. The fiber is thinner and naturally sparse around the perineum, sternum, ventrum, axilla, and inguinal regions. (See Figures 28.1–28.4.) These areas provide access to visualize skin appearance and integrity. The axillary region is the site for performing intradermal tuberculin skin testing. The pinna of the ears and bridge of the nose are common sites for alopecia to arise from rubbing during insect season. In addition, the ears and face may be affected by hair loss associated with hormonal changes during gestation in some females, which spontaneously resolve during gestation or after parturition. With generalized poor hair growth, breakage, and/ or alopecia consider metabolic problems such as micro and macromineral disparities such as copper, molybdenum, and protein/energy mismatches.

Unique integument characteristics should be recognized. The skin is relatively thick, especially in the cervical region of intact males, as well as tense and nonpliable. (See Figure 28.5.) Camelids have functional sweat and sebaceous glands that can initiate abnormal growths in addition to their normal thermoregulatory functions. They also possess normal glandular structures seen at both the medial and lateral metatarsal regions, which are long, thick, scaly skinned areas, and should not be confused with "equine chestnuts" or pathology. (See Figure 28.6.) Also note a similar appearance of the dorsal interdigital space; these are interdigital glands. (See Figure 28.7.) Unlike cloven-hooved species where interdigital pododermatitis commonly affects the interdigital cleft of the hoof, camelids are affected by an infectious pododermatitis that will commonly

Veterinary Techniques in Llamas and Alpacas, Second Edition. Edited by David E. Anderson, Matt Miesner, and Meredyth Jones.

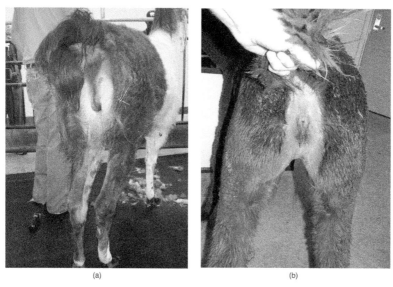

Figure 28.1 Normally thin hair distribution in the perineum and medial thigh.

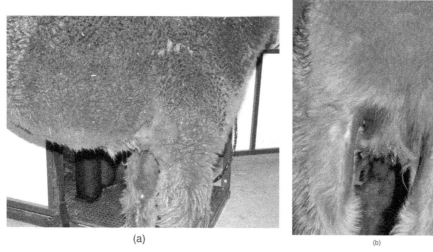

Figure 28.2 (a, b) Thin fiber coat is seen in the axilla. This is the indicated site for tuberculin skin testing in camelids.

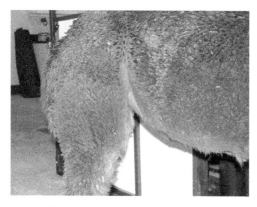

Figure 28.3 Normal thin fiber distribution along ventral abdomen.

cause a central, circular, necrotic lesion in the bottom of the foot pad. Generalized crusty, thickened skin may be associated with other dietary deficiencies, such as a zinc responsive dermatosis, immune-mediated or infectious dermatitis and others (Lamm et al. 2009; Van Saun 2006).

Skin problems from ectoparasites are recognized in camelids, causing variable syndromes of alopecia, erythema, hyperkeratosis, pruritis, and skin excoriation (Lusat et al. 2009). Both subclinical and clinical manifestations exist to various mange mites, including demodicosis

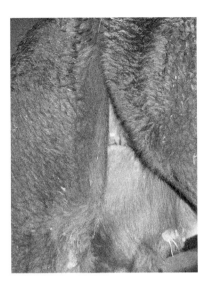

Figure 28.4 Thinner fiber covering in the caudal abdomen and groin regions is normal.

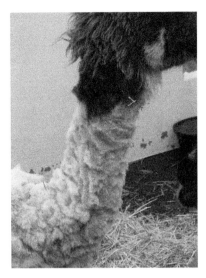

Figure 28.5 Thick cervical skin is expected in camelids, especially intact males. Sometimes venous cutdown is necessary for jugular catheterization.

(Kyung-Yeon et al. 2010). The fiber of the dorsal midline should be parted to look for evidence of lice and dermatophytosis. Skin lesion distribution for mite infestation is often seen in the perineum and inguinal regions; however, skin scrapings in these areas are often negative. With suspected mange cases, consider skin scraping between the patient's toes. Skin scraping techniques are presented elsewhere in this manual.

A great amount of information regarding camelid dermatologic conditions has arisen over the past couple of decades, but dermatology in general still often remains a frustrating complaint. As with any species, full thickness skin biopsy and

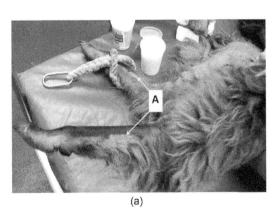

(a)

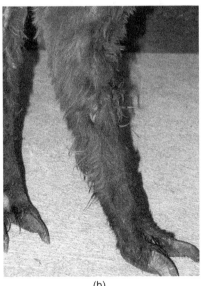

(b)

Figure 28.6 (a, b) The metatarsal glands (**A**) are thick, crusty areas of the mid metatarsals and should not be confused with pathology or equine "chestnuts."

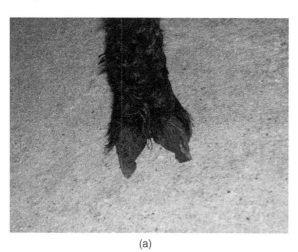

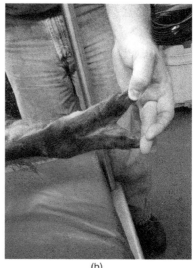

(a)   (b)

Figure 28.7 (a, b)   Normal appearance of the dorsal interdigital space of camelids is hairless and scaly.

microscopic exam of deep scrapings are essential for accurate diagnosis of disease. Refer to the biopsy chapter (Chapter 30) in this text for techniques. Recognize the common areas for disease distribution and areas of normal skin variance.

Recommended Reading

Atlee BA, Stannard AA, Fowler ME, et al. 1997. The histology of normal llama skin. *Vet Derm*; 8(3):165–176.

Kyung-Yeon E, Kwak D, Shin T, et al. 2010. Skin lesions associated with demodex sp. in a llama (lama peruana). *J Zoo Wildlife Med*; 41(1):178–180.

Lamm CG, Love BC, Rogers LL, et al. 2009, Apr 15. Pathology in practice. *J Am Vet Med Assoc*; 234(8):1013–1015.

Lusat J, Morgan ER, Wall R. 2009. Mange in alpacas, llamas and goats in the UK: incidence and risk. *Vet Parasit*; 163:179–184.

Van Saun RJ. 2006. Nutritional diseases of South American camelids. *Sm Rum Res*; 61:153–164.

29

Skin Scraping

Meredyth L. Jones and Patricia Payne

Purpose or indication for Procedure

This procedure is for the detection of ectoparasites and to aid in the diagnosis of integumentary disease.

Equipment needed

Glass slide, coverslip, scalpel blade, and mineral oil are needed.

Restraint/Position

Standing or recumbent, haltered, chute restraint, or sedated positions may be used.

Technical Description of procedure/Method

Superficial scrapings (e.g., for *Sarcoptes* sp. mites) may be taken by stretching the skin to be scraped between the thumb and forefinger, and firmly raking the blade along the skin surface until flakes and cells are exfoliated. (See Figure 29.1.) These exfoliated cells and debris are scraped along the edge of the glass slide and moved to the center of the slide. Then, the sample is immersed and mixed in mineral oil,

and a coverslip is then placed on top of the sample. The sample is then sequentially examined using 4×, 10×, and 40× objectives on a microscope. *Sarcoptes* sp. mites are easily seen at 4× and 10× and are a cause of severe dermatitis in alpacas. (See Figure 29.2.) These mites are recognized by their characteristic round bodies and short, wide limbs.

Deep scrapings (e.g., for *Chorioptes* sp, mites) are done in similar fashion, but the affected skin is squeezed upward using digital pressure, and the scraping is performed until bleeding occurs. One of the most consistent sites in camelids for detection of Chorioptic mange is the dorsal interdigital spaces. The interdigital space is scraped with a scalpel blade until light bleeding occurs (Figure 29.3). Exfoliated debris is picked up with the blade (Figure 29.4), deposited on the slide, immersed in mineral oil, and covered with a coverslip. *Chorioptes* mites are easily recognizable under 4× and 10× power and are characterized by round bodies and long, slender legs. (See Figure 29.5.)

Psoroptes and *Demodex* spp. mites have also been reported in camelids, but have less clinical significance than *Sarcoptes* and *Chorioptes* spp. *Psoroptes* is identified by having round bodies with long, wide legs, while *Demodex* spp. has an elongated cigar-shaped body. These mites are most often associated with clinical disease affecting the pinna, dorsum, perineum, axillae, neck, and legs.

Veterinary Techniques in Llamas and Alpacas, Second Edition. Edited by David E. Anderson, Matt Miesner, and Meredyth Jones.

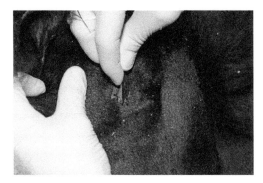

Figure 29.1 Superficial skin scraping of an alpaca. The operator uses a scalpel blade, held horizontally to the skin and at a slight angle to scrape the skin's surface. For deep scrapings, this procedure is done firmly and repeatedly, with the sample area squeezed between scrapings to extrude deep mites.

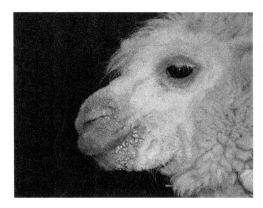

Figure 29.2 A male alpaca severely affected by sarcoptic mange. This animal was primarily affected around the eyes, ears, muzzle, inguinal region, perineum, and feet.

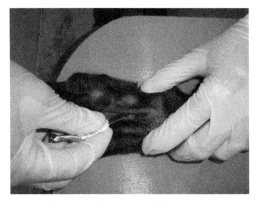

Figure 29.3 The dorsal interdigital space being scraped for suspected *Chorioptes* spp. mites.

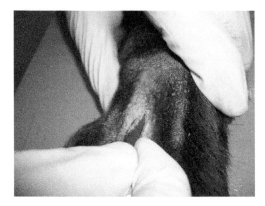

Figure 29.4 Exfoliated skin cells and debris collected from the interdigital space for microscopic examination.

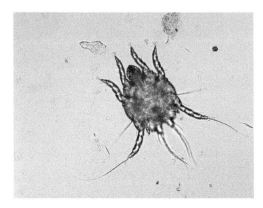

Figure 29.5 A *Chorioptes* spp. mite as seen microscopically with mineral oil immersion.

Practice Tip to Facilitate Procedure

Depending on the location of lesions, and particularly if they are on the head, animals may need to be sedated in order to provide sufficient restraint for quality scraping samples. Sedation and placement of the patient in lateral recumbencymay facilitate interdigital skin scraping.

Potential Complications

Minimal bleeding should occur with deep scrapes. Accidental incision into the animal or operator may occur with inadequate restraint. Accidental penetration of vital structures such as joints, tendons, etc., should be addressed immediately.

Patient monitoring/Aftercare

Monitor sites of skin scraping for swelling, pain, discharge, or lameness.

Recommended Reading

Ballweber LR. 2009. Ectoand endoparasites of New World camelids. *Vet Clin N Am Food Anim Pract*; 25(2):295–310.

D'Alterio GL, Batty A, Laxon K, et al. 2011. Psoroptes species in alpacas. *Vet Rec*; 149(3):96.

D'Alterio GL, Jackson AP, Knowles TG, et al. 2005. Comparative study of the efficacy of eprinomectin versus ivermectin, and field efficacy of eprinomectin only, for the treatment of chorioptic mange in alpacas. *Vet Parasitol*; 130(3–4):267–275.

Kyung-Yeon E, Kwak D, Shin T, et al. 2010. Skin lesions associated with *Demodex* sp. in a llama (lama peruana). *J Zoo Wildlife Med*; 41(1):178–180.

Lau P, Hill PB, Rybnicek J, et al. 2007. Sarcoptic mange in three alpacas treated successfully with amitraz. *Vet Dermatol*; 18(4):272–277.

Plant JD, Kutzler MA, Cebra CK. 2007. Efficacy of topical eprinomectin in the treatment of Chorioptes sp. infestation in alpacas and llamas. *Vet Dermatol*; 18(1):59–62.

Rosychuk RA. 1989. Llama dermatology. *Vet Clin N Am Food Anim Pract*; 5(1):203–215.

Rosychuk RA. 1994. Llama dermatology. *Vet Clin N Am Food Anim Pract*; 10(2):228–239.

Twomey DR, Birch ES, Schock A. 2009. Outbreak of sarcoptic mange in alpacas (Vicugna pacos) and control with repeated subcutaneous ivermectin injections. *Vet Parasitol*; 159(2):186–191.

30

Skin Biopsy
Meredyth L. Jones

Purpose or Indication for Procedure

A skin biopsy can provide a diagnosis for bacterial, viral, neoplastic, metabolic (nutritional) (Figure 30.1), and parasitic (Figure 30.2a and 30.2b) skin conditions. Punch biopsy instruments may also be used for excision of small lesions.

Equipment Needed

Clippers, exam gloves, biopsy punch, 20-gauge needle, syringe, 1 mL 2% lidocaine, 6- to 8-mm diameter punch biopsy instrument, scissor or scalpel blade, specimen container with and without formalin, thumb forceps, and 2–0 skin suture and needle drivers or skin stapler will be needed.

Restraint/Position

Standing, haltered, and chute restraint positions may be used.

Technical Description of Procedure/Method

If the area to be sampled has fiber, clip the region without scraping skin, in order to maintain the integrity of the skin surface for histopathology. The skin surface should not be scrubbed or prepared with antiseptic. (If a sample is to be taken aseptically for bacterial culture, a second region should be aseptically prepared and the biopsy performed.) One mL of 2% lidocaine is injected subcutaneously by introducing the needle 8 to 10 mm away from the proposed biopsy site and injecting the lidocaine beneath the proposed site. If there is a discrete skin lesion, the biopsy site should be at the junction of normal/abnormal skin. Some histopathologists advocate placing the lidocaine remote to the skin being biopsied because lidocaine can cause vasodilation and edema in the sample. Alternatives to injection of lidocaine include topical lidocaine gel or hypothermia (ice packing) to numb skin prior to biopsy. These are somewhat less effective at achieving analgesia.

After allowing approximately 5 minutes for lidocaine onset of action, the skin is stretched using the thumb and forefinger, and the biopsy punch is centered perpendicularly over the desired site (Figure 30.3). The punch is then rotated back and forth to "drill" into the skin (Figure 30.4). A release will be felt when the punch has entered the subcutaneous space and incised fully through the skin (Figure 30.5). The punch is removed and the circular sample will remain. The edge of the sample is gently grasped with thumb forceps (Figure 30.6) so the cellular

Veterinary Techniques in Llamas and Alpacas, Second Edition. Edited by David E. Anderson, Matt Miesner, and Meredyth Jones.
© 2023 John Wiley & Sons, Inc. Published 2023 by John Wiley & Sons, Inc.

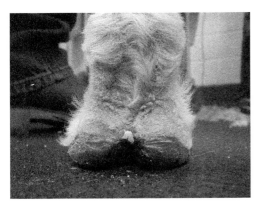

Figure 30.1 Photo of the palmar aspect of an alpaca affected by zinc responsive dermatosis. Histopathology confirms the diagnosis, along with trace mineral testing.

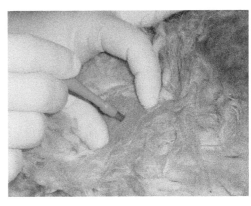

Figure 30.3 Initial insertion of skin biopsy punch with slight skin stretching to facilitate the procedure.

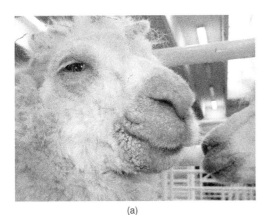

(a)

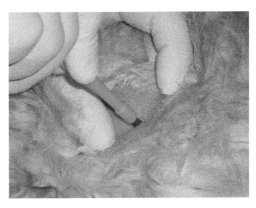

Figure 30.4 The biopsy instrument is twisted as it passes through the skin.

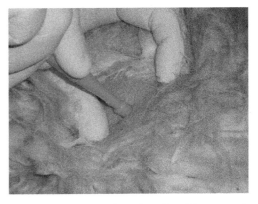

(b)

Figure 30.2a and 30.2b Alpaca affected by *Sarcoptes*. *Sarcoptes* can be difficult to confirm on skin scraping, but mites may be demonstrated on histopathology.

Figure 30.5 The cutting edge of the biopsy punch is completely through the skin and is the subcutis.

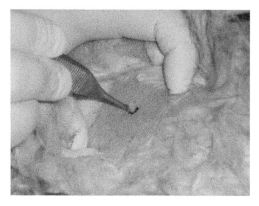

Figure 30.6 Thumb forceps are used to gently grasp the biopsy specimen by the edge.

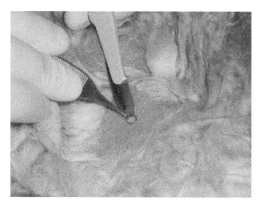

Figure 30.7 Scissors or a scalpel may be used to release the tissue specimen from the subcutaneous tissue.

structure of the sample is not crushed or altered. The sample is then lifted, and the subcutaneous connection is cut with Metzenbaum scissors or a scalpel blade (Figure 30.7).

The sample should be placed in formalin for histopathology or in a sterile container for culture.

The biopsy site may be closed with a simple interrupted suture or a single skin staple, to be removed in 10 days.

Practice Tip to Facilitate Procedure

Biopsy punches may be resterilized or disinfected and reused. They do become dull over time, however, particularly when used repeatedly on abnormal skin, and they should be replaced regularly.

Potential Complications

Accidental deep biopsy of underlying tissues and infection at biopsy site may occur. Minor hemorrhage is expected, particularly due to the vasodilative effects of lidocaine.

Patient Monitoring/Aftercare

The biopsy site should be monitored for swelling or abnormal drainage. Nonabsorbable suture or skin staples should be removed in 10 days.

Recommended Reading

Atlee BA, Stannard AA, Fowler ME, et al. 1997. The histology of normal llama skin. *Vet Dermatol*; 8:165–176.

Ballweber LR. 2009. Ectoand endoparasites of New World camelids. *Vet Clin N Am Food Animal Pract*; 25(2):295–310.

Clauss M, Lendl C, Schramel P, et al. 2004. Skin lesions in alpacas and llamas with low zinc and copper status—a preliminary report. *Vet J*; 167(3):302–305.

D'Alterio GL, Jackson AP, Knowles TG, et al. 2005. Comparative study of the efficacy of eprinomectin versus ivermectin, and field efficacy of eprinomectin only, for the treatment of chorioptic mange in alpacas. *Vet Parasitol*; 130(3–4):267–275.

Kyung-Yeon E, Kwak D, Shin T, et al. 2010. Skin lesions associated with *Demodex* sp. in a llama (lama peruana). *J Zoo Wildlife Med*; 41(1):178–180.

Plant JD, Kutzler MA, Cebra CK. 2007. Efficacy of topical eprinomectin in the treatment of Chorioptes sp. infestation in alpacas and llamas. *Vet Dermatol*; 18(1):59–62.

Pollock J, Bedenice D, Jennings SH, Papich MG. Pharmacokinetics of an extended-release formula of eprinomectin in healthy adult alpacas and its use in alpacas confirmed with mange. *J Vet Pharm Therap*; 40:192–199.

Rosychuk RA. 1989. Llama dermatology. *Vet Clin N Am Food Anim Pract*; 5(1):203–215.

Rosychuk RA. 1994. Llama dermatology. *Vet Clin N Am Food Anim Pract*; 10(2):228–239.

Waldridge BM, Pugh DG. 1997. Managing trace mineral deficiencies in South American camelids. *Veterinary Medicine*; August:744–750.

31

Toenail Trimming
Meredyth L. Jones

Purpose or Indication for Procedure

Toenail trimming maintains the structural alignment of the foot and prevents infectious diseases of the foot.

Equipment Needed

The following equipment is needed: toenail trimmers or pruning shears (Figure 31.1), ± sedation, and ± restraint chute.

Restraint/Position

Standing, haltered, chute restraint, and shearing restraints may be used. Toenail trimming can easily be done during shearing if the camelid is laid in recumbency with the limb securely attached to stretch ropes or a shearing table.

Technical Description of Procedure/Method

For the standing animal, the operator uses their foot to abduct the animal's leg (Figure 31.2) and then leans into the animal while picking

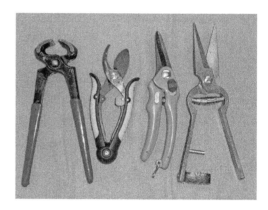

Figure 31.1 Various nail trimming instruments useful for camelid feet.

up the foot and flexing it at the carpus (tarsus) and fetlock (Figure 31.3a and 31.3b). Camelids have a "v"-shaped toenail (Figure 31.4a and 31.4b), rather than a hoof, making trimming rapid and simple. Using trimmers and entering the toenail from the palmar or plantar side parallel to the footpad, make cuts to level the nail with the footpad. Depending on the exact conformation of the nail, a single cut may be made across both sides of the nail or two "v" cuts may be made (Figure 31.5) with an additional cut to level out the apex. For severely overgrown toes, extensive cuts (Figures 31.6a, 31.6b, 31.6c) may be required. Although the quick does not grow out significantly into the nail, bleeding may occur in some cases.

Veterinary Techniques in Llamas and Alpacas, Second Edition. Edited by David E. Anderson, Matt Miesner, and Meredyth Jones.

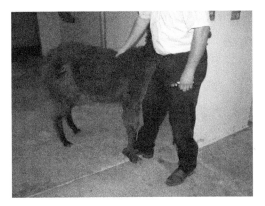

Figure 31.2 The operator places his hand on the animal's back and abducts the animal's forelimb.

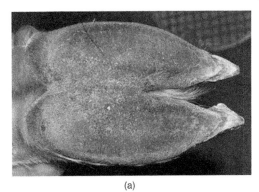

(a)

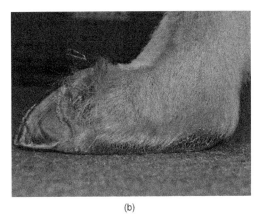

(b)

Figure 31.4a and 31.4b Well-trimmed toenail showing the "v"-shaped nail and proper relation to the footpad.

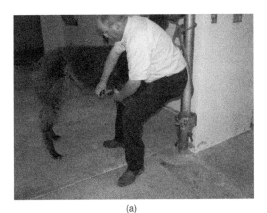

(a)

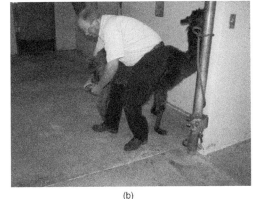

(b)

Figure 31.3a and 31.3b The operator leans into the animal and picks up the front foot, flexing the limb at the carpus and fetlock to expose the palmar surface for trimming. The procedure is repeated for the hind feet.

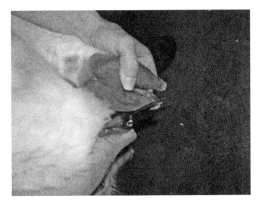

Figure 31.5 Using pruning shears to trim one side of the nail at a time.

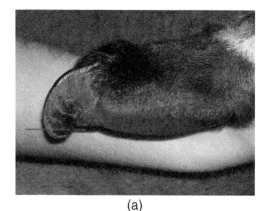

(a)

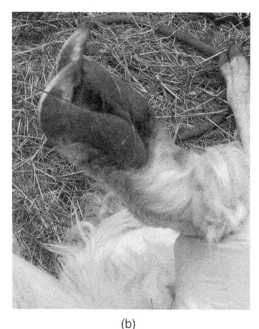

(b)

Figure 31.6a, 31.6b, and 31.6c Overgrown toenails. These are easily shortened to the proper level following the red line.

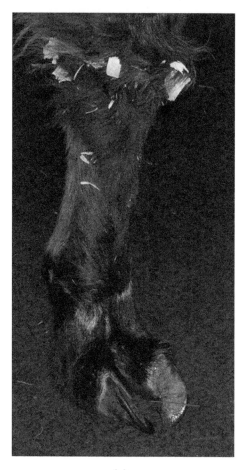

(c)

Potential Complications

Minor bleeding may occur when the nail is trimmed too short. When using sharp-pointed shears, an animal struggling may result in gouging of the operator's hand.

Patient Monitoring/Aftercare

Monitor for lameness.

Recommended Reading

Jones M, Boileau M. 2009. Camelid herd health. *Vet Clin N Am Food Anim Pract*; 25(2):239–263.

Practice Tip to Facilitate Procedure

When picking up camelid feet, keep the foot low to the ground and in as close to a normal standing position as possible. Also, keep the limb close into the patient's body to minimize altering balance. These will greatly reduce struggling. Sedation may be required in fractious animals.

Section VII

Respiratory

32

Thorax Anatomy and Auscultation

Matt D. Miesner

Purpose or Indication for Procedure

Use this procedure to evaluate the patient for cardio-respiratory disease or pathology.

Equipment Needed

A stethoscope is needed.

Restraint/Position

The standing position is ideal for auscultation.

Technical Description of Procedure/Method

Comprehensive knowledge of the borders of the cardiac and pulmonary fields should be understood and considered during auscultation as well as anatomical considerations during necropsy or procedures.

Camelid lungs are separated left and right with a complete mediastinum, and the only distinct lobe is an accessory lobe on the right side around the caudal vena cava. Lung regions are defined by three primary bronchial branches at the apical, cardiac, and diaphragmatic levels.

Camelids have 12 ribs. (See Figure 32.1.) The caudal border of the line of diaphragmatic reflection courses from caudodorsal, just caudal to the last rib, cranio-ventral to about the level of the seventh rib. (See Figure 32.1.) The auscultation field is a much smaller area from the olecranon and caudal triceps cranially triangulated to a point caudodorsal about the level of the 8 to 9th intercostal space. (See Figures 32.2 and 32.3.) A normal gradation of very quiet vesicular sounds in the caudal-dorsal fields to more pronounced bronchial sounds cranio-ventrally are expected, but the overall intensity of lung sounds in camelids is diminished compared to other large animal species. Pathophysiology of disease is typical,

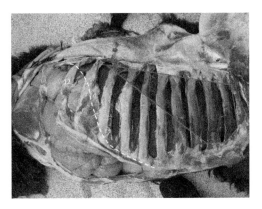

Figure 32.1 Postmortem specimen in left lateral recumbency. The twelfth rib is labeled. The approximate line of pleural reflection is indicated by the dashed white line. The shaded area outlined in red is the lung field of auscultation.

Veterinary Techniques in Llamas and Alpacas, Second Edition. Edited by David E. Anderson, Matt Miesner, and Meredyth Jones.
© 2023 John Wiley & Sons, Inc. Published 2023 by John Wiley & Sons, Inc.

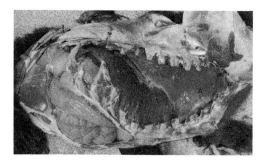

Figure 32.2 Postmortem specimen in left lateral recumbency with ribs resected, showing the orientation of the thoracic organs. The cardiac notch of the right lung is labeled (**A**).

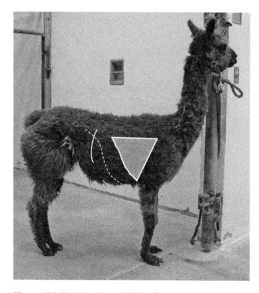

Figure 32.3 The last rib in this photograph is designated as the solid white line. The approximate line of diaphragmatic reflection is the dashed white line. The auscultable lung field is the shaded area.

resulting in abnormal sounds such as wheezing, crackles, and friction rubs due to narrowed or inflammatory airways, edema, fluid/mucus accumulation, and pleural inflammation. Absence of lung sounds, with additional clinical signs such as tachypnea and exercise intolerance, should be further investigated with ultrasound and radiographs for evidence of pleural effusion and lung consolidation. Normal respiratory rate at rest is between 10 and 30 breaths per minute.

The heart is situated in the cranial thorax, draped by the cardiac notch of the left and right lungs. (See Figure 32.2.) The normal heart rate is between 60 and 90 beats per minute with sinus arrhythmia common. A variety of toxic, neoplastic, and congenital cardiac diseases are described in camelids. Careful auscultation is warranted during all routine physical examinations.

Recommended Reading

Adolf JE, Dykes NL, Semevolos S, et al. 2001. The diagnosis and treatment of a thoracic abscess in an alpaca. *Aust Vet J*; 79(10):675–679.

Firshman AM, Wünschmann A, Cebra CK, et al. 2008. Thrombotic endocarditis in 10 alpacas. *J Vet Intern Med*; 22(2):456–461.

Fowler ME. 1998. Chapter 4: clinical diagnosis and examination. In: *Medicine and Surgery of South American Camelids*, Second Edition. Fowler ME, Ed., Blackwell Publishing, Ames, IA, p. 72.

Fowler ME. 1998. Chapter 12: respiratory system. In: *Medicine and Surgery of South American Camelids*, Second Edition. Fowler ME, Ed., Blackwell Publishing, Ames, IA, p. 295–303.

Gall DA, Zekas LJ, Van Metre D, et al. 2006. Imaging diagnosis-pulmonary metastases in new world camelids. *Vet Rad Ultrasound*; 47(6):571–573.

McLane MJ, Schlipf JW, Margiocco ML, et al. 2008. Listeria associated mural and valvular endocarditis in an alpaca. *J Vet Cardiol*; 10(2):141–145.

33

Tracheotomy/Tracheostomy

Matt D. Miesner

Purpose or Indication for Procedure

Tracheotomy provides emergency airway access in patients with upper airway obstruction. Camelids are obligate nasal breathers and distress occurs with complete nasal obstruction demonstrated by heritable choanal atresia seen occasionally in the species. (Prader et al. 2017) Physiologic disease (Dykgraaf et al. 2006), soft palate displacement, traumatic upper airways due to herd fighting or predator attacks are possible. Compressive hematomas from vascular bleeding from inadvertent carotid puncture or failed catheterization attempts have been seen by the author. Tracheotomy/tracheostomy may also be necessary for endotracheal intubation, bypassing the oronasopharynx, for complex procedures involving the upper airway, nasal passages, or oral cavities.

Equipment Needed

The following equipment is needed: clippers, scrub, local anesthetic, #10 scalpel blade, basic surgical instrument pack, tracheotomy tube, lidocaine, suture, umbilical tape, and roll gauze and bandage material. Tracheotomy tubes come in a variety of models, shapes, and sizes and are made from either silicone or metal. Self retaining "Y-type" tracheotomy tubes are easier to clean and less likely to obstruct, but they have poor fit in camelids and may cause excess trauma to the tracheal mucosa. If a cuffed tube is used, it is best not to inflate the cuff or to use minimal inflation. Double bore tubes with an inner sleeve are easy to clean, but the lumen is greatly narrowed, and the entire tube needs to be cleaned daily. Choose a tube that will most closely match the tracheal lumen.

Restraint/Position

The position to use is standing or sternal with head and neck extended dorsally. It is best to have the patient restrained in a chute or head catch with halter straps to prevent head and neck movement and to protect the clinician from the patient's front limbs. In most cases, sedation is not recommended due to preexisting respiratory compromise, which could be exacerbated with sedation.

Technical Description of Procedure/Method

The fiber covering the ventral neck, spanning just dorsal to the palpable transverse cervical vertebral processes of the proximal one-third of the neck, should be clipped and surgically prepped.

Veterinary Techniques in Llamas and Alpacas, Second Edition. Edited by David E. Anderson, Matt Miesner, and Meredyth Jones.

In emergency cases, a minimum of clipping fiber and aseptic prep should be performed. Infuse 2 to 4 mL of 2% lidocaine subcutaneously, superficial to trachea in the area to be incised.

Due to the tight skin and prominent transverse vertebral processes in this region of camelids, grasping the trachea prior to skin incision is difficult. Span the trachea with the middle and index fingers and put equal pressure on the ventral aspect of the transverse vertebral processes. (See Figure 33.1.) This will help isolate the trachea from the esophagus and cervical vasculature during the skin incision. A sharp surgical incision in made through the skin directly on midline over the trachea, using the #10 scalpel blade. (See Figures 33.1 and 33.2.) Make the skin incision 5- to 10-cm long depending on patient size. Next, make the best attempts to separate the paired sternohyoideus and sternothyroideus muscles along their median raphe. (See Figure 33.3.) Avoid excess tissue trauma and inflammation caused by incising directly through the muscle bellies. Make sure the incision is long enough to visualize several tracheal rings to facilitate manipulation and incision between the rings. (See Figure 33.4.)

Grasp the trachea and make a sharp stab incision between two tracheal rings through the

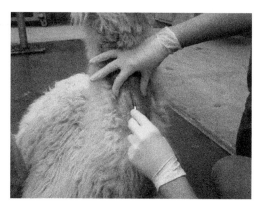

Figure 33.2 Sharp dissection is used to continue the incision to the cervical musculature. Make the incision sufficient to easily visualize and grasp the trachea.

annular ligament and tracheal mucosa. Extend the tracheal incision far enough to place a tracheostomy tube, but avoid incising more than one-third to one-half the circumference of the trachea. (See Figure 33.4.) Overaggressive tracheal incisions may exacerbate tracheal collapse after healing.

Place the tracheostomy tube through the incision after temporarily widening the opening between the tracheal rings with tissue forceps, Gelpi retractors, or the like. Avoid traumatizing the tracheal mucosa during insertion. (See Figures 33.4 and 33.5.) The tube should then be secured in place, either by suturing it to the skin or tying it in place around the neck. Suturing

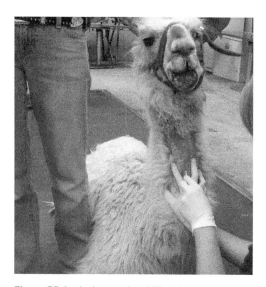

Figure 33.1 Isolate and stabilize the trachea from the esophagus and cervical vasculature with the index and middle finger for initial incision.

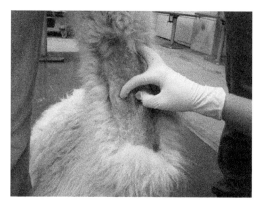

Figure 33.3 The paired sternohyoideous and sternothyroideus muscles should be separated along the median raphe if possible to avoid excessive muscle trauma and subsequent inflammation.

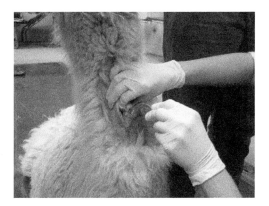

Figure 33.4 Sufficient length of incision has allowed the clinician to grasp and support the trachea for incision between the annular ligament and insertion of the tracheotomy tube. Avoid incising more than one-third to one-half the circumference of the annular ligament to reduce the chance of tracheal collapse.

to the tense and sometimes thick skin of camelids is difficult. Tying the tube in is also preferable to facilitate daily care and cleaning. (See Figure 33.6.) Suture the skin dorsal and ventral to the tracheotomy site with a nonabsorbable monofilament suture in an interrupted or cruciate pattern. (See Figure 33.7.)

Direct tracheal intubation for general anesthesia using the tracheotomy site may be used. (See Figure 33.8.) Take note of the length of tube to be introduced into the tracheal lumen so that it is not inserted too far resulting in bronchial intubation. Inflate the cuff of endotracheal tube as usual, taking care to

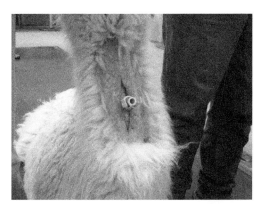

Figure 33.5 The tracheotomy tube has been inserted into the trachea. Note: This is a double bore, cuffed tube with an inner sleeve to facilitate cleaning. See text on pros and cons of tube type.

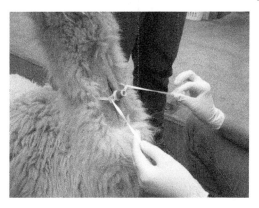

Figure 33.6 The tracheostomy tube is being secured in place by tying it in place with lace around the neck. This facilitates removal for routine cleaning, versus suturing in place.

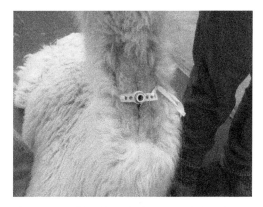

Figure 33.7 The skin is being sutured dorsal and ventral to the tracheotomy tube with nonabsorbable suture material.

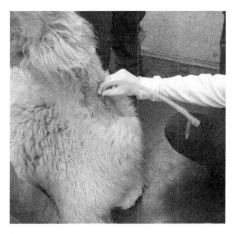

Figure 33.8 Direct tracheal intubation through tracheotomy site may be necessary during surgical correction of upper airway diseases. Consider length of endotracheal tube used, to avoid bronchial intubation.

avoid overinflation that may result in excessive lateral wall pressure and tracheal damage.

Practice Tip to Facilitate Procedure

Assure the length of the skin incision is sufficient to visualize multiple tracheal rings facilitating isolation of the trachea. A petrolatum-based ointment applied around the tracheotomy site after completing the procedure will help keep the surgery site free from mucus and debris.

Potential Complications

Complications in camelids may be more commonly encountered in the author's opinion, and the tracheotomy should only be maintained for as short amount of time as is necessary. As with any species, localized infection as well as pulmonary disease is a potential sequelae to tracheostomy. Exuberant granulation may develop during healing. Subcutaneous emphysema, tracheal mucosa undermining, septic fasciitis, and tracheal collapse may develop occasionally. In addition, the author and other colleagues have discussed a sudden death phenomenon without obvious postmortem evidence of causation, which warrants recognition.

Patient Monitoring/Aftercare

Monitor closely for a sudden increase in respiratory difficulty, especially if a cuffed endotracheal tube was used. If a cuffed type tube is used, the author recommends not inflating it, to allow for some air passage around the tube if it obstructs before being cleaned. The tracheal tube and tracheotomy site should be cleaned a minimum of twice daily, and mucus buildup on the tube should be evaluated, possibly indicating more frequent cleaning. Systemic antimicrobials should be started at the time of the procedure and continued 5 to 7 days after removal of the tube.

Recommended Reading

Dykgraaf S, Pusterla N, Van Hoogmoed LM. 2006. Rattlesnake envenomation in 12 New World camelids. *J Vet Intern Med*; 20(4):998–1002.

Mason TE, Dowling BA, Dart AJ. 2005. Surgical repair of a cleft soft palate in an alpaca. *Aust Vet J*; 83(3):145–146.

Nichols S. 2008. Tracheotomy and tracheostomy tube placement in cattle. *Vet Clin N Am Food Anim Pract*; 24(2):307–317.

Prader K, Burns PM, Brisville A-C, etal. 2017. Use of a novel surgical approach for treatment of complete bilateral membranous choanal atresia in an alpaca cria. *Javma*; 250(9):1036–1041.

34

Field Diagnosis of Choanal Atresia

David E. Anderson

Purpose or Indication for Procedure

Congenital defects are relatively common among camelids compared to horses and cattle. The high prevalence of congenital defects has been blamed on the relatively narrow range of genetic diversity in the native populations in South America. This was associated with severe decreases in populations of llamas and alpacas in the sixteenth century. Although these species are not endangered, this may have caused dramatic narrowing of the genetic base upon which the thriving camelid industry in South America of today is based. The veterinarian's role in counseling owners of camelids with congenital defects centers around the difference between congenital and heritable defects. Many veterinarians have taken the position that all congenital defects in llamas and alpacas should be considered to be heritable until proven otherwise because of the seemingly high prevalence of congenital defects in these two species. Choanal atresia is considered to be a heritable genetic defect. Offspring affected with choanal atresia were successfully produced by researchers at Oregon State University. Recently, a candidate gene, chromodomain helicase DNA-binding protein 7 gene (CHD7), has been identified in alpacas as having similarity to the human regulatory gene associated with CHARGE (Coloboma, Heart malformation, choanal

Atresia, Retardation of growth and (or) development, Genital anomalies, and Ear anomalies) syndrome. Camelids are a semi-obligate nasal breather and thus, accurate diagnosis of choanal atresia is critical to decisions that must be made soon after the birth of the affected cria. Affected cria should not be utilized in breeding programs and are most often euthanatized because of the poor prognosis for normal life.

Choanal atresia refers to the failure of the nasopharynx and pharynx to unite. A tissue barrier (membranous, cartilaginous, or osseous) obstructs the lumen of the nasopharynx and prevents air passage (Figure 34.1). This forces the cria to attempt to mouth breathe. Clinical signs of choanal atresia include flared nostrils, open mouth breathing, puffing of the cheeks

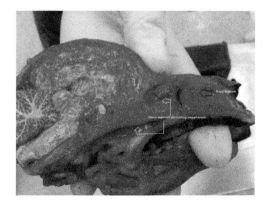

Figure 34.1 Sagittal section through the head of an alpaca cria demonstrating the atretic tissue occluding the nasopharynx.

Veterinary Techniques in Llamas and Alpacas, Second Edition. Edited by David E. Anderson, Matt Miesner, and Meredyth Jones.

during expiration, bluish discoloration of the mucous membranes, and distress (Figure 34.2 and Video 34.1: Choanal Atresia Breathing). Respiratory rate in increased and shallow, and an obstructive pattern is present (thoracic wall falls as abdominal wall expands and vice versa).

Equipment Needed

The following equipment is needed: 12-mL syringe, red rubber feeding tube (10 to 14 French), loose cotton, mirror, normal saline, pediatric bronchoscope (optional), radiographic equipment (optional), and radiopaque contrast material (optional).

Restraint/Position

Sternal recumbency (cushed posture) or lateral recumbency is used. Sedation is not recommended unless orotracheal intubation also is done.

Technical Description of Procedure/Method

Crias suspected of being affected with choanal atresia can be difficult to make an accurate diagnosis because of the small size of the head

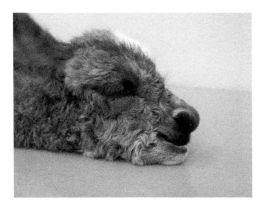

Figure 34.2 Obstruction of the nasopharynx results in breathing patterns associated with flaring of the nostrils and opening of the mouth.

and nasopharynx and because of the location of the obstruction. The obstruction is normally located 8- to 10-cm caudal to the nares and at the level of the medial canthus of the eye. If clinical signs are consistent with choanal atresia, then confirmatory tests should be done before euthanasia is opted. There are six readily performed clinical tests to determine if complete obstruction of the nasal passageway is present. These tests are most useful when complete (bilateral) choanal atresia exists. In the rare cases of unilateral choanal atresia, false test results can easily occur with the exception of endoscopy.

Follow these steps:

1) Hold loose cotton fibers (pulled from a cotton ball) in front of the nares and observe for movement. This test has a high risk of false negatives (air movement present) and false positives (air movement absent) because of ambient conditions.
2) Place a mirror immediately in front of each nares and observe for fogging on the mirror. This test has a high risk of false positives (fogging absent) because of ambient conditions.
3) Pass a small red rubber feeding tube (catheter) along the ventral and common meatus of the nasopharynx (Video 34.2: Red rubber catheter test for choanal atresia). If the nasopharynx is open, the tube can be passed into the esophagus or trachea. If the nasopharynx is obstructed, the tube will stop, usually at the level of the eye. This test has a risk of false negatives (tube coils up in the nasopharynx and gives impression of being passed) and false positives (tube displaces into the dorsal meatus and stops in the dorsal pharyngeal recess).
4) With the cria in sternal posture, hold the cria's head and neck upward and extended. Then instill 5 to 10 mL of sterile saline in each nasal passageway. If the nasopharynx is open, the cria will swallow the saline or cough as a result of aspiration. If the nasopharynx is closed, the cria will not respond, and the saline will run back out of the

nostril when the head is lowered. This test has a risk of false negatives (saline does not come back out and may have moved into the sinuses) and false positives (saline comes back out after being trapped in conchae and pharyngeal recess).

5) A horizontal beam, positive contrast radiograph can be taken to determine presence of an obstructing tissue barrier. With the cria in sternal posture, hold the cria's head and neck upward and extended. Then instill 5 to 10 mL of radiopaque contrast material in each nasal passageway. If the nasopharynx is open, the cria will swallow the contrast or cough as a result of aspiration. Radiographs will show no contrast except for small amounts coating the mucosae. If the nasopharynx is closed, the cria will not respond, and the contrast will pool rostral to the tissue barrier. This will be easily seen on radiographs, and the contrast will run back out of the nostril when the head is lowered. This test has a risk of false negatives (contrast does not pool as a result of poor head positioning or cria struggling).

6) Endoscopic examination of the nasopharynx is a definitive test for choanal atresia (Figures 34.3 and 34.4). This test can be inconclusive if the endoscope cannot be passed via the nasopharynx. In many cases,

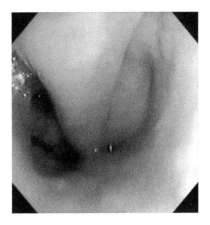

Figure 34.4 Endoscopic image of unilateral choanal atresia. The left nasopharynx is obstructed, and the right nasopharynx is normal.

an endoscope that is 6.0-mm in diameter or less can be successfully passed for complete examination.

Practice Tip to Facilitate Procedure

Test performance relies upon restraint and control of the cria. Care must be taken not to force closure of the mouth because asphyxiation may ensue. Restraint is facilitated by placing the cria in a cushed position on a table, extending the head and neck, and applying pressure on the neck immediately caudal to the base of the skull. Temporary tracheostomy alleviates respiratory distress and is tremendously beneficial for restraint and conduction of the tests (excepting the cotton fiber and mirror tests). Temporary tracheostomy can be done by making a 4-cm-long incision on the ventral midline of the neck and inserting a tracheostomy tube or endotracheal tube (4–8 OD size range). (See Figures 34.5–34.7).

Computer tomography (CT scan) or MRI imaging are definitive antemortem tests for choanal atresia, but these tests lack cost effectiveness and practicality, and are not able to be applied on the farm at this time.

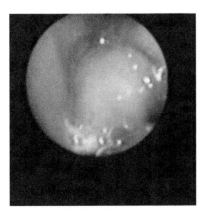

Figure 34.3 Endoscopic image of the atretic tissue obstructing the nasopharynx in a cria with complete choanal atresia.

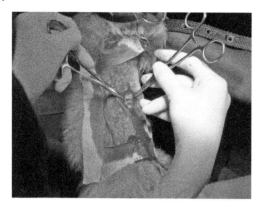

Figure 34.5 Ventral midline incision in the mid-cervical region of the neck. The trachea is exposed and isolated using forceps.

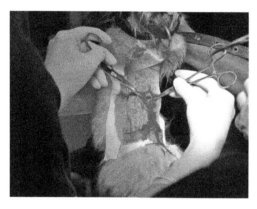

Figure 34.6 Temporary tracheostomy is done via a transverse incision through the annular ring between tracheal cartilages. A tracheostomy tube is inserted at this point.

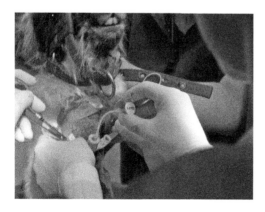

Figure 34.7 Placement of a temporary tracheostomy tube.

Potential Complications

Acute collapse and respiratory failure, acute death, and false test results may result from this procedure.

Patient Monitoring/Aftercare

Crias diagnosed with choanal atresia are most often euthanatized because of the poor quality of life and high mortality rate. Death is most often associated with septicemia, aspiration pneumonia, asphyxiation, or malnutrition and dehydration. Permanent tracheostomy or rhinoplasty can be done for research purposes. Clinical use of these procedures is restricted to pet camelids or neutered fiber production animals.

Recommended Reading

Nykamp SG, Dykes NL, Cook VL, et al. 2003. Computed tomographic appearance of choanal atresia in an alpaca cria. *Vet Rad & Ultrasound*; 44(5):534–536.

Reed KM., Bauer MM, Mendoza KM., Armien AG. 2010. A candidate gene for choanal atresia in alpaca. *Genome*; 53(3):224–230.

Reed KM, Mendoza KM, Fleege EC, Damerow JA, Armién AG. 2013 Oct. Evaluation of CHD7 as a candidate gene for choanal atresia in alpacas (Vicugna pacos). *Vet J*; 198(1):295–8. doi: 10.1016/j.tvjl.2013.07.006. Epub 2013 Aug 9. PMID: 23932654.

Bertin FR, Squires JM, Kritchevsky JE, Taylor SD. 2015 Jan. Clinical findings and survival in 56 sick neonatal New World camelids. *J Vet Intern Med*; 29(1):368–74. doi: 10.1111/jvim.12478. Epub 2014 Oct 15. PMID: 25319312; PMCID: PMC4858106.

35

Transtracheal Wash

Matt D. Miesner

Purpose or Indication for Procedure

Transtracheal wash (TTW) is a relatively simple procedure performed for cytology and sterile airway culture.

Equipment Needed

Sterile surgical gloves, 2% lidocaine, suture material, #10 or #15 scalpel blade, 3 to 4 meters of sterile polyethylene tubing, nested trocar set or 12- to 14-gauge needle, 40 to 60 mL of sterile saline solution in 35-mL syringes, and sterile sample containers for culture and cytology.

Restraint/Position

Light sedation with xylazine or butorphanol is helpful. If available, restraint in a chute designed for camelids facilitates handling. The head and neck should be extended and supported dorsally to expose access to the trachea. The patient can either be maintained in standing or sternal positions.

Technical Description of Procedure/Method

Clip the fiber covering the ventral neck, spanning just dorsal to the palpable transverse cervical vertebral processes of the proximal one-half to one-third of the neck and surgically prep the area. Before final scrub, infuse 2 to 4 mL of 2% lidocaine subcutaneously, superficial to trachea where the stab skin incision and trachea puncture with the trocar will occur. Prefill two sterile 35-mL syringes with 30-mL of sterile saline and place in sterile field. Insert a 20-gauge needle into the exterior end of the tubing for syringe attachment during the wash stage of the procedure.

Due to the tight skin and prominent transverse vertebral processes in this region of camelids, grasping the trachea prior to skin incision is difficult. Span the trachea with the middle and index fingers and put equal pressure on the ventral aspect of the transverse vertebral processes. (See Figure 35.1.) This will help isolate the trachea from the esophagus and cervical vasculature during the skin incision and helps stabilize the trachea during needle puncture.

Veterinary Techniques in Llamas and Alpacas, Second Edition. Edited by David E. Anderson, Matt Miesner, and Meredyth Jones.

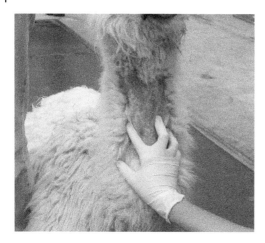

Figure 35.1 Span the trachea with the index and middle fingers and put pressure on the ventral aspect of the transverse processes of the cervical vertebrae. This allows the clinician to stabilize the trachea and protect the cervical vasculature and esophagus.

Stabilize the trachea and make a small stab skin incision with a scalpel blade through the skin. (See Figures 35.1 and 35.2.) If using a

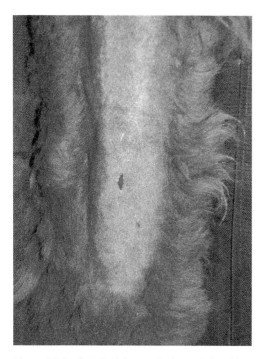

Figure 35.2 Stab incision made through the skin for insertion of nested trocar. Stab incision is not necessary when using a needle as the entry port to tracheal lumen.

hypodermic needle instead of a nested trocar, the stab incision is not necessary; however, see cautions regarding needle use at the end of this text. Insert the nested trocar through the incision and an annular ligament between the tracheal rings into the lumen of the trachea and remove the inner stylette, leaving the cannula in place. (See Figure 35.3.) Attach a sterile syringe and aspirate to determine correct lumen positioning by no resistance of plunger withdrawal. Pass the polyethylene tubing through the stylette into the lumen of the trachea and advance until resistance is apparent. (See Figures 35.4 and 35.5.)

Attach one of the 35-mL syringes and swiftly infuse the saline through the tubing. (See Figure 35.6.) Aspirate immediately after infusion. Only a small percentage of the original volume of fluid will be retrieved due to pulmonary absorption and dispersion of the fluid within the lower airway. Coughing will be noted. Set the syringe aside or pass to an assistant to transfer the fluid to culture containers and Ethylenediaminetetraacetic acid (EDTA tubes for cytology. Reposition the tubing and repeat the procedure with the second syringe.

Remove the tubing prior to removal of the trocar. Place one or two interrupted skin sutures to close the wound. Broad-spectrum antibiotic

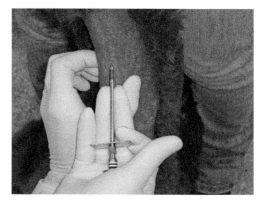

Figure 35.3 Nested trocar set used for insertion into the tracheal lumen between annular rings. The stylette is removed after penetrating the lumen, the catheter is passed, a syringe is attached and suction applied by withdrawing the plunger. Intraluminal placement is proper when air can be withdrawn without resistance.

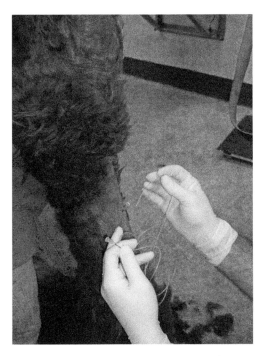

Figure 35.4 The polyethylene tubing is being placed through the bore of the needle. Note that the 20-gauge needle has been inserted in the lumen of the tubing for syringe attachment.

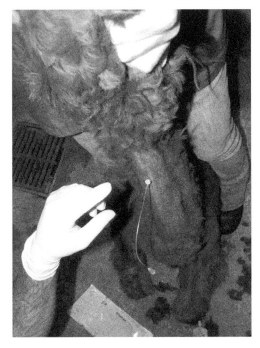

Figure 35.5 Advance the tubing until resistance is met at the lower airway.

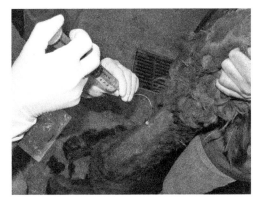

Figure 35.6 The syringe containing the saline is attached to the needle and rapidly flushed into the airway, then aspirated immediately to collect the sample. Most of the infused fluid will not be recovered.

therapy is indicated for 5 to 7 days, and a non-steroidal anti-inflammatory is administered once or twice after the procedure.

Practice Tip to Facilitate Procedure

Advanced preparation of multiple lavage syringes greatly helps in completion of the procedure. Use of a three-way stop-cock on the tracheal catheter aids in ease of aspiration and change of syringes.

Potential Complications

Complications are infrequent but may occur depending upon the nature of the respiratory disease in question. Patient demeanor and cooperation may be a hindrance but can be overcome through combination of chemical and physical restraint. Classification of the disease through sample analysis for accurate diagnosis and targeted treatment is the goal.

If using a large bore hypodermic needle instead of a nested trocar, caution should be used. It is generally easier to insert the needle into the trachea lumen; however, there is a greater risk of cutting the polyethylene tubing during manipulation, particularly during withdrawal from the trachea.

Patient Monitoring/ Aftercare

Monitor for signs of respiratory distress immediately after the procedure. The incision site should be monitored for evidence of infection or subcutaneous emphysema. Some mild localized emphysema around the incision and intermittent coughing are common but should resolve within 24 to 48 hours. Skin sutures can be removed within 7 to 10 days.

Recommended Reading

Bohn AA, Callan RJ. 2007. Cytology in food animal practice: evaluation of airway washes. *Vet Clin N Am Food Anim Pract*; 23(3):457–459.

Cooper VL, Brodersen BW. 2010. Respiratory disease diagnostics of cattle. *Vet Clin N Am Food Anim Pract*; 26(2):409–416.

Gerros TC, Andreasen CB. 1999. Analysis of transtracheal aspirates and pleural fluid from clinically healthy llamas (Llama glama). *Vet Clin Path*; 28(1):29–32.

Section VIII

Abdomen

36

Anatomical Comments on the Camelid Abdomen

Matt D. Miesner

The clinician should be aware of the orientation of major abdominal organs for basing decisions on surgical approaches and performing diagnostic tests. The following description should serve as an overview for better understanding of other topics described in this text.

The forestomachs are unique from true ruminants yet still occupy the majority of the abdomen (Alzola et al. 2004; Vallenas et al. 1971). Where the rumen, reticulum, and omasum fill the left hemiabdomen in ruminants, this area is occupied by the first two of three stomach compartments in South American camelids. The first two stomach compartments are termed as Compartments 1 and 2 (C-1 and C-2), serving fermentation, nutrient and water absorption, and feed transit functions similar to that of true ruminants. (See Figure 36.1.) C-1 has two ventral compartments, and the ingesta is homogenous, unlike the striated fluid-fiber mat- gas arrangement in the rumen. Glandular saccules are associated with the compartments of C-1 serving both absorptive and secretory functions. (See Figure 36.1.) The spleen lies lateral to C-1 with a broad mesenteric attachment at the base similar to that in true ruminants (Smith and Dallap 2005). Unlike ruminants, the spleen does not have a capsule and thus can rotate about its mesenteric attachment. Clinical cases of splenic torsion have been reported to occur. Also, the spleen is located along the caudal aspect of C-1

in the area of the caudal abdomen, caudal to the last rib. This is important when performing diagnostic procedures such as C-1 paracentesis and left lateral abdomen laparotomy. C-2 follows in line between C-1 and the third compartment (C-3) providing further fermentation, absorption, and passage of smaller fiber particles. (See Figure 36.1.) C-3 is a long cylindrical compartment performing similar functions as C-1 and C-2 as well as acting as the true gastric stomach with enzymatic digestion at its terminal pyloric region prone to ulceration. (Cebra et al. 2003; Smith et al. 1994) The ratio of

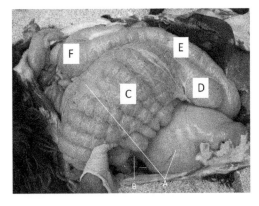

Figure 36.1 Postmortem photograph of specimen in left lateral recumbency with right ribs resected. The cranial and caudal sacs of C-1 (**A**), the serosal surface of the vertical pillar (**B**), the glandular saccules (**C**), compartment 2 (**D**), the nongladular portion of C-3 (**E**), and the glandular portion of C-3 entering the pyloric antrum (**F**), are shown.

nonglandular to glandular segments of C-3 is about 80:20 respectively. (See Figures 36.2 and 36.3.) Although a distinct margo plicatus is not observed at necropsy or endoscopy of C-3, gastric ulcers most commonly occur at this junctional area. When performing diagnostic tests, such as ultrasonography or laparoscopy, or during necropsy examination, the lesser curvature of the distal aspect of C-3 should be carefully examined for the presence of ulceration.

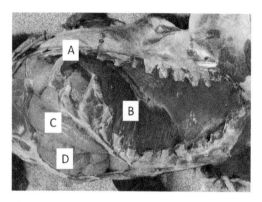

Figure 36.2 Postmortem photograph of specimen in left lateral recumbency to view approximate orientation of viscera viewed through the right abdomen. The twelfth rib (**A**), the diaphragm (**B**), C-3 (**C**), and saccules of C-1 (**D**), are shown.

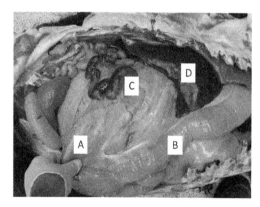

Figure 36.3 Postmortem photograph of specimen in left lateral recumbency showing orientation of C-3 and duodenum. The glandular portion of C-3 (**A**), the nonglandular C-3 (**B**), and the proximal portion of the duodenum (**C**), are shown. The liver is labeled (**D**).

The small intestinal tract courses along to fill the right ventral quadrant of the abdomen. The duodenum exits the pylorus of C-3 (See Figure 36.3.), where a prominent ampulla, or luminal dilatation, is present. This normal duodenal dilatation can be mistaken for pathologic dilatation, diverticula, or stricture. The duodenum and pylorus are common sites for trichobezoars to become lodged and cause obstruction. The duodenum first courses cranial-dorsal to the liver before returning distal to the jejunum then finally transitioning into the ileum, which terminates in the ceco-colic orifice in the central abdomen. Camelids do not have a distinct ileocecal junction or ceco-colic junction.

The large intestinal tract consists of a cecum, proximal ascending colon, spiral-ascending colon, distal ascending colon, transverse colon, descending colon, and rectum. The apex of the cecum is directed caudally toward the pelvis, followed by a long proximal loop of ascending colon entering a tighter spiral colon situated in the mid to ventral abdomen. Feces exit by way of the distal loop of the ascending colon into the transverse colon (right to left), descending colon, rectum, and anus. The spiral colon is a common site for fecaliths to become lodged and cause obstruction of the flexure of the central loop. The elongated proximal loop of the ascending colon may become displaced causing impaction or obstruction.

The anatomic association of the llama liver has been investigated (Castro et al. 2009). The liver is situated in the right cranial abdomen. (See Figure 36.3.) The caudo-dorsal border is at the level of the twelfth rib and the caudo-ventral border extends to about the fifth or sixth rib, covering C-2 and all but a small ventral portion of C-3. The liver is a solid, lobulated organ, and the caudal border may appear rough or fimbriated. (See Figure 36.4.) Camelids do not have a gall bladder, but dilatations of the bile duct have been observed during necropsy in rare cases.

Nonlobulated kidneys of equal size are located ventral to the fourth to seventh

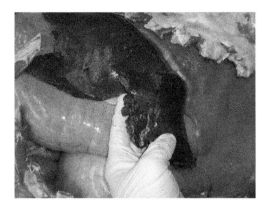

Figure 36.4 The edge of the liver margin may appear irregular or fimbriated and is considered normal.

transverse processes of the lumbar vertebrae. The right kidney is located slightly cranial to the left kidney and is most easily accessed through the right dorsal abdominal wall, immediately cranial to the wing of the ileum and immediately ventral to the transverse processes. The left kidney lies just caudal to C-1, ventral or cranial to the wing of the ileum, and ventral to the transverse processes. (See Figure 36.5.) Transabdominal ultrasound examination of both kidneys is easily performed through the dorsal paralumbar region.

Recommended Reading

Alzola RH, Ghezzi MD, Gimeno EJ, et al. 2004. Topography and morphology of the llama stomach (Lama glama). *J Int Morphol*; 22(2):155–164.

Castro ANC, Ghezzi MD, Dominguez MT, et al. 2009. Conformation and anatomical relations of the liver of llama (Lama glama). *Anat Histol Embryol*; 38(2):108–111.

Cebra CK, Tornquist SJ, Bildfell RJ, et al. 2003. Bile acids in gastric fluids from llamas and alpacas with and without ulcers. *J Vet Intern Med*; 17(4):567–570.

Smith BB, Pearson EG, Timm KL. 1994, Jul. Third compartment ulcers in the llama. *Vet Clin N Am Food Anim Pract*; 10(2):319–330.

Smith JJ, Dallap BL. 2005. Splenic torsion in an alpaca. *Vet Surg*; 34(1):1–4.

Vallenas A, Cummings JF, Munnell JF. 1971. A gross study of the compartmentalized stomach of two New World camelids, the llama and guanaco. *J Morphol*; 134(4):399–424.

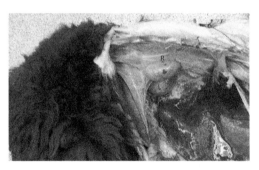

Figure 36.5 The right and left kidneys are closely situated at the dorsal midline.

151

37

Abdominal Ultrasound
Matt D. Miesner

Purpose or Indication for Procedure

The abdominal ultrasound procedure is used for noninvasive evaluation of abdominal contents for case decision making and workup.

Equipment Needed

The following equipment is needed: ultrasound machine, 3.5- and 5.0-MHz probes, hair clippers, isopropyl alcohol, and ultrasound gel. Probes may be sector scanners, which provide an optimal viewing window for abdominal viscera, or linear probes, which can serve as multipurpose probes including transrectal uses.

Restraint/Position

Standing most accurately places the abdominal viscera in the correct positions for evaluation. Camelids may resist touching of the abdomen and will often cush or lay in sternal recumbency. Neonates are often placed in lateral or dorsal recumbency for evaluation.

Technical Description of Procedure/Method

Percutaneous or transabdominal ultrasound is a routine procedure for clinical evaluation of camelids during physical examination, especially in cases presenting for colic or having abnormal diagnostic tests suggestive of liver disease or kidney disease. Valuable information can also be gained regarding questionable organ health and ultrasound guided biopsy for organs such as the liver, spleen, or kidney. See Chapter 50 on ultrasound examination of the urinary tract for more information on that topic. Many chapters throughout this book will refer to ultrasound guidance and methods for major system techniques. A 5-MHz linear probe is sufficient for evaluating the abdomen routinely for the majority of clinical presentations. A 3.5-mHz curvilinear or sector probe will provide greater penetration depth for imaging of more centrally located organs, especially in adults.

A mental image of the anatomical structures of the abdomen should be formed to understand the image generated by the ultrasound. (See Figure 37.1.) This author prefers to begin

Veterinary Techniques in Llamas and Alpacas, Second Edition. Edited by David E. Anderson, Matt Miesner, and Meredyth Jones.
© 2023 John Wiley & Sons, Inc. Published 2023 by John Wiley & Sons, Inc.

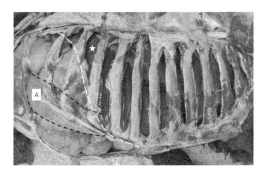

Figure 37.1 Postmortem photograph of specimen in left lateral recumbency with flank and intercostal muscles resected showing the line of pleural reflection (*dashed white line*). The approximate position of C-3 is shown (**A** and *dashed black lines*). The tenth intercostal space is labeled (*white star*).

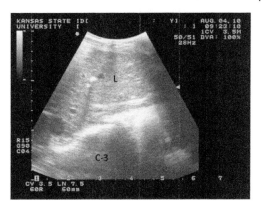

Figure 37.3 This ultrasound image shows the liver and a proximal portion of C-3.

scanning the right abdomen at about the tenth intercostal space, about 5-cm ventral to the origin of the rib. (See Figure 37.2.) At this point, the plane of imaging is through the caudodorsal lung fields, the diaphragm, and into the middle to dorsal aspect of the liver. Air within this region will often obscure clear views of the organs, but as the probe is moved ventrally, the liver is visualized. (See Figure 37.3.) The probe is gradually moved ventrally following the intercostal space along the right lobe of the liver. The duodenum and dorsal portion of C-3,

near the area where the glandular and nonglandular regions of this compartment converge, can consistently be examined. (See Figure 37.4.) Ten to 20 cm of C-3 can be followed by moving the probe caudally and cranially along its length. The triangle formed by the liver, duodenum, and C-3 and pylorus are closely assessed for evidence of C-3 ulcers. When ulcers are suspected, slowly rotate the probe looking for evidence of fluid or gas accumulation as well as wall integrity disruption or edema. Repeat the process of intercostal imaging at the ninth and eleventh intercostal space to the right paramedian region to visualize the duodenum, pylorus, and pyloric antrum. (See Figure 37.5.) The liver provides a reference point in most of these images in contrast to the bowel and compartment viscera. Occasionally,

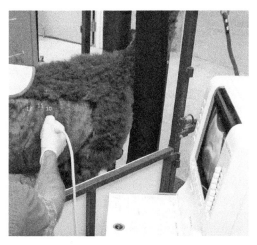

Figure 37.2 The probe is placed in the dorsal portion of the tenth intercostal space then moved ventrally.

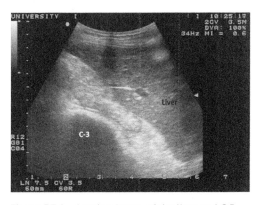

Figure 37.4 Another image of the liver and C-3 near the glandular portion of the pyloric antrum.

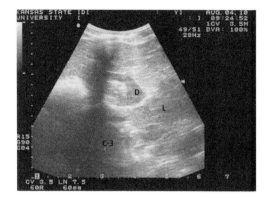

Figure 37.5   An ultrasound image of the liver (**L**), C-3, and a proximal loop of duodenum (**D**).

intraluminal obstructions, such as those caused by trichobezoars, can be visualized in the proximal duodenum and pyloric antrum. These lesions are suspected when intraluminal fluid accumulation, mixed-echogenicity intraluminal matter, and ileus are noted in the duodenum.

Continue imaging the right ventral quadrant of the abdomen to view the small bowel. Motility patterns and ultrasonographic appearance of the small bowel in normal camelids have been described (Cebra et al. 2002). The right paralumbar area will produce images of the ascending colon and large bowel. Segments of small bowel have a more hypoechoic intraluminal ingesta and more frequent motility patterns than large intestinal segments. Nonmotile, distended loops of small intestine, possibly with a plicated appearance and containing static ingesta, are indicative of obstruction. Ultrasound guided abdominocentesis can be performed to collect and analyze peritoneal fluid. This must be done cautiously in cases with significant distention of intestines or forestomach compartments. Aside from ascites and uroabdomen, *Streptococcus zooepidemicus* infection has been noted to result in significant peritoneal effusion (Hewson et al., 2001; Jones et al. 2009).

The ventral surface of the cranial and caudal portions of the first compartment can be imaged via the left ventral abdomen. Compartment motility can be evaluated, however, due to the

glandular saccules and orientation of the compartment, ingesta consistency is not able to be defined unless there has been profound dissipation of the fiber content and reduction of gas production. The saccules have a characteristic appearance to orient the clinician on position within the abdomen. (See Figure 37.6.) Small volumes of free peritoneal fluid may be seen in this area.

The right kidney can be imaged through the right paralumbar fossa ventral to the transverse process of the caudal lumbar vertebrae. (See Figures 37.7 and 37.8.) The left kidney

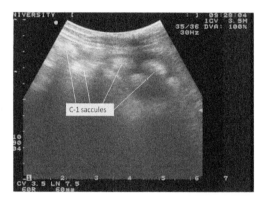

Figure 37.6   An ultrasound image of the left ventral abdomen just caudal to the xyphoid showing the appearance of the saccules of the first compartment.

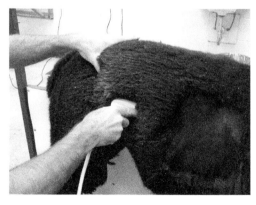

Figure 37.7   Positioning of the ultrasound probe for imaging the right kidney. The clinician's left thumb is at the level of the tuber coxae and the probe is ventral to the transverse processes of the lumbar vertebrae.

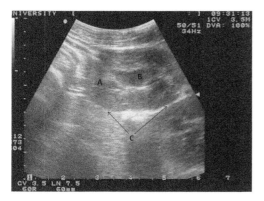

Figure 37.8 Image of the right kidney showing the smooth capsular appearance (**C**), the renal cortical parenchyma (**A**), and pelvis (**B**).

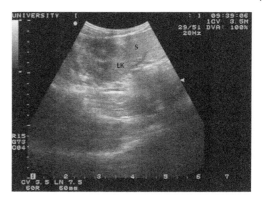

Figure 37.10 An ultrasound image of the left kidney (**LK**), showing the close approximation to the spleen (**S**). Splenic vasculature can be seen coursing through the parenchyma.

and spleen can be imaged through the left paralumbar region. (See Figure 37.9.) The left kidney is positioned slightly more caudal in the abdomen than the right kidney. After finding the left kidney, the clinician can image the base of the spleen just anterior to it. (See Figure 37.10.) Various pathological and incidental findings involving the spleen have been reported.

Images of the liver can be obtained through the right intercostal areas previously mentioned. (See Figures 37.3 to 37.5.) Camelids are affected with multiple ailments leading to liver disease, yet many are not able to be definitively confirmed on ultrasonographic appearance alone. Other ancillary diagnostics, possibly including liver biopsy, should be used in conjunction with ultrasound for diagnosis. See Chapter 39 on liver biopsy in this text. Focal or distributed lesions due to abscessation, neoplasia, and parasite migration often lead to hyperechoic foci within the liver parenchyma. An incidental finding of multiple hyperechoic foci throughout the hepatic parenchyma due to *Sarcocystis spp.* may be noted in animals from endemic regions. (See Figure 37.11.)

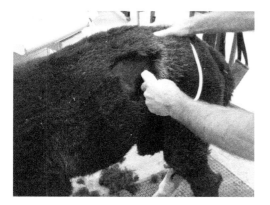

Figure 37.9 Approximate probe positioning for imaging the left kidney is more caudal than the right. By positioning the probe face cranial to the left kidney, the spleen can be located.

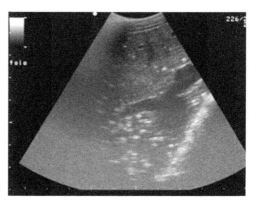

Figure 37.11 Ultrasound image of an alpaca showing wide distribution of hyperechoic lesions within the parenchyma. Finding may be incidental or pathologic depending on the cause.

Practice Tip to Facilitate Procedure

Clipping fiber is not necessary for imaging abdominal structures, however, it is recommended for added detail. Soak the fiber with alcohol, and part the fibers at the base of the hair, before placing the probe on the skin. Ultrasound gel may provide additional imaging quality.

Recommended Reading

Cebra CK, Watrous BJ, Cebra ML. 2002. Transabdominal ultrasonographic appearance of the gastrointestinal viscera of healthy llamas and alpacas. *Vet Rad Ultrasound*; 43(4):359–366.

DeWitt SF, Bedenice D, Mazan MR. 2004. Hemolysis and Heinz body formation associated with ingestion of red maple leaves in two alpacas. *J Am Vet Med Assoc*; 225(4):578–583.

Hamir AN, Timm KI, Smith BB. 2000. Thrombosis of the splenic vein in llamas (Lama glama). *Vet Rec*; 146:226–228.

Hewson J, Cebra CK. 2001. Peritonitis in a llama caused by Streptococcus equi subsp. Zooepidemicus. *Can Vet J*; 42(6):465–467.

Johnson AL, Stewart JE, Perkins GA. 2009. Diagnosis and treatment of Eimeria macusaniensis in an adult alpaca with signs of colic. *Vet J*; 179(3):465–467.

Jones M, Miesner M, Grondin T. 2009. Outbreak of Streptococcus equi ssp zooepidemicus polyserositis in an alpaca herd. *J Vet Intern Med*; 23(1):220–223.

King AM. 2006. Development, advances and applications of diagnostic ultrasound in animals. *Vet J*; 171(3):408–420.

Oevermann A, Pfyffer GE, Zanolari P, et al. 2004. Generalized tuberculosis in llamas (Lama glama) due to Mycobacterium microti. *J Clin Microbiol*; 42(4):1818–1821.

Smith JJ, Dallap BL. 2005. Splenic torsion in an alpaca. *Vet Surg*; 34(1):1–4.

Zanolari P, Robert N, Lyashchenko KP, et al. 2009. Tuberculosis caused by Mycobacterium microti in South American camelids. *J Vet Intern Med*; 23(6):1266–1272.

38

Abdominocentesis

Matt D. Miesner

Purpose or Indication for Procedure

The abdominocentesis procedure is used for evaluating and classifying abdominal fluid.

Equipment Needed

The following equipment is needed: 2% lidocaine HCl, 3-cc syringe, metal bovine teat cannula or 18-gauge, 3.81 cm long hypodermic needles, #15 scalpel blade, sterile teat cannula, Ethylenediaminetetraacetic acid (EDTA) blood tubes, and sterile culture container. An ultrasound machine is recommended for locating areas for fluid collection and to determine potential risks associated with distended viscera.

Restraint/Position

Standing is recommended when possible, but sternal positioning is also successful. Standing position allows for ventral or paracostal aspiration; sternal position allows for paracostal aspiration. Also, it may be necessary to securely restrain the patient in a position to allow ultrasound-guided access for fluid aspiration. This may require sedation.

Technical Description of Procedure/Method

A safe and effective method for routine collection and analytic parameters of peritoneal fluid from normal llamas and alpacas has been described (Cebra et al. 2008). One location described for routine collection in healthy camelids is the right paracostal area, 1- to 2-cm dorsal and 3- to 5-cm caudal to the costochondral junction of the twelfth rib (Cebra et al. 2008). (See Figure 38.1.) An alternative location is ventral

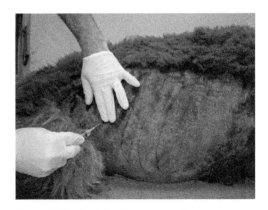

Figure 38.1 Location for paracostal abdominocentesis is about 3- to 5-cm caudal and 1- to 2-cm dorsal to the costochondral junction of the twelfth (last) rib. The middle finger of the clinician is placed over the line drawn at the twelfth rib in this image. Inject 1 to 3 mL of 2% lidocaine subcutaneously and into the deeper soft tissues. Note that this patient is in sternal recumbency.

midline from the linea alba at the level of the umbilicus. (See Figure 38.2.) When possible, especially in compromised patients, utilize ultrasound to detect the location of fluid accumulation as well as any abnormal appearance of fluid consistency. Guidelines for changes in fluid parameters with various abdominal diseases have been described (Fowler 1998).

For paracostal or midline abdominocentesis utilizing a teat cannula, clip, and surgically prep the skin over the area to be aspirated. Inject 2 to 3 mL of 2% lidocaine subcutaneously and into the soft tissues. A small (0.5-cm) stab incision is made with the #15 scalpel blade through the skin only. (See Figure 38.3.) Insert the teat cannula perpendicular to the body

wall and through the soft tissues and the peritoneum. (See Figure 38.4.) A firm thrust is necessary to penetrate the peritoneum, and the operator will sense a sudden release of pressure. Peritoneal fluid may flow freely, and adjustments of depth and rotation of the cannula may facilitate flow. (See Figure 38.5.) Care must be taken not to introduce the cannula into a distended viscus. For this reason, ultrasonographic examination of the target region is encouraged immediately prior to insertion of the cannula. After collecting the sample, remove the teat cannula. The small stab incision may be left to heal by second

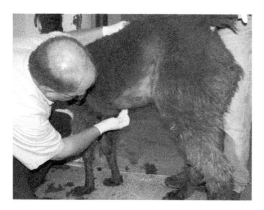

Figure 38.2 The depression of the linea alba can be palpated just caudal or cranial to the umbilicus.

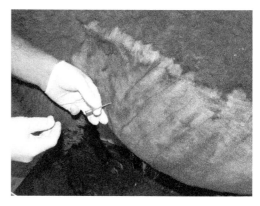

Figure 38.4 A teat cannula is inserted through the stab skin incision and the deeper soft tissues perpendicular to the abdominal wall. A quick thrust is necessary to penetrate the peritoneum.

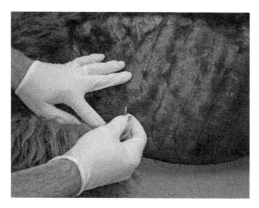

Figure 38.3 A #15 scalpel blade is used to make a stab incision through the skin when utilizing a teat cannula for abdominocentesis.

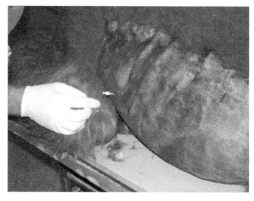

Figure 38.5 Peritoneal fluid is seen flowing from the teat cannula in this image, and could be collected in a suitable container for analysis.

intention, or a single skin suture or skin staple may be placed.

Alternatively, an 18-gauge hypodermic needle may be used for collection of peritoneal fluid at the midline location. The abdominal muscles, peritoneum, and soft tissues converge at the linea and provide a natural trough for fluid accumulation (See Figure 38.6). Llamas and alpacas deposit considerable fat into the retroperitoneal space. This "fat pad" often interferes with paramedian attempts to obtain abdominal fluid. The attachment of the peritoneum to the linea alba creates a window of access free of this fat interference. The anatomical trough that is created is most prominent cranial to the umbilicus and tapers considerably caudal to the umbilicus.

Clip and prep an area surrounding the umbilicus, and extend 10 cm cranial to it. Local anesthesia in the area is optional but recommended. Insert the needle directly on midline through the linea alba, approximately 0.5-cm deep, and just cranial to the umbilicus. (See Figure 38.7.) If peritoneal fluid does not flow freely, adjust the depth carefully and rotate the needle to facilitate flow. (See Figure 38.8.) Also, the author has found that placing a second needle about 1-cm to 2-cm caudal or cranial to the first has improved success in some cases. This should be avoided if subsequent diagnostic

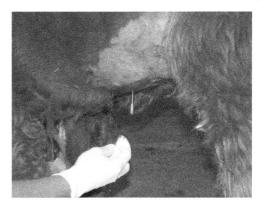

Figure 38.7 Abdominal fluid can be seen flowing from the hub of this 18-gauge needle inserted through the linea alba near the umbilicus.

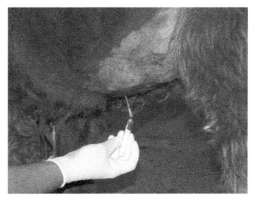

Figure 38.8 Approximately 1 mL of peritoneal fluid has been collected in this EDTA tube, which is sufficient for cytology and protein analysis.

procedures (such as ultrasonography or radiography) of the abdomen are anticipated. Collect the sample and remove the needle(s).

Practice Tip to Facilitate Procedure

Restraint will greatly facilitate the procedure. If a llama or alpaca chute is not available, chemical sedation is encouraged if the animal's condition allows for the use of these drugs. Light sedation with butorphanol tartrate (0.05 to 0.1 mg/kg IV) will help patient cooperation and provide analgesia. If needed, xylazine (0.2 mg/kg IV) will provide a more profound sedative effect. Ultrasonographic
(Continued)

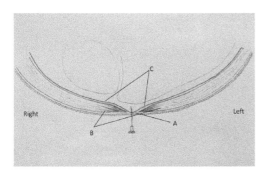

Figure 38.6 Cross-sectional abdominal diagram viewed from cranial to caudal. Linea alba (**A**), abdominal musculature (**B**), and peritoneum (**C**). A natural linear depression (trough) is formed where the abdominal musculature and soft tissues converge at the linea alba. Peritoneal fluid can be collected with a hypodermic needle.

(Continued)
examination of the site of abdomino-centesis is encouraged to minimize the risk of perforation of a viscus (intestine, uterus, bladder) or viscera (spleen, liver, kidney).

Potential Complications

Localized soft-tissue infection and peritonitis are possible. A blind needle aspiration using a hypodermic needle is not recommended in the paracostal location. Ultrasound is recommended in cases with abdominal distention and suspected intestinal obstruction cases. In most cases, inadvertent perforation of a viscus or viscera will not result in detriment to the patient. Exceptions include disease conditions that compromise the integrity of these organs (e.g., urethral obstruction, uterine torsion, intestinal obstruction).

Patient Monitoring/Aftercare

Monitor patient closely for 24 hours for signs of abdominal pain, fever, abdominal distention, and adverse changes in behavior (e.g., lethargy, inappetence, diminished fecal or urine output) and leakage from the site of needle or cannula insertion. If such changes are noted, a complete examination and appropriate diagnostic investigation (e.g., ultrasonography, hematology, serum biochemistry) are indicated.

Recommended Reading

Cebra CK, Tornquist SJ, Reed SK. 2008. Collection and analysis of peritoneal fluid from healthy llamas and alpacas. *J Am Vet Med Assoc*; 232(9):1357 1361.
Fowler ME. 1998. Chapter 13, digestive system. In: *Medicine and Surgery of South American Camelids*, Second Edition. Fowler ME, Ed., Blackwell Publishing, Ames, IA, p. 341.

39

Liver Biopsy

Meredyth L. Jones

Purpose or Indication for Procedure

Percutaneous liver biopsy is useful for diagnosis of a variety of individual or herd-level hepatobiliary diseases, including toxic, infectious, developmental, or metabolic diseases. Biopsy samples can be used for metabolic profiles, including trace mineral evaluation and hepatic adipose quantification.

Equipment Needed

The following equipment is needed: ultrasound with 3.5mHz probe (strongly encouraged), clippers with #40 blade, sterile gloves, gauze, iodine or chlorhexidine scrub solution, isopropyl alcohol, 2% lidocaine, syringe, 18- to 20-gauge 1-inch (2.54-cm) needle, scalpel, 18- to 14-gauge liver biopsy instrument, skin suture or staples, sterile evacuated tubes, formalin container, and ± ultrasound. If trace mineral analysis including zinc will be performed, royal blue top tubes must be used as other tube types contain zinc in the rubber stopper.

Restraint/Position

The following restraint or positions may be used: standing, chute restraint, ± standing sedation, or sternal recumbency.

Technical Description of Procedure/Method

The liver of camelids resides on the right side of the abdomen and is contained under the ribcage (Figure 39.1). To perform the procedure, clip and clean a region along the right thoracic wall extending from the eighth to eleventh intercostal spaces. This area is within the prime fleece region, so it may be appropriate to ask the owner if they want to keep the sheared fiber. The area to be clipped can be minimized by using adhesive tape to reflect the fiber along a line appropriate for the biopsy procedure. Ultrasound guidance is strongly encouraged. Scan can dorsal to ventral in the intercostal

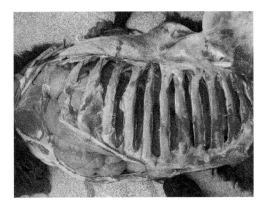

Figure 39.1 Necropsy specimen of an alpaca showing the location of the liver beneath the ribs on the right side of the body.

Veterinary Techniques in Llamas and Alpacas, Second Edition. Edited by David E. Anderson, Matt Miesner, and Meredyth Jones.
© 2023 John Wiley & Sons, Inc. Published 2023 by John Wiley & Sons, Inc.

spaces (Figure 39.2) to identify a target lesion or to identify a region free of large vessels and of sufficient depth to perform the biopsy. (See Figure 39.3.) The right lobe and caudate lobes of the liver are expected to lie at the junction of the dorsal and middle thirds of the abdomen (as judged by a distance from the dorsal midline to the ventral midline). The easiest window of access is often through the ninth or tenth intercostal spaces. Measurements may be made as to depth of insertion and correlated to cm markers on the biopsy instrument. After the site is selected, the site should be blocked subcutenously with 2 mL of 2% lidocaine HCl

and aseptically prepared. If performing the biopsy by the blind technique, select an area in the tenth intercostal space (camelids have 12 ribs) at the intersection of a line drawn from the ileal wing to the mid-humerus (Figure 39.4). In general, blind liver biopsy in camelids is discouraged because of the small size of the liver and anatomical differences from cattle.

After preparation of the ultrasound guided or blind site, make a small stab skin incision (0.5 cm) may be made and insert the closed biopsy instrument in the intercostal space immediately cranial to the rib. This is selected because the vasculature and intercostal nerve courses along the caudal border of each rib. Direct the needle in a ventromedial direction until the liver is penetrated (Figure 39.5). At this location, the instrument penetrates the caudal thoracic cavity, the pleura, and the diaphragm prior to entering the liver. Caution should be used in tachypneic camelids because extreme caudal excursion of the lung may result in inadvertent penetration by the biopsy instrument.

The operator will have a sense of the instrument entering a dense, spongy tissue. Some describe it as a gritty or coarse feel. Occasionally,

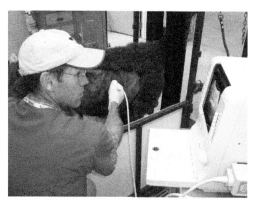

Figure 39.2 Proper animal restraint and ultrasound placement for visualization of the liver and for subsequent biopsy.

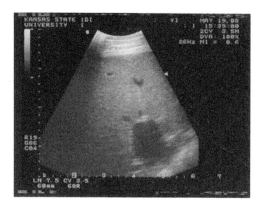

Figure 39.3 Ultrasound image of liver. Note the depth of the body to the liver surface and the depth to major blood vessels. The cm guides on the biopsy instrument can be used to ensure that the sample is taken within the hepatic parenchyma.

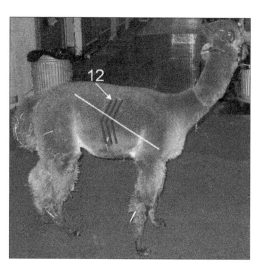

Figure 39.4 The site for blind liver biopsy is at the intersection of a line drawn from the ileal wing to the mid-humerus on the right side and the ninth or tenth intercostal space.

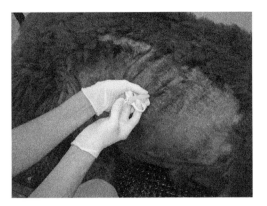

Figure 39.5 Use of an automatic biopsy instrument in an alpaca. The instrument is placed off the cranial border of the rib and is directed ventromedially.

the patient will involuntarily and suddenly move when the peritoneum and/or capsule of the liver is penetrated. Once into the liver parenchyma, trigger the automatic instrument and withdraw. For manual instruments, extend the obturator, advance the handle to close the sheath over the obturator, and remove the instrument. The liver sample should be within the chamber. (See Figure 39.6.) If liver tissue is not present in the chamber, repeat the procedure by redirecting the instrument slightly until a sample is obtained. Place samples in evacuated royal blue top tubes for trace mineral analysis (and frozen if necessary), formalin containers for histopathology or sterile tubes for bacterial, viral, or fungal culture.

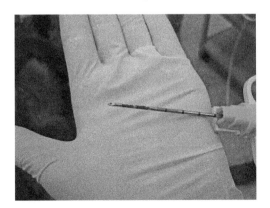

Figure 39.6 Typical appearance of liver tissue within the chamber of a biopsy instrument. This is best removed from the chamber using a needle.

Laboratories often desire significant amounts of liver tissue for full trace mineral panels. The clinician should contact the laboratory for specifications as needed. Most 14-gauge tissue biopsy needles have a channel dimension that harvests approximately 10 mg of wet-weight tissue when fully engaged. Thus, laboratories requiring 30 mg of tissue would need three biopsy samples with standard biopsy instruments to yield a sufficient sample mass.

Practice Tip to Facilitate Procedure

To minimize the amount of prime fiber clipped for liver biopsy, a small amount may be sheared and the remaining fiber held back with adhesive tape. (See Figure 39.7.)

A coagulation profile is recommended prior to liver biopsy. A convenient field test of coagulation is to perform a modified Lee-White clotting time. Collect 5 mL of venous blood and inject this into a red top (serum) tube. Normally, blood will clot within 5 minutes; the normal range is <10 minutes. Blood that is not clotted at 10 minutes should be considered to have an abnormal clotting time. One study in horses, however, indicated that, even with coagulation profile abnormalities, complications of liver biopsy were rare and mild.

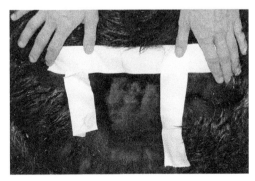

Figure 39.7 Use of bandage tape to hold fiber away from a prepared site to minimize the amount of fiber removed.

Refer to the following biopsy instrument sources: manual Tru-Cut (Baxter Travenol, St. Louis, MO) and automatic biopsy instrument (Bard Medical, Covington, VA).

Potential Complications

Hemorrhage, intestinal perforation, subcutaneous abscess, pneumothorax, bile or infectious peritonitis, clostridial hepatitis, and excess internal hemorrhage may occur. Suspected liver abscesses should not be sampled using a biopsy instrument. Rather, suspected abscesses should be sampled by fine needle aspiration (22-gauge × 6-inch [15.2-cm] needle inserted through an 18-gauge guide needle) under ultrasound guidance in order to reduce the likelihood of introducing bacteria into the abdominal cavity. Focal lesions (abscesses, granulomas, neoplasias, flukes) may be missed by single liver biopsy especially when using the blind technique.

Patient Monitoring/Aftercare

In some cases antimicrobial therapy and a vaccination booster of appropriate clostridial vaccines may be indicated. Animals should be monitored for attitude, appetite, and abdominal contour for 1 week post-procedure, and compromised animals should have a rectal temperature performed daily for 3 days after the procedure.

Notes: Liver tissue analysis may offer useful insight into the trace mineral status of animals. This is particularly true for copper (Cu), selenium (Se), zinc (Zn), iron (Fe), phosphorus (P), and cobalt (Co), for which liver is the primary pool or blood concentrations that may be altered by various pathologic and physiologic states. Blood concentrations of copper, zinc, and selenium may additionally be affected by stress, infection, pregnancy, and hemolysis. For herd testing, at least 10 animals should be sampled and ideally should be resampled after intervention for any deficiencies.

Recommended Reading

Johns IC, Sweeney RW. 2008. Coagulation abnormalities and complications after percutaneous liver biopsy in horses. *J Vet Intern Med*; 22:185–189.

Puls R. 1994. *Mineral Levels in Animal Health*, 2nd Edition. Clearbrook BC: Sherpa.

Tournquist SJ, Van Saun RJ, Smith BB, et al. 1999. Hepatic lipidosis in llamas and alpacas: 31 cases (1991–1997). *J Am Vet Med Assoc*; 214(9):1368–1372.

Van Saun RJ. 2006. Nutritional diseases of South American camelids. *Sm Rum Res*; 661(2):153–164.

Van Saun RJ. 2009. Nutritional requirements and assessing nutritional status in camelids. *Vet Clin N Am Food Anim Pract*; 25(2):265–279.

Waldridge BM, Pugh DG. 1997, August. Managing trace mineral deficiencies in South American camelids. *Vet Med*; 92(8):744–750.

40

First Compartment Paracentesis (Rumenocentesis) and Fluid Evaluation

Meredyth L. Jones

Purpose or Indication for Procedure

First compartment (C-1) fluid aspiration and examination is a diagnostic aid for animals suspected of having forestomach dysfunction, especially of the first compartment, and in camelids exhibiting abdominal distension, colic, reduced fecal output, anorexia, and abnormal first compartment texture or motility.

Equipment Needed

The following equipment is needed: halter and chute ± standing sedation, exam gloves, clippers with #40 blade, gauze, lidocaine HCl 2%, iodine or chlorhexidine scrub solution, 16 or 18-gauge × 2- to 3-inch (5.1- to 7.6-cm) needle, specimen vials and glass tubes, microscope slides, microscope, 0.03% methylene blue, pH paper or meter, and Gram's staining solutions.

Restraint/Position

Halter with standing sedation or chute restraint can be used.

Technical Description of Procedure/Method

First-compartment fluid may be obtained by passage of an orogastric tube with aspiration by a dosing syringe or reversed stomach pump. This method, in cattle, has been shown to result in salivary contamination, which can significantly affect some analytes, including pH, sodium (Na), potassium (K), and methylene blue reduction time.

First-compartment (C-1) paracentesis avoids salivary contamination and is the preferred method for pH determination when accuracy is critical. However, this method usually results in a small sample volume. Caution is advised because this technique risks septic peritonitis, subcutaneous abscessation, and death in extreme cases. This procedure should be avoided in females in late gestation.

To obtain fluid in adult llamas, the site for insertion is on the left side of the abdomen, 20-cm caudal to the last costochondral junction. Another method of determining the insertion point is to choose a point halfway between the last rib and the stifle along the body wall, at the level of the stifle. (See Figure 40.1.) This point should be clipped and disinfected, and

Veterinary Techniques in Llamas and Alpacas, Second Edition. Edited by David E. Anderson, Matt Miesner, and Meredyth Jones.
© 2023 John Wiley & Sons, Inc. Published 2023 by John Wiley & Sons, Inc.

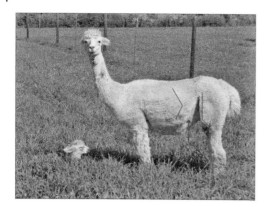

Figure 40.1 First-compartment fluid may be obtained at the point of the arrow, at a distance halfway between the last rib and the stifle, at the level of the stifle.

numerous protozoa should be seen moving rapidly across the slide. (See Figure 40.2; Video 40.1: Protozoa low power.) Three sizes of protozoa are normally present (small, medium, and large) and can be easily discerned using high magnification (Video 40.2: Protozoa high power). The large protozoa are the most sensitive to lactic acidosis and will be the first to be lost in cases of first compartment acidosis. This slide may then be dried and Gram stained to assess ratios of Gram-positive and Gram-negative bacteria. (See Figure 40.3.) Recall that Gram's staining was designed for use on pure cultures of bacteria, and staining can be misleading with a very heterogenous population such as rumen flora.

the animal should be well restrained. A 16 or 18-gauge × 2- to 3-inch (5.1- to 7.6-cm) needle should then be directed dorsomedially and thrust into the first compartment. Gentle aspiration should yield 4 to 5 mL of first-compartment fluid.

Once collected, the fluid should be placed in a clean vial and either analyzed immediately or kept at body temperature until timely analysis can be performed (Table 40.1).

C-1 fluid pH is best measured using a pH meter as they are less affected by the color of the fluid than litmus papers. A drop of fluid may be placed on a warm glass slide and examined using a microscope. On low power,

Methylene blue reduction time, a test of microbial function, is determined by mixing 1 drop of 0.03% methylene blue to 20 drops of fresh fluid in a clear tube. The time taken for the C-1 fluid to be decolorized back to its original color is then determined. The decolorization is the result of normal anaerobic bacterial reduction of the methylene blue (Figures 40.4a and 40.4b).

Sedimentation time is determined by placing C-1 fluid into a clear tube and observing for feed particles to sink to the bottom of the tube. With active fermentation, gas bubbles cause the feed to float. Samples that sediment quickly (<2 to 6 minutes in cattle) have abnormal fermentation.

Table 40.1 Normal first compartment fluid values in llamas.

	Mean	Range
Volume (mL)	4.1 ± 2.1	2 to 9
Color	Brown to green	Yellow to green
Odor	Slightly acidic	
Consistency	Moderate to thick	
pH	6.67 ± 0.02	6.30 to 6.89
Protozoa/100X field	20 to 30	10 to > 30 Small predominate
Gram's Stain	Gram-negative > Gram-positive	
Methylene Blue Reduction Time (sec)	173	75 to 266
Chloride (mmol/L)	14	

Llama normal values adapted from Navarre et al., JAVMA, (Navarre et al. 1999).

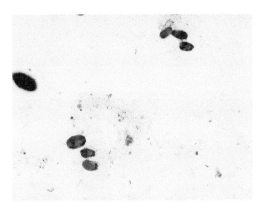

Figure 40.2 Iodine-stained protozoa. These can be observed in fresh fluid rapidly moving, and a population of small, medium, and large should be seen.

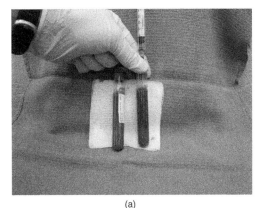

(a)

Figure 40.3 Gram stained first-compartment fluid. Many "artifacts" of C-1 fluid take up stain and make Gram staining difficult to interpret.

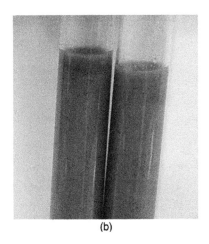

(b)

Figure 40.4a and 40.4b The addition of methylene blue turns C-1 fluid bright green, and the anaerobic activity of normal C-1 flora will decolorize the stain rapidly. It is useful to retain a tube of unstained fluid for comparison to know when decolorization is complete.

First compartment fluid chloride concentration is a useful test to help localize gastrointestinal disease. Third-compartment (C-3, abomasal) HCl reflux into C-1 can occur with vagal indigestion, small intestinal obstruction, or ileus. Because of highly effective C-1 buffering systems and volume, this HCl will not cause the C-1 pH to change, but will alter [Cl$^-$]. Standard chemistry analysis methods are not accurate for analyzing Cl- concentration in rumen fluid because of interference from other molecules in the fluid. Thus, specialized equipment at a reference laboratory is needed to ensure accuracy. Standard benchtop and hand-held analyzers are not suitable for C-1 chloride determination. [Cl$^-$] also cannot be interpreted easily in animals that have received oral electrolytes.

Practice Tip to Facilitate Procedure

Excellent restraint should be employed to prevent patient movement or kicking, which increases the risk of GI content leakage. Rapid thrusting of the needle into C-1, with rapid withdrawal (with the negative pressure released) also decreases this risk. When aspirating fluid, feed particles may become lodged against the needle bevel, preventing fluid flow. To correct this, simply depress the syringe plunger to expel the blockage and continue to aspirate more slowly.

Potential Complications

Potential complications include septic peritonitis, laceration or slit-shaped perforation of C-1, subcutaneous abscess, and inability to obtain fluid.

Patient Monitoring/Aftercare

The animal should be monitored for alterations in attitude, appetite, or abdominal contour. Daily rectal temperature monitoring is advised for early detection of peritonitis. The body wall should be examined daily for evidence of swelling or drainage.

Recommended Reading

Cebra C 2009. Abdominal discomfort in llamas and alpacas: diagnosis and treatment. *Proceedings of the Am Coll Vet Intern Medicine Forum*. Montreal, Quebec.

Cebra CK, Cebra ML, Garry FB, et al. 1996. Forestomach acidosis in six New World camelids. *J Am Vet Med Assoc*; 208(6):901–904.

Lakritz J, Gerspach C. 2009. Gastrontestinal disorders in camelids—clinical evaluation and treatment. *Proceedings of the Am Coll Vet Intern Medicine Forum*. Montreal, Quebec.

Navarre CB, Pugh DG, Heath AM, et al. 1999. Analysis of first compartment fluid collected via percutaneous paracentesis from healthy llamas. *J Am Vet Med Assoc*; 214(6):812–815.

Newman KD, Anderson DE. 2009. Gastrintestinal surgery in alpacas and llamas. *Vet Clin N Am Food Anim Pract*; 25(2):495–506.

Smith JA. 1989. Noninfectious diseases, metabolic diseases, toxicities, and neoplastic disease of South American camelids. *Vet Clin N Am Food Anim Pract*; 5(1):101–143. (Contains sections on bloat, indigestion, forestomach perforation, vagal indigestion, colic, and others).

41

Intubation of the First Forestomach Compartment ("C1" or "Pseudorumen")

David E. Anderson

Purpose or Indication for Procedure

Intubation of the C1 or rumen is indicated to either administer oral fluids (e.g., water, electrolytes) or medications, (e.g., anthelmintics, bismuth subsalicylate) and for collection of C1 fluid for analysis (e.g., "rumen" chloride, protozoal assessment, pH determination, bacterial fermentation activity). This procedure also can be done to alleviate bloat (also known as "rumen" tympany) that may occur during grazing, especially of clover, or during sedation or anesthesia because of drug induced atony of the forestomachs.

Equipment Needed

The following equipment is needed:

- Nasogastric: Small size (ideally <1-cm diameter) tube such as a stallion urinary catheter or foal nasogastric tube, and lubricant (either sterile lubricant or lidocaine 2% gel)
- Orogastric: Mouth speculum, small to medium (<2-cm diameter) size tube such as a foal nasogastric tube or equine nasogastric tube, and lubricant (obstetrical lubricant or sterile lubricant)

Restraint/Position

Positions to be used include standing in a camelid chute or using manual head and neck restraint, or sternal recumbency.

Technical Description of Procedure/Method

Nasogastric Intubation

Nasogastric intubation requires firm restraint, and sedation facilitates this procedure if the condition of the patient is suitable to the use of sedatives (e.g., butorphanol at 0.1 mg/kg IV or xylazine at 0.2 mg/kg IV). In adult camelids, the nasal passages will accommodate a tube approximately 1 cm in diameter when passed along the ventral and common meatus. In young llamas and alpacas, the diameter of the tube should be no larger than 5 to 6 mm in diameter. The handler must restrain the head so that movement is minimized. The operator then places the index finger of one hand into the nasal passage (Figure 41.1). This will allow the tube to be directed ventrally into the ventral meatus of the nasal passage (Figure 41.2). The ventral meatus unites at the termination of the nasal septum into a common meatus about

Veterinary Techniques in Llamas and Alpacas, Second Edition. Edited by David E. Anderson, Matt Miesner, and Meredyth Jones.

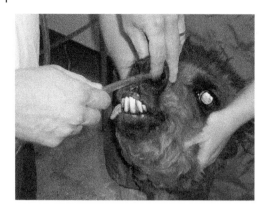

Figure 41.1 Nasogastric intubation is done by inserting the index finger through the nares and directing the tube ventrally into the ventral meatus of the nasopharynx.

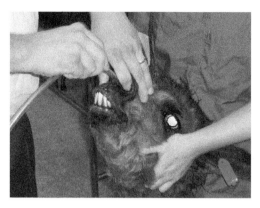

Figure 41.3 Resistance to passage diminishes considerably after the tube has traversed the nasopharynx into the pharynx.

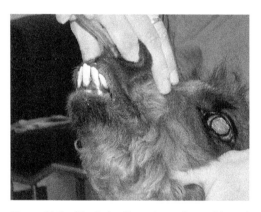

Figure 41.2 The index finger is used to guide and verify correct placement of the tube prior to firm insertion.

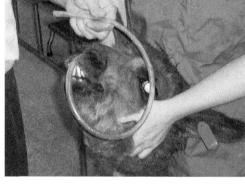

Figure 41.4 Intubation is facilitated by swallowing, and correct placement is verified by palpation of the tube in the esophagus, aspiration resulting in negative pressure in the tube, and auscultation of bubbles in the C1 during infusion of air into the tube.

8-cm caudal to the nares. Thus, this is the largest passageway through the nose. The nasogastric tube is lubricated and inserted through the nares and directed ventrally to ensure passage into the common meatus. Most camelids strongly resist passage of the tube through the rostral 8- to 10-cm of the nasal passageway (Figure 41.3). Lidocaine 2% HCl gel may be used as a lubricant to diminish the stimulation associated with passage of the tube. The tube is advanced until swallowing is observed, at which time the tube can be advanced into the esophagus and C1 (Figure 41.4). If the progress of the tube stops or a significant increase in resistance is noted without any swallowing

reflex, then the position of the tube must be re-evaluated to ensure proper placement in the ventral meatus.

Orogastric Intubation

Orogastric intubation requires firm restraint, and sedation facilitates this procedure if the condition of the patient is suitable to the use of sedatives (e.g., butorphanol at 0.1 mg/kg IV or xylazine at 0.2 mg/kg IV). In adult camelids, the oral cavity will accommodate a tube approximately 2.54 cm (1 inch) in diameter.

The oral cavity of pre-weaned crias will allow tubes of approximately 1 cm in diameter. Oral feeding tubes up to 5-mm in diameter can be used in neonates (<30 days old). The handler must restrain the head so that movement is minimized. An oral speculum is placed into the mouth and held firmly in place to prevent the patient from biting the tube (Figure 41.5). PVC pipes cut to appropriate length and coated with rubber or elastic tape are suitable for use as mouth speculums (adult = 3- to 5-cm diameter; pre-weaned crias 1.5- to 2.5-cm diameter; neonates 1-cm diameter). The tube is advanced until swallowing is observed, at which time the tube can be advanced into the esophagus and C1 (Figure 41.6). If the progress of the tube stops or a significant increase in resistance is noted without any swallowing reflex, then the position of the tube must be re-evaluated to ensure proper placement in the oral cavity and that the tube has not become lodged between the teeth. Passage of the tube can be facilitated by blowing air through the tube throughout passage (Figure 41.7).

Assessment of Tube Placement

The correct placement of the tube into the esophagus can be confirmed by palpation of the ventral aspect of the neck immediately to

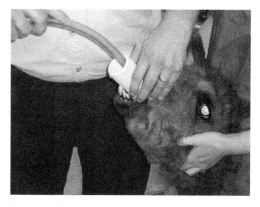

Figure 41.6 Orogastric intubation is achieved by firmly advancing the tube along the midline of the tongue until passage into the esophagus is achieved. Proper positioning of the tube must be ascertained before administration of any drugs or fluids.

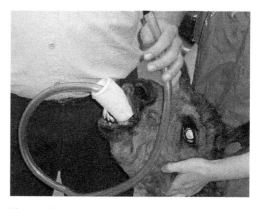

Figure 41.7 Infusing air through the tube can stimulate a swallowing reflex and ease passage of the tube.

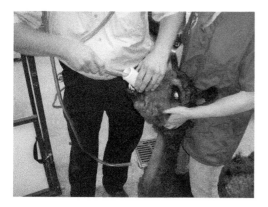

Figure 41.5 An oral speculum constructed of a short length of PVC pipe covered with adhesive tape is used to keep the mouth open during insertion of an orogastric tube.

the left side of the trachea. The tube can be felt passing along the esophagus deep to the skin. Alternatively, a stethoscope can be placed on the cranial left abdominal wall overlying the C1. While ausculting C1, air is blown through the tube. The sound of air bubbles being blown through to tube into C1 confirms correct placement. The contents of C1 of camelids are not stratified in the same way as that of the rumen of cattle. Rather, the liquid, gas, and fibrous contents are more uniformly distributed and mixed. This stratification interferes with collection of C1 fluid.

Simple aspiration of contents by applying suction to the tube is often unsuccessful. If fluid is not readily obtained, air should be blown through the tube to clear any obstructing debris that might have become lodged in the tube during attempts at aspiration, and then the tube should be advanced into C1 as far as possible. The tube is then gently advanced and retracted, while staying within the C1 chamber, several times to encourage passive fluid entry into the tube. Finally, the free end of the tube is plugged or suction applied to prevent out flow of fluid during removal of the tube. This procedure is expected to glean 10 to 30 mLs of fluid.

Practice Tip to Facilitate Procedure

Nasogastric tubes should be soft and pliable to prevent injury to the nasal mucosa and to make passage into the ventral meatus easier. An index finger placed as far caudally as possible helps to force the tube into the ventral meatus. Entry and advancement of the tube is most difficult at the nares and rostral nasal passageway. Orogastric tubes must be sufficiently stiff to allow the operator to control the direction of the tube caudally through the oral cavity, past the dental arcades, and beyond the base of the tongue. Adult swine oral speculums are more easily maintained in the mouth during passage of the tube compared to tubular mouth specula.

Potential Complications

The nasal mucosa is easily damaged during nasogastric intubation, and nasal hemorrhage is not uncommon. This complication is normally self-limiting unless a coagulation disorder is present. Passage of the tube into the trachea, especially during nasogastric intubation, must be corrected prior to administration of any fluids or medications. Cough reflex alone should not be used as an indicator of placement into the trachea. Similarly, absence of a cough reflex alone does not indicate correct placement into the esophagus.

Patient Monitoring/Aftercare

Patients should be monitored for nasal or oral bleeding, difficulty eating, dyspnea, or clinical deterioration after these procedures. When present, clinical signs of these complications are expected to occur within several hours of the procedure but could be delayed up to 72 hours in the case of aspiration pneumonia.

42

Laparotomy—Lateral Approach

David E. Anderson

Purpose or Indication for Procedure

Laparotomy may be performed as a diagnostic or therapeutic procedure. Acute, severe, or continuous pain is an indication for exploratory surgery, but mild, intermittent, and persistent pain also justify laparotomy. Physical and laboratory examination findings supportive of laparotomy include abnormal rectal palpation findings, abnormal peritoneal fluid, failure to pass feces for more than 24 hours, urinary outflow obstruction, ultrasound identification of severe intestinal or urinary bladder distention, or serum biochemistry changes suggestive of visceral compromise.

Equipment Needed

The following equipment is needed: clippers, preparation for aseptic surgery (povidone iodine scrub, alcohol rinse, gauze pads), surgery cap and mask, sterile drapes, sterile gloves, sterile gowns, suction apparatus, sterile saline or lactated Ringer's solution (LRS) rinse, soft tissue surgery instruments, intestinal forceps, tissue retractors (e.g., Balfour or Richardson retractors), suture materials, bandaging material (cotton sheets, brown roll gauze, elastic non-adhesive tape, adhesive tape), anesthesia, IV fluids, antibiotics, and nonsteroidal anti-inflammatory drugs.

Restraint/Position

Laparotomy may be performed with the patient sedated (e.g., butorphanol tartrate at 0.1 mg/kg IV; xylazine at 0.2 mg/kg IV) and after local anesthesia, but these procedures are most efficiently done after induction of general anesthesia. The author prefers to perform exploratory laparotomies under gas anesthesia because of optimal patient management and surgeon comfort. Ideally, orotracheal or nasotracheal intubation should be performed to optimize breathing and protect the airways from regurgitation. Lateral laparotomy can be performed with the patient standing, placed in sternal (cushed) recumbency, or restrained in lateral recumbency. Llamas are more amenable than alpacas to remaining standing during laparotomy, but this is appropriate for few procedures, and patient selection is critical. Standing laparotomy is best reserved for laparoscopic procedures where the integrity of the abdominal cavity is better protected.

Sternal recumbency increases intra-abdominal pressure and limits access to the lateral

Veterinary Techniques in Llamas and Alpacas, Second Edition. Edited by David E. Anderson, Matt Miesner, and Meredyth Jones.

abdominal wall because of the positioning of the limbs. Positioning in lateral recumbency or with a pad positioned so that the patient can be maintained in a 30-degree off dorsal-lateral position (Figure 42.1) are preferred because of the safety and efficiency of this approach.

Technical Description of Procedure/Method

Preparation

The hair should be clipped with #40 clipper blades and aseptically prepared for surgery. The clipped and prepared area should be four times the surface area of the operative site in order to provide wide margins for maintenance of a sterile field. In general, the preparation site should extend from the ventral midline to the dorsal midline.

Approach

A ventral midline approach to the abdomen is the standard method used in monogastric species for access to abdominal viscera. Anatomic

differences require paralumbar fossae laparotomy for many problems in ruminant species. South American camelids have many clinical and anatomical similarities to ruminants. However, llamas and alpacas do not possess a distinct paralumbar fossa as is found in cattle, sheep, and goats. In camelids, the abdominal wall is tapered without a pronounced flank. Thus, laparotomy is described as being done from a lateral approach. The laparotomy incision may be made perpendicular to the spine (mid-lateral laparotomy), may follow the curvature of the last rib (paracostal laparotomy), or may be angled along the border of the internal abdominal oblique muscle at approximately a 30-degree angle caudal to the mid-lateral laparotomy site (caudal oblique laparotomy; Figure 42.2). The decision for left versus right-sided lateral approach is based on the viscera to which access is needed (Table 42.1). The tissue layers involved in the approach to the abdomen through a lateral abdominal approach include the skin, minimal subcutaneous tissues, external abdominal oblique muscle (Figure 42.3), internal abdominal oblique muscle (Figure 42.4), transversus abdominus muscle, and peritoneum (Figure 42.5). From the right

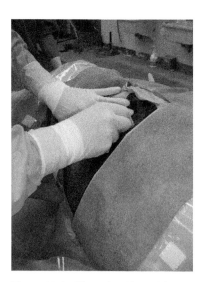

Figure 42.1 The animal is positioned in sternolateral recumbency so that the position of the spine is maintained 30-degrees toward lateral.

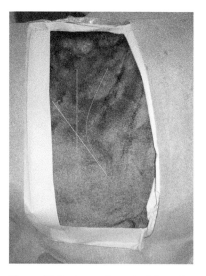

Figure 42.2 Laparotomy incisions through the lateral abdominal wall may be made via a perpendicular incision, paracostal incision, or a 30-degree oblique position.

Table 42.1 Differences in desired incision site for visceral access in llamas and alpacas.

	Right Side	Left Side
Paracostal Laparotomy	Liver Right crus of diaphragm Pyloric antrum of third forestomach compartment (C3) Pylorus and duodenal ampulla Duodenum Pancreas	First forestomach compartment Left crus of diaphragm
Midlateral Laparotomy	Pyloric antrum and fundus of third forestomach compartment Duodenum Jejunum Ileum Cecum Spiral Colon Right kidney Uterus Right ovary	First forestomach compartment Spleen Left kidney Uterus Left ovary
Caudal Oblique Laparotomy	Uterus	Uterus

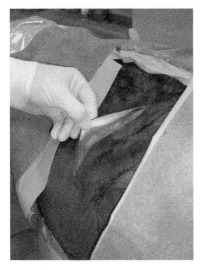

Figure 42.3 After the skin incision has been made, the external abdominal oblique muscle is visible.

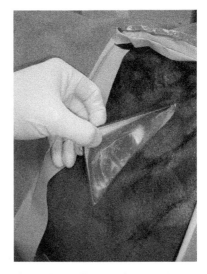

Figure 42.4 The muscle layers in alpacas and llamas are thin with minimal fascial coverage compared with other livestock.

lateral abdominal approach, the pyloric antrum of C3 (Figure 42.6), jejunum and ileum (Figure 42.7), and cecum and spiral colon (Figure 42.8) can be readily exteriorized. As compared to the ventral midline approach, the most significant advantage of the right lateral abdominal approach is the ease of access to the duodenum (Figure 42.9), pancreas (Figure 42.10), and right kidney (Figure 42.11). The left lateral approach gives ready access to the spleen, C1, and left kidney.

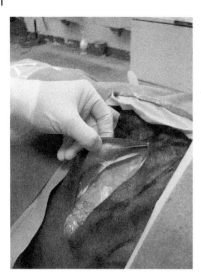

Figure 42.5 The abdomen is exposed after incising the external abdominal oblique, internal abdominal oblique, and transversus abdominus muscles.

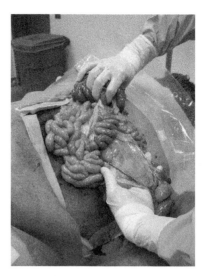

Figure 42.7 The jejunum and ileum can be exteriorized via a right lateral abdominal incision.

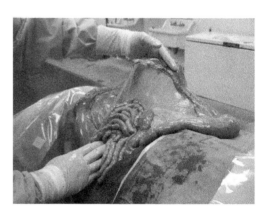

Figure 42.8 The proximal loop of the spiral colon and the spiral colon can easily be exteriorized via a right flank approach.

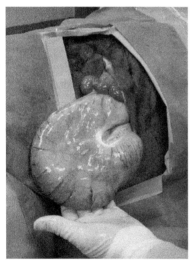

Figure 42.6 The distal portion (pyloric fundus) of C3 can be exteriorized from the abdomen and inspected for impaction, gastric ulcers, and other pathology.

Wound Closure

The muscular wall of the lateral abdomen is thin and contains minimal fascial support (Figure 42.5). Therefore, the abdominal wall must be carefully reconstructed with close attention to detail. Suture size and selection should be made with consideration for tissue holding, knot security, absorption times, and bulkiness of knots (Table 42.2). These incisions may be more prone to postoperative hernia formation compared with ventral midline incisions because of the relatively poor holding power of the muscles for suture materials. Closure of all muscles (transversus m, internal abdominal oblique m, and external abdominal oblique m) in one layer may increase the holding power of sutures so that each muscle layer

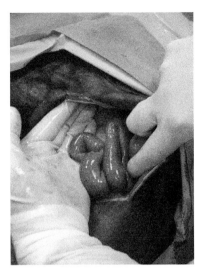

Figure 42.9 The duodenum can be viewed but minimally exteriorized via a right paracostal incision.

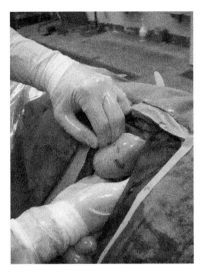

Figure 42.11 The right kidney can be inspected via a right paracostal incision.

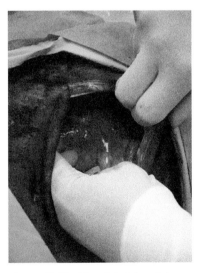

Figure 42.10 The right lobe of the pancreas can be inspected via a right paracostal incision.

provides support for adjacent layers. However, the authors prefer to close the peritoneum, transversus abdominus m, and internal abdominal oblique m together in one layer and then close the external abdominal oblique muscle as a separate layer. Simple continuous suture patterns with suture bites taken a minimum of 1.5 cm from the margin and no more than 1.5 cm apart provide for accurate reconstruction and minimal risk of dehiscence. When significant tension is present on the abdominal wall, tension relieving interrupted suture patterns may be used (e.g., cruciate pattern). Absorbable suture materials should be used, and either monofilament or braided suture materials are appropriate. Camelids lack a substantial subcutaneous layer, extensive undermining of the skin is rarely needed, and, therefore, subcutaneous sutures are rarely used. Skin can be closed using continuous or interrupted suture patterns or stainless-steel skin staples. This author prefers to use a Ford Interlocking pattern (also known as forward interlocking pattern), but suture bites should not be taken more than 1 cm from the skin margin and should be spaced no more than 1 cm apart to maintain accurate alignment of the skin edges.

Operative Techniques for Correction of Intestinal Obstruction

Enterotomy

When obstruction of the duodenum, jejunum, or spiral colon is present, the site of obstruction can be found by exteriorizing a segment of

Table 42.2 Suture selection and suture patterns for reconstruction of the lateral abdominal wall of llamas and alpacas after laparotomy.

	Suture	Size
Peritoneum/Transversus abdominus muscle/internal abdominal oblique muscle	Polydioxanone Polyglactin 910 Polyglycolic acid	Adult: Alpaca: #1; Llama: #2 Weanlings: Alpaca: #0; Llama: #1 Neonates: Alpaca: #0; Llama: #0
External abdominal oblique muscle	Polydioxanone Polyglactin 910 Polyglycolic acid	Adult: Alpaca: #1; Llama: #2 Weanlings: Alpaca: #0; Llama: #1 Neonates: Alpaca: #0; Llama: #0
Skin	Nylon Polypropylene Polymerized caprolactam	Adult: Alpaca: #1; Llama: #2 Weanlings: Alpaca: #0; Llama: #1 Neonates: Alpaca: #0; Llama: #0

normal or distended intestine and tracing this segment orad or aborad respectively, until the obstruction is found. The intestines of llamas and alpacas are relatively easily traumatized, and the surgeon should take precautions not to cause injury to the bowel. The author prefers to apply carboxymethylcellulose jelly (without preservative) to the intestine as a lubricant to prevent unintended intestinal irritation. For intraluminal obstructions, such as trochophytobezoars, the obstructed segment of intestine should be exteriorized from the abdomen, isolated using moistened surgical towels, and an enterotomy performed. A common site for trichophytobezoars to become obstructed is the distal duodenum, followed by the spiral colon. The duodenum cannot be fully exteriorized from the abdomen, but a paracostal incision provides direct access to the segment of interest. Moistened surgical towels or laparotomy sponges can be used to pack off the area, and suction is used during the enterotomy to prevent or minimize contamination of the enterotomy site. After removal of the foreign body, the enterotomy is closed with absorbable suture material (e.g., polydioxanone, polyglactin 910) using one or two lines of an appositional or inverting suture pattern. Sutures of small sizes (e.g., #3–0) with swaged-on needles of small dimension (taper only) should be used so the margins of the affected intestine are not

damaged and the suture tracks do not leak. This will minimize the risk of postoperative leakage or dehiscence. The author prefers to close the enterotomy transversely in an attempt to maximize the lumen of the affected segment of intestine and minimize the tension endured by the suture line during cycles of contraction and distension of the intestinal wall.

Intestinal Resection
When an intestinal segment has lost integrity, such as with strangulations or intussusception, surgical removal by resection and anastomosis is the treatment of choice. The intestinal segment is exteriorized from the abdomen and isolated using a barrier drape and moistened towels. The margins for excision are selected in healthy-appearing intestine. Only the portion to be resected and immediately adjacent bowel should be exteriorized to avoid excessive traction and contamination during the resection-anastomosis. The relevant mesenteric vessels (arteries and veins) are ligated with absorbable suture material (e.g., #3–0 or #2–0 poliglecaprone) being sure not to compromise the blood supply to the intestine to be preserved. After completion of mesentery ligation and transection, Doyen intestinal forceps are used to occlude the lumen of the normal and abnormal bowel. Then, the associated bowel is resected and discarded. The proximal segment

of bowel is carefully exteriorized to its maximum length, and the two segments of intestine are reunited by end-to-end or side-to-side anastomosis with an absorbable suture material (#3– 0 polydioxanone or polyglactin 910) using a simple interrupted or cruciate suture pattern. The initial sutures should be placed at the mesenteric attachment because this is the most likely site for leakage to occur. A second suture is placed at the antimesenteric border to ensure proper alignment of the intestine during closure. Then, rows of sutures are placed and leakage assessed by releasing the proximal Doyen forceps and allowing some ingesta to flow into the segment. Slight pressure is applied and the incision line inspected. When needed to support the primary closure, a second row of interrupted sutures or a continuous oversew using an inverting Cushing suture pattern may be placed into the seromuscular layer to ensure that no leakage occurs at the site of the anastomosis. The affected intestine is thoroughly rinsed with sterile isotonic fluids, again checked for the presence of leakage, and replaced into the abdomen.

Practice Tip to Facilitate Procedure

General anesthesia with intubation and the ability to administer fluids, monitor blood pressure, and assess oxygen saturation greatly improves the safety and efficacy of intestinal surgery. Balfour self-retaining abdominal retractors greatly facilitate exposure of viscera that cannot be exteriorized. In cases having excessive distention of the intestine, visceral retainers (also referred to as "fish") are useful to retain and protect the intestines during suture closure of the first layer of the abdominal wall.

Potential Complications

Incisional infection, hernia, peritonitis, intestinal adhesions, and death are potential complications of intestinal surgery and laparotomy. These complications most often manifest clinically within 3 to 5 days after surgery.

Patient Monitoring/Aftercare

Camelids appear to be fairly tolerant of intestinal surgery when performed early in the progression of the disease, but ileus and adhesions are prominent concerns. Antibiotics, non-steriodal anti-inflammatory drugs, and ulcer prophylaxis are routinely administered after abdominal surgery.

Recommended Reading

Anderson DE. 2009 Jul. Uterine torsion and cesarean section in llamas and alpacas. *Vet Clin North Am Food Anim Pract*; 25(2):523–538. doi: 10.1016/j.cvfa.2009.02.002. PMID: 19460653.

Cebra CK, Cebra ML, Garry FB, Larsen RS, Baxter GM. 1998 Mar-Apr. Acute gastrointestinal disease in 27 New World camelids: clinical and surgical findings. *Vet Surg*; 27(2):112–21. https://doi.org/10.1111/j.1532-950x.1998.tb00106.x. PMID: 9525025.

Newman KD, Anderson DE. 2009 Jul Gastrointestinal surgery in alpacas and llamas. *Vet Clin North Am Food Anim Pract*; 25(2):495–506. https://doi.org/10.1016/j.cvfa.2009.02.007. PMID: 19460651.

43

Laparotomy—Ventral Midline

David E. Anderson

Purpose or Indication for Procedure

Ventral midline laparotomy is most often performed for exploration of the abdomen or when access to the uterus or both ovaries is needed. Exploratory laparotomy may be performed as a diagnostic or therapeutic procedure in patients having acute, severe, or continuous pain or suffer mild, intermittent, and persistent pain. This procedure is useful to obtain diagnostic samples when tissue segments are inaccessible via percutaneous biopsy needles or when substantial amount of tissue are required for the tests.

Equipment Needed

The following equipment is needed: clippers, preparation for aseptic surgery (povidone iodine scrub, alcohol rinse, gauze pads), surgery cap and mask, sterile drapes, sterile gloves, sterile gowns, suction apparatus, sterile saline, or lactated Ringer's solution (LRS) rinse, soft tissue surgery instruments, intestinal forceps, tissue retractors (e.g., Balfour or Richardson retractors), suture materials, bandaging material (cotton sheets, brown roll gauze, elastic non-adhesive tape, adhesive tape), anesthesia, IV fluids, antibiotics, and nonsteroidal anti-inflammatory drugs.

Restraint/Position

Ventral midline laparotomy should be performed with the patient under general anesthesia; however, ventral laparotomy may be performed with the patient sedated and after local anesthesia. Gas anesthesia with orotracheal or nasotracheal intubation minimizes the risk of complications such as aspiration pneumonia, hypoxia, hypercapnia, sudden movements, and patient pain. Orotracheal or nasotracheal intubation is advised to ensure adequate breathing and protect the airways from regurgitation as well as the ability to provide assisted ventilation if needed. After induction of sedation or anesthesia, the alpaca or llama is rolled onto the back into dorsal recumbency. For most procedures, standard dorsal recumbency is used. In patients having significant space occupation with weight (e.g., term pregnancy, C1 impaction, intra-abdominal abscess), a 30-degree deviation from perpendicular to dorsal (60-degree deviation from angle to the ground) may help to maintain hemodynamic stability by preventing interference with central venous return from the abdomen by lessening compression of the caudal vena cava.

Veterinary Techniques in Llamas and Alpacas, Second Edition. Edited by David E. Anderson, Matt Miesner, and Meredyth Jones.

Technical Description of Procedure/Method

Preparation

The hair should be clipped with #40 clipper blades and aseptically prepared for surgery. The clipped and prepared area should be four times the surface area of the operative site to provide wide margins for maintenance of a sterile field. In general, the preparation site should be centered on the ventral midline and extend from the sternum to the pelvis and from the junction of the ventral and lateral abdominal walls.

Approach

A ventral midline approach to the abdomen is the standard method used in monogastric species for access to abdominal viscera. South American camelids have many anatomical similarities to ruminants, and lateral abdominal approach to the abdomen is recommended for those procedures in which more immediate access is needed (e.g., nephrectomy, splenectomy, duodenotomy). The tissue layers involved in the ventral midline approach to the abdomen include the skin, subcutaneous tissues, linea alba, and peritoneum. Surgical procedures involving the bladder, uterus or ovaries, and large intestine require a caudal ventral midline incision. This incision is made starting at the umbilicus cranially and extending to the brim of the pelvis caudally. Surgical procedures involving the C1, C2, C3, spleen, liver, or proximal small intestine require a cranial incision. An incision is made at the umbilicus caudally, and the incision is extended cranially to the xyphoid. General exploratory laparotomies may be performed with the incision centered on the umbilicus and extended cranially or caudally as needed based on the operative findings (Figure 43.1). The author uses a #10 scalpel blade to divide the linea alba for a length of 2 cm, then manual digital pressure is applied until the peritoneum is penetrated as denoted by a sudden release of resistance (Figure 43.2). Then, the surgeon's index finger and middle finger are inserted into the abdomen, and the ventral abdominal wall is inspected and

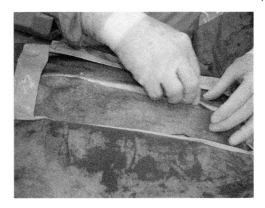

Figure 43.1 The alpaca is positioned in dorsal recumbency and the incision centered on the umbilicus and extended cranially or caudally as needed based on the operative findings.

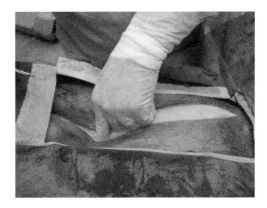

Figure 43.2 A #10 scalpel blade is used to divide the linea alba for a length of 2 cm, then manual digital pressure is applied until the peritoneum is penetrated as denoted by a sudden release of resistance.

elevated to facilitate the remainder of the incision (Figure 43.3). A ventral midline laparotomy should provide access to the ventral compartment of C1 (Figure 43.4), fundus of C3 (Figure 43.5), jejunum, cecum, and spiral colon (Figure 43.6), and reproductive tract. In camelids, the cecum is contiguous with the proximal loop of the spiral colon. However, the cecum can be identified by inspection of the blind end and the ileocecal ligament (Figure 43.7). With difficulty, the bladder can be exteriorized (Figure 43.8). Although not exteriorized, the spleen, liver (Figure 43.9), and kidneys can be inspected and biopsies performed.

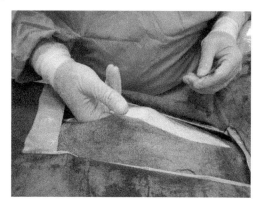

Figure 43.3 The surgeon's index finger and middle finger are inserted into the abdomen and the ventral abdominal wall elevated to facilitate the remainder of the incision.

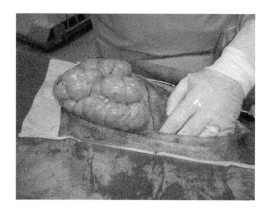

Figure 43.4 The ventral sacs of C1 are easily viewed and can be partially exteriorized via a ventral midline laparotomy incision.

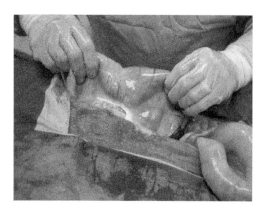

Figure 43.5 The main body (fundus) of C3 can be partially exteriorized and inspected via ventral midline.

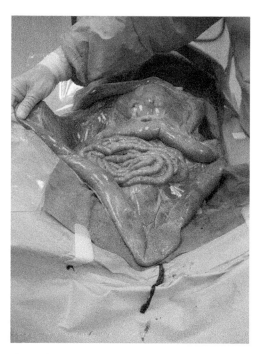

Figure 43.6 The proximal loop of the spiral colon and the spiral colon can easily be exteriorized via a ventral midline approach.

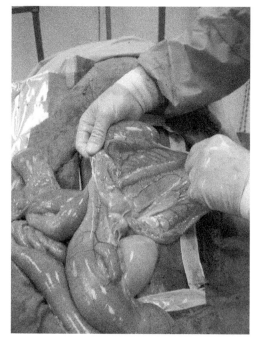

Figure 43.7 The ileocecal ligament has been exteriorized for examination.

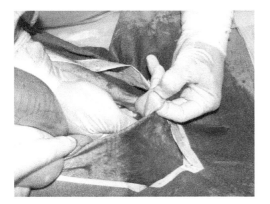

Figure 43.8 The bladder can be palpated and only partially exteriorized when not distended.

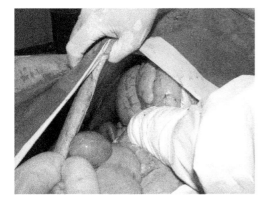

Figure 43.9 The liver can be viewed but not exteriorized via ventral midline.

Wound Closure

The wall of the ventral abdomen is relatively thin and must be carefully reconstructed with close attention to detail. Incisions contained within the linea alba provide for good suture holding power and minimal postoperative complication. Incisions that deviate to the rectus abdominus are more prone to herniation and the external rectus sheath must be accurately reconstructed to minimize this risk. Suture size and selection should be made with consideration for tissue holding, knot security, absorption times, and bulkiness of knots (Table 43.1). Suture patterns with suture bites taken approximately 1.5 cm from the margin and no more than 1.5 cm apart provide for accurate reconstruction and minimize risk of dehiscence. Either simple continuous or interrupted suture patterns are acceptable. Appositional suture patterns are preferred to facilitate rapid tissue healing. When significant tension is present on the abdominal wall, tension-relieving interrupted suture patterns may be used (e.g., cruciate pattern). Absorbable suture materials should be used, and either monofilament or braided suture materials are appropriate. The subcutaneous layer is more substantial along the ventral midline and a subcutaneous suture closure is recommended. Skin can be closed using continuous or interrupted suture patterns or stainless steel skin staples. The

Table 43.1 Suture selection and suture patterns for reconstruction of the ventral midline abdominal wall of llamas and alpacas after laparotomy.

	Suture	Size
Linea alba/rectus abdominus muscle	Polydioxanone	Adult: Alpaca: #1; Llama: #2
	Polyglactin 910	Weanlings: Alpaca: #0; Llama: #1
	Polyglycolic acid	Neonates: Alpaca: #0; Llama: #0
Subcutaneous tissue	Polydioxanone	Adult: Alpaca: #2–0; Llama: #0
	Polyglactin 910	Weanlings: Alpaca: #2–0; Llama: #2–0
	Polyglycolic acid	Neonates: Alpaca: #3–0; Llama: #2–0
Skin	Nylon	Adult: Alpaca: #1; Llama: #2
	Polypropylene	Weanlings: Alpaca: #0; Llama: #1
	Polymerized caprolactam	Neonates: Alpaca: #0; Llama: #0

author prefers to use a Ford Interlocking pattern (also known as forward interlocking pattern), but suture bites should not be taken more than 1 cm from the skin margin and should be spaced no more than 1 cm apart to maintain accurate alignment of the skin edges.

Operative Techniques for Correction of Intestinal Obstruction

Exploratory Examination for Simple Intraluminal Obstruction
When obstruction of the duodenum, jejunum, or spiral colon is present, the site of obstruction can be found by exteriorizing a segment of normal or distended intestine and tracing this segment orad or aborad, respectively, until the obstruction is found (Video 43.1: Obstruction). The intestines of llamas and alpacas are relatively easily traumatized, and the surgeon should take precautions not to cause injury to the bowel. The author prefers to apply carboxymethylcellulose jelly, without preservative, to the intestine as a lubricant to prevent unintended intestinal irritation. For intraluminal obstructions, such as trochophytobezoars, the obstructed segment of intestine should be exteriorized from the abdomen, isolated using moistened surgical towels, and an enterotomy performed.

Practice Tip to Facilitate Procedure

General anesthesia with intubation and the ability to administer fluids, monitor blood pressure, and assess oxygen saturation greatly improves the safety and efficacy of intestinal surgery. Balfour self-retaining abdominal retractors greatly facilitate exposure of viscera that cannot be exteriorized. In cases having excessive distention of the intestine, visceral retainers (also referred to as "fish") are useful to retain and protect the intestines during suture closure of the first layer of the abdominal wall. Camelid possess a significant ventral, retroperitoneal fat pad.

These fat pads end where the peritoneum fuses with the ventral midline. Incisions made accurately along the ventral midline provide ready access to the abdomen. Incisions that deviate from ventral midline risk entry into the fat pads. This error complicates laparotomy and may increase the risk of postoperative hernia.

Potential Complications

Incisional infection, hernia, peritonitis, intestinal adhesions, and death are potential complications of intestinal surgery and laparotomy. These complications most often manifest clinically within 3 to 5 days after surgery.

Patient Monitoring/Aftercare

Camelids appear to be fairly tolerant of intestinal surgery when performed early in the progression of the disease, but ileus and adhesions are prominent concerns. Antibiotics, non-steriodal anti-inflammatory drugs, and ulcer prophylaxis are routinely administered after abdominal surgery.

Recommended Reading

Anderson DE. 2009 Jul. Uterine torsion and cesarean section in llamas and alpacas. *Vet Clin North Am Food Anim Pract*; 25(2):523–38. doi: 10.1016/j.cvfa.2009.02.002. PMID: 19460653.

Cebra CK, Cebra ML, Garry FB, Larsen RS, Baxter GM. 1998 Mar-Apr. Acute gastrointestinal disease in 27 New World camelids: clinical and surgical findings. *Vet Surg*; 27(2):112–21. doi: 10.1111/j.1532-950x.1998.tb00106.x. PMID: 9525025.

Miller BA, Brounts SH, Anderson DE, Devine E. 2013 Mar 1. Cesarean section in alpacas and llamas: 34 cases (1997–2010). *J Am Vet Med*

Assoc; 242(5):670–4. doi: 10.2460/ javma.242.5.670. PMID: 23402415.

Newman KD, Anderson DE. 2009 Jul. Gastrointestinal surgery in alpacas and llamas. *Vet Clin North Am Food Anim Pract*; 25(2):495–506. doi: 10.1016/j.cvfa.2009.02.007. PMID: 19460651.

44

Laparoscopy

David E. Anderson

Purpose or Indication for Procedure

Accurate differentiation of medical and surgical lesions in the abdomen of camelids often is difficult because of their stoic nature. Peritoneal fluid samples can be difficult to obtain, and changes in peritoneal fluid constituents may not be specific to surgical or medical conditions. Laparoscopy provides a rapid, minimally invasive method for examination of the abdomen with reduced morbidity compared to that for exploratory laparotomy. Laparoscopy also is an effective tool for evaluation of reproductive structures in llamas and alpacas. The abdominal anatomy in camelids is markedly different from that of horses and cattle, and knowledge of these differences is important to accurate placement of portals and interpretation of findings.

Equipment Needed

The following equipment is needed: laparoscope (30-cm long × 10-cm diameter); laparoscopic instruments including forceps, scissors, retractors (5-mm to 12-mm diameter); cannulas with trochars (5- to 12-mm range); insufflation tubing and gas source (filtered air or carbon dioxide); light cables and source; minor surgery pack (scalpel, scissors, needle driver, sterile gauze); sterile drapes; gowns; gloves; cap and mask; and aseptic preparation set (povidone iodine or chlorhexidine, alcohol).

Restraint/Position

Distention of viscera with ingesta—but especially gas—is the principle impediment to performing laparoscopy. Distended viscera may prevent successful laparoscopy if viewing is obstructed or if there is interference to instrument access. Whenever possible, feed and water should be withheld for a minimum of 24 hours prior to laparoscopy. Antibiotics and non-steroidal anti-inflammatory drugs are routinely administered prior to surgery.

Lateral Abdominal Approach

Diagnostic laparoscopy can be performed in llamas with the animal standing and sedated. However, alpacas frequently assume sternal recumbency during preparation and during surgery. Alpacas should be placed in a sternal (cushed) position for conscious laparoscopy. Operative laparoscopy is often associated with pain or noxious stimuli and is more efficiently and effectively performed with the patient under general anesthesia. Short procedures can be completed using injectable anesthesia alone, but inhalational anesthesia is ideal for procedures requiring more than 30 to 45 minutes.

Ventral Abdominal Laparoscopy

The patient is placed in dorsal recumbency and tilted to accommodate viewing the region of interest. For caudal abdomen viewing and procedures, the patient is positioned in a 30-degree head down (Trendelenburg) position. For cranial abdomen procedures, the patient is positioned in a 30-degree head up (reverse Trendelenburg) position. This assists in displacement of viscera away from the area of interest and minimizes interference with the field of view.

Technical Description of Procedure/Method

Laparoscopy generally includes a viewing portal (cannula and camera) and an instrument portal (cannula and endoscopic instruments). Additional instrument portals can be added based on the procedure being done (e.g., when a grasping and cutting instrument are needed simultaneously). Each additional portal and instrument adds to the complexity of the procedure and increases the need for accurate placement to prevent interference from one cannula or instrument to another.

Lateral Abdominal Approach

The lateral abdomen, defined caudally by the area of the stifle, cranially by the last palpable rib, dorsally by the transverse processes of the lumbar vertebrae, and ventrally by the tapered aspect of the abdominal wall, is clipped and prepared for aseptic surgery. A 2-cm skin incision is made in the dorsal, central aspect of the prepared area, and a trochar and cannula are placed into the peritoneal cavity. The skin incision should be made through the external and internal abdominal oblique muscles. Then, a blunt (rounded conical tip) trochar and cannula are inserted, using steady pressure, into the abdomen, as evidenced by sudden release of resistance to pressure. Correct placement within the abdominal cavity must be confirmed prior to insufflation. Placement of the cannula retroperitoneally or within the omentum or mesentery will interfere with completion of the procedure and increase risk of morbidity for the patient. Correct placement can be assured by viewing of the serosal surface of viscera. Carbon dioxide gas or filtered air is insufflated to a pressure of 15 to 20 mm Hg, and the pressure is maintained at <22 mm Hg. Only enough air to complete the procedure should be insufflated. Unnecessary insufflation increases the risk of morbidity. A 30-cm-long rigid laparoscope is sufficient to perform a systematic examination of the abdomen. A 10-mm-diameter scope provides a larger view and is adequately sturdy to allow manipulation of the scope and viscera.

Left lateral laparoscopy allows viewing of the first forestomach compartment (C1), spleen, and diaphragm in the cranial region of the abdomen. The left kidney can be observed caudal and medial to the dorsal attachment of C1. Perirenal fat may obscure the kidney from direct view. The small intestine can be observed dorsal and caudal to C1, but differentiation of specific segments of the small intestine is more difficult. Often, the proximal loop of the spiral colon is observed caudal to C1. The spiral colon is identified by the inter-serosal mesentery. The urinary bladder is viewed in the caudal region of the abdomen and is evident by its dark color and characteristic musculature. The left inguinal ring can be observed in most standing animals without additional instruments, but recumbent animals require use of an endoscopic retractor to reflect viscera out of the field of view. The left ovary and uterine horn are more easily viewed with the patient in standing or sternal (cushed) posture, but they may be viewed in lateral recumbency with the assistance of an endoretractor.

Right lateral laparoscopy provides viewing of the third forestomach compartment (C3), which includes the duodenum and pancreas. The ventral margin of C1 may be visible in laterally recumbent patients. The liver and diaphragm are seen in the cranial and middle region of the abdomen. The first forestomach compartment can be observed during laparoscopy in a recumbent position and is identified by the longitudinal rows of small saccules protruding from its ventromedial surface. The third forestomach compartment has a long tubular appearance, with a prominent serosal vascular pattern and omental attachments on the greater curvature. The second forestomach compartment (C2), spherical and covered by omentum, is rarely identified. The right kidney is observed in the dorsal region of the abdomen protruding into the peritoneal cavity and surrounded by perirenal fat. The caudate and right lobes of the liver are observed cranial and lateral to C3. The small intestine, including the proximal portion of the jejunum and duodenum, are easily found. The proximal loop of the spiral colon (ascending colon) can be viewed in the caudoventral region of the abdomen and is identified as a large, tubular viscera without associated omentum or large serosal vessels. The spiral colon is identified by the interserosal mesentery. The urinary bladder is viewed in the caudal region of the abdomen and evident by its dark color and characteristic musculature. The inguinal ring is similarly viewed as described for the left approach. The right ovary and right uterine horn are more easily viewed with the patient in standing or sternal (cushed) posture, but may be viewed in lateral recumbency with the assistance of an endoretractor.

After completion of laparoscopy, the fascia of the external abdominal oblique muscle is apposed using #2–0 polyglactin 910 or polydioxanone in an interrupted cruciate pattern. Skin edges are closed using #0 or #1 nylon, polypropylene, or stainless-steel skin staples.

Ventral Abdomen Approach

The viewing portal for ventral abdominal laparoscopy is most often placed through, or immediately cranial or caudal to, the umbilicus. A 2-cm long skin incision is made on the ventral midline and a trocar and cannula placed into the abdomen. The initial incision should be made through the skin and linea alba but not the peritoneum. Then, a blunt (rounded conical tip) trochar and cannula are inserted, using steady pressure, into the abdomen. Successful entry into the abdomen is evidenced by sudden release of resistance to pressure. Correct placement within the abdominal cavity must be confirmed prior to insufflation to ensure that insufflation of the retroperitoneal space or omental bursa does not occur. Carbon dioxide gas or filtered air is insufflated as previously described with careful attention to limit the intra-abdominal pressure to <22 mm Hg. Insufflation should only be maintained sufficient to complete the procedure to minimize the risk of overinflation.

Ventral midline laparoscopy provides viewing of the ventral aspect of C1, liver, spleen, and diaphragm in the cranial region of the abdomen (Video 44.1: Laparoscopy caudal abdomen). Rows of individual saccules are observed protruding from the ventral aspect of C1. The caudoventral edge of the liver is fimbriated and can be found near the attachment of the right crus of the diaphragm to the abdominal wall. The third forestomach compartment can be identified in the right hemiabdomen and the small intestine is observed in the caudal abdomen (Video 44.2: Laparoscopy caudal abdomen). The proximal loop of the ascending colon and the spiral colon also observed caudal to C3 and C1.

After completion of laparoscopy, the linea alba is apposed using #0 or # 1 polyglactin 910 or PDS in an appositional pattern (e.g., cruciate or simple interrupted). Skin edges are apposed using #0 or #1 nylon, polypropylene or stainless-steel skin staples.

Operative Laparoscopy

Laparoscopic-guided biopsy of the liver, spleen, and kidneys may be useful for evaluation of these tissues. Laparoscopic examination of reproductive structures is readily accomplished including ovariectomy, cryptochidectomy, and vasectomy. Laparoscopy has also been used successfully to resolve clinical adhesions to the uterus, ovaries, and intestine. Laparoscopic reduction or fenestration has been used to resolve ovarian cysts, endometrial cysts, ovarian neoplasia, and for ovariohysterectomy.

Practice Tip to Facilitate Procedure

With practice, good working equipment, proper patient selection, and preparation, laparoscopy can be rapidly and efficiently performed. The key elements to successful laparoscopy include appropriate equipment and sufficient light source and insufflation. Versatile laparoscopic ports that allow the user to switch between 10- and 5-mm- diameter instruments greatly facilitate procedures when the viewing port and instrument ports need to be changed. Also, ports that have an inflatable cuff on one end allow secure retention of the cannula in the abdominal wall while retaining little length of the cannula within the abdomen (Figures 44.1–44.5). Dual cannulas that serve both as a viewing port and an instrument port provide flexibility when space limitations of the anatomical window limits the number of ports that can be inserted.

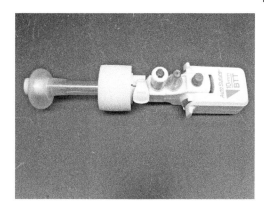

Figure 44.2 Cuff inflated on disposal laparoscopy portal.

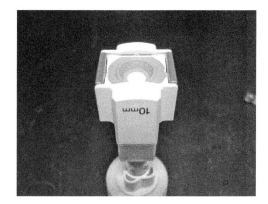

Figure 44.3 Adjustable ports are useful to minimize port manipulation and optimize instrument seal (10-mm main port shown).

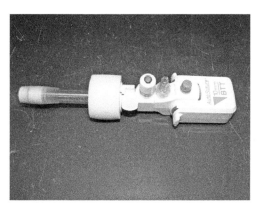

Figure 44.1 Disposable laparoscopy portal with inflatable cuff and sliding lock washer.

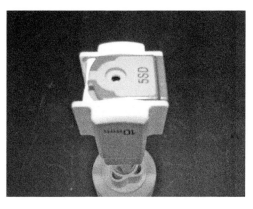

Figure 44.4 Adjustable ports are useful to minimize port manipulation and optimize instrument seal (5-mm port shown).

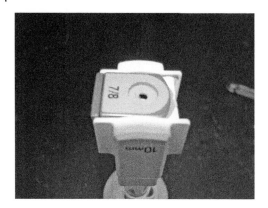

Figure 44.5 Adjustable ports are useful to minimize port manipulation and optimize instrument seal (7- to 8-mm port shown).

Potential Complications

Suboptimal placement of portals is a common mistake. If the lateral abdominal incision is made too far dorsal, retroperitoneal placement of the laparoscope is possible. Gas insufflation of the retroperitoneal space can prevent successful completion of laparoscopy. Hemorrhage into the abdomen, usually caused by inadvertent trauma to viscera, can obscure the view and could pose the risk of death for the patient. Of the more than 1,000 published laparoscopy procedures in camelids for manipulation of reproductive structures in llamas and alpacas, only 1 (0.08%) resulted in inadvertent penetration of viscera (C1) (Bravo and Sumar 1989; 1991). Hemorrhage can be sufficient to cause the procedure to be aborted. Another common error is placement of instrument cannulas too close to the viewing portal or too far from the target tissue for instrument use. This may require repositioning of the portal, which complicates or impedes the ability to maintain gas inflation of the abdominal cavity. Complications observed after surgery have been minor (e.g., emphysema, hematoma, seroma) and resolve without treatment.

Patient Monitoring/Aftercare

Patients should be closely observed for 24 hours after laparoscopy for signs of abdominal pain, abdominal distension, straining to urinate or defecate, apparent depression, lethargy, recumbency, or inappetence.

Recommended Reading

Anderson DE, Gaughan EM, Baird AN, Lin HC, Pugh DG. 1996, Jan 1. Laparoscopic surgical approach and anatomy of the abdomen in llamas. *J Am Vet Med Assoc*; 208(1):111–116. PMID: 8682698.

Anderson DE, Schulz KM., Rousseau M. 2010, Aug. Laparoscopic cystotomy for removal of a large bladder polyp in a juvenile alpaca with polypoid cystitis. *Vet Surg*; 39(6):733–736. doi: 10.1111/j.1532-950X.2010.00693.x. Epub 2010 May 6. PMID: 20459501.

Bravo PW, Sumar J. 1989. Laparoscopic examination of the ovarian activity in Alpacas. *Anim Reprod Sci*; 21:271–281.

Carpenter EM, Hendrickson DA, Anderson DE. 2000, Aug. Laparoscopic ovariectomy and ovariohysterectomy in llamas and alpacas. *Vet Clin North Am Equine Pract*; 16(2):363–375, vii. doi:10.1016/s0749-0739(17)30111-6. PMID: 14983913.

Lin HC, Baird AN, Pugh DG, Anderson DE, Gaughan EM. 1997, Sep-Oct. Effects of carbon dioxide insufflation combined with changes in body position on blood gas and acid-base status in anesthetized llamas (Llama glama). *Vet Surg*; 26(5):444–450. doi: 10.1111/j.1532-950x.1997.tb01703.x. PMID: 9381667.

Sumar J, Bravo PW. 1991. In situ observation of the ovaries of llamas and alpacas by use of a laparoscopic technique. *J Am Vet Med Assoc*; 199(9):1159–1163.

45

Creation of Stoma into First Forestomach Compartment ("Rumenostomy")

David E. Anderson

Purpose or Indication for Procedure

This procedure is performed for repeated access to the C1 or when emergency decompression of severely distended C1 is needed. In severe cases, rumenostomy has been used to decompress C1 tympany associated with gastrointestinal disease prior to induction of anesthesia for laparotomy and when decompression via orogastric tube is not possible. Rumenostomy has also been used for hyperalimentation in chronically debilitated camelids and camelids having severe disease of the head and/or neck.

Equipment Needed

The following equipment is needed: clippers with #40 blades, preparation for aseptic surgery (povidone iodine scrub, alcohol rinse, gauze pads), surgery cap and mask, sterile drapes, sterile gloves, sterile gowns, suction apparatus, sterile saline or lactated Ringer's solution (LRS) rinse, soft tissue surgery instruments including #10 scalpel blade, tissue retractors, and suture materials.

Restraint/Position

C1 stoma can be done with the llama or alpaca standing, in sternal recumbency, or in lateral recumbency. This procedure is readily performed with the patient sedated and after infusion of local anesthesia (2% lidocaine HCl). Minimal to no sedation is advised in patients severely debilitated or with extreme tympany. Nasotracheal intubation may be performed to optimize breathing and protect the airways from regurgitation during the procedure.

Technical Description of Procedure/Method

Preparation

The hair should be clipped with #40 clipper blades and aseptically prepared for surgery. The clipped and prepared area should be four times the surface area of the operative site to provide wide margins for maintenance of a sterile field. In general, the preparation site should extend from the left costochondral arch dorsally to the dorsal midline and from the tenth rib to the tuber coxae (Figure 45.1). Aseptic preparation of the skin should be done using a standard 5-minute scrub technique to achieve aseptic surgical field.

Procedure

The incision for this procedure is centered in the lateral abdominal wall approximately 6- to 8-cm caudal to the last rib and 6- to 8-cm ventral

Veterinary Techniques in Llamas and Alpacas, Second Edition. Edited by David E. Anderson, Matt Miesner, and Meredyth Jones.

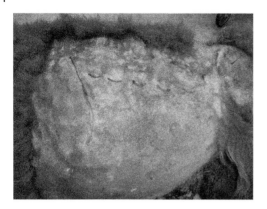

Figure 45.1 The left lateral abdominal wall is clipped for rumenostomy.

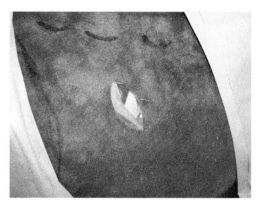

Figure 45.3 An incision is continued through the muscles of the lateral abdominal wall using Metzenbaum scissors by separating the muscle parallel to the direction of the muscle fibers.

to the transverse processes of the lumbar vertebrae. For temporary C1 stoma, a linear skin incision is made perpendicular to the spine. For permanent or long-term use C1 stomas, an elliptical skin incision is made approximately 3 cm in length and 2 cm in width (Figure 45.2). Larger stomas are possible, and permanent C1 cannulas may be placed in camelids (using commercially available cannulas designed for use in goats), but these are associated with greater morbidity and risk of death. The incision is continued through the muscles of the lateral abdominal wall using Metzenbaum scissors by separating the muscle parallel to the direction of the muscle (external abdominal oblique cranial-dorsal to caudal-ventral; internal abdominal oblique caudal-dorsal to

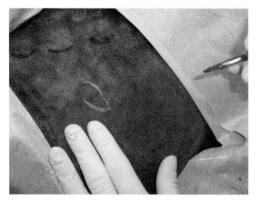

Figure 45.2 An elliptical skin incision is made approximately 3 cm in length and 2 cm in width.

cranial-ventral; transversus abdominus dorsal to ventral). (See Figure 45.3). The peritoneum is grasped using Brown-Adson forceps and penetrated using Metzenbaum scissors. The surgeon should take extreme care to avoid injury to the spleen. The spleen is freely movable (no encapsulation in C1) and lies deep to the left abdominal wall. The dorsal-lateral aspect of the C1 grasped using Allis tissue forceps or a penetrating towel clamp and exteriorized from the abdomen. Stay sutures (e.g., #0 PDS or PGA-910) are placed through the external abdominal oblique muscle and seromuscular layer of the C1 at 4 equidistant places along the circumference of the stoma site (e.g., using a clock-face template, these sutures would be placed at the 12, 3, 6, and 9 o'clock positions; Figures 45.4 and 45.5). These stay sutures help to protect the stoma suture from tension. The C1 stoma is made using simple continuous sutures placed through the skin and seromuscular layer of C1 (Figure 45.6). The simple continuous patterns are interrupted at 120-degree arcs around the circumference of the stoma (e.g., using a clock-face template, three segments of simple continuous suture would be done from 12 to 4 o'clock, 4 to 8 o'clock, and 8 to 12 o'clock). (See Figure 45.7.) Interruption of the simple continuous suture lines prevents formation of a purse string and allows better

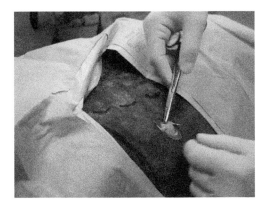

Figure 45.4 Stay sutures are placed through the seromuscular layers of the C1 and the muscular layers of the abdomen.

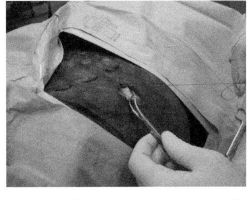

Figure 45.6 Simple continuous suture is placed in the skin and seromuscular layer of C1 to create an air- and water-tight seal.

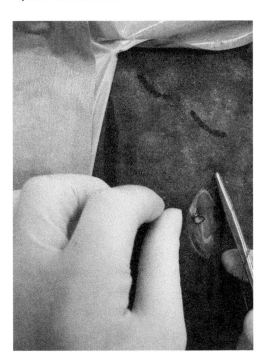

Figure 45.5 Stay sutures are placed at four quadrant intersection points around the circumference of the incision.

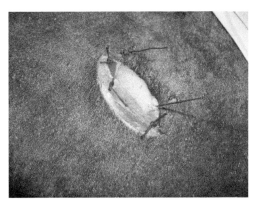

Figure 45.7 The simple continuous suture should establish an air- and water-tight seal so that the peritoneal cavity is protected and the wound is not contaminated.

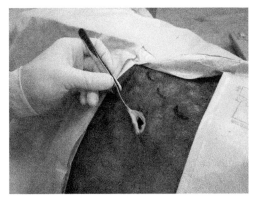

Figure 45.8 The C1 is opened by making a vertical incision in the midpoint of the surgery site being careful not to compromise the preplaced sutures.

control of the tension along the suture lines. Finally, a vertical incision is made into the lumen of C1 being careful not to compromise any of the prior placed sutures (Figure 45.8). These stomas are expected to heal closed within 4 to 6 weeks unless maintained open by use of indwelling cannulas. If the stoma does not heal closed, these stomas can be surgically reconstructed by en bloc resection of the stoma and careful reconstruction of each tissue layer. Surgical reconstruction is most easily done with the patient under general anesthesia. For permanent stomas, the C1 stoma can be made first and then the cut edge of the C1 sutured to the cut edge of the skin in such a way that these tissues heal together to form a permanent fistula from the skin to C1. These procedures require careful attention to detail to prevent contamination of the abdomen.

Practice Tip to Facilitate Procedure

The wall of severely distended C1 is thin and placement of seromuscular sutures difficult. In these cases, exteriorization of C1 and drainage through a small stoma may be required prior to any suture placement.

Potential Complications

The most significant risk with this procedure is septic peritonitis as a result of leakage of ingesta into the abdomen or migration of bacteria along suture tracts into the abdomen or incision site. Other complications include incision site infection or abscess formation, ulceration of C1 around stoma site, chronic leakage from the stoma, cosmetic blemish at the surgery site, chronic weight loss associated with C1 dysfunction, and death.

Patient Monitoring/Aftercare

Llamas and alpacas must be carefully monitored for evidence of peritonitis or interference with forestomach motility or function. Anti-inflammatory drugs, antibiotics, and supportive care are routinely done for 7 to 10 days after stoma formation.

Section IX

Musculoskeletal

46

Musculoskeletal Anatomy and Ambulation

David E. Anderson

Discussion Of Functional Anatomy

Foot Anatomy

Llamas and alpacas possess two digits or toes on each foot. Of the phalanges in the foot (P1, P2, and P3), P2 and P3 are most distal on the limb, are horizontal to the ground, and are both weight bearing. This is different from other livestock and horses in which only P1 contacts the ground via a hoof. The proximal phalanx, P1, is oriented at a 45-degree angle to the ground (Figure 46.1). The splayed digits contribute to stability and traction via the foot pad, which is thick and comparable to that of carnivores (Figure 46.2). The foot pad also can be referred to as the sole or slipper (Figure 46.3). In llamas and alpacas, the foot pad associated with each digit unites at the palmar/plantar aspect of the foot to form a common digital pad (Figure 46.4). At the tip of each digit is a small toenail that is non-weight bearing and is attached to P3 via the corium (Figure 46.5). The toenail may contribute to traction and locomotion. The foot is joined to the leg at the fetlock joint.

Ambulation

Llamas and alpacas have several gaits including the walk, pace, trot, and gallop. Juvenile camelids have an unusual hopping gait that may be

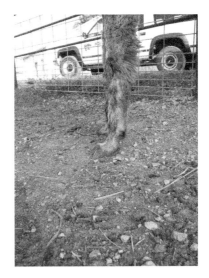

Figure 46.1 Alpacas stand on P2 and P3 with the proximal phalanx, P1, oriented at a 45-degree angle to the ground.

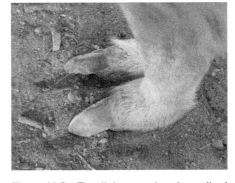

Figure 46.2 The digits are splayed contributing to stability and traction.

Veterinary Techniques in Llamas and Alpacas, Second Edition. Edited by David E. Anderson, Matt Miesner, and Meredyth Jones.

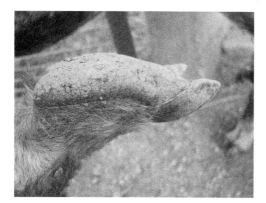

Figure 46.3   The foot pad, or slipper, covers the weightbearing surface. The toenail contributes to traction but not weight bearing.

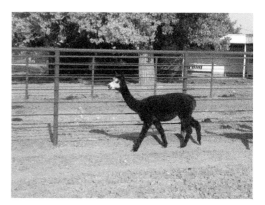

Figure 46.6   Some camelids walk with a pacing gait, but many walk with a diagonal gait.

and hind limbs) swinging in unison rather than a forelimb on one side swinging with the contralateral hind limb as is seen with the typical quadruped gaits (Figure 46.6).

Leg Conformation

Correct leg conformation is important for bone and joint health throughout the life of the animal. Abnormal angulation of the limbs detracts from balance and can cause degenerative joint disease with advancing weight and age. Llamas and alpacas should have straight limbs when viewed from the front or rear. In the front limb and viewed from the front, a straight line should bisect the shoulder, carpus, fetlock, and toes. In the rear limb as viewed from behind the animal, a straight line should bisect the hip, stifle, tarsus (hock), fetlock, and toes. The toes should point forward.

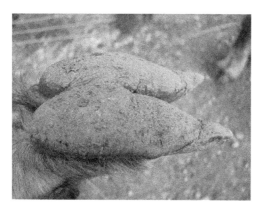

Figure 46.4   The foot pads of each digit are connected at the heel region of the foot.

Equipment Needed

Halter and lead rope, and non-adhesive bandage material are needed for this procedure.

Restraint/Position

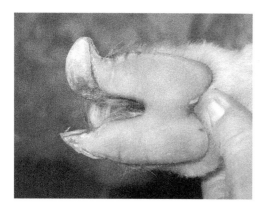

Figure 46.5   The non-weight-bearing toenail may overgrow causing distortion of the P3.

described as "prancing" or "pronging." Although not always present, the pacing gait can be recognized by both limbs on one side (ipsilateral fore

The animal may stand or may be restrained in a chute or with a halter with lead rope.

Technical Description of Procedure/Method

Conformation and structure should be done on a clean, level surface.

Practice Tip to Facilitate Procedure

Limb conformation can be difficult to assess in llamas and alpacas because of the long hair coverage of the limbs. Conformation is most easily assessed in alpacas immediately after shearing, but llamas infrequently have their legs sheared. In animals with long hair on the limbs, examination can be facilitated by wrapping the limbs firmly with non-adhesive, elastic bandages. Questions of long-bone alignment can be quantitatively assessed by obtaining radiographic images of the limbs (dorsal to caudal and lateral to medial views).

Potential Complications

A variety of congenital defects and conformational defects have been identified in llamas and alpacas. Failure to make sound breeding and genetic selections regarding these defects is likely to result in further expression of unwanted traits in musculoskeletal structures.

Patient Monitoring/Aftercare

Monitor feet including digital pads and toenails. Monitor conformation of breeding pairs and offspring to ascertain unwanted traits.

Recommended Reading

Clemente CJ, Dick TJM, Glen CL, Panagiotopoulou O. 2020 Mar 2. Biomechanical insights into the role of foot pads during locomotion in camelid species. *Sci Rep*; 10(1):3856. doi: 10.1038/s41598-020-60795-9. PMID: 32123239; PMCID: PMC7051995.

Fowler M. Llama medicine. Conformation and soundness. *Vet Clin North Am Food Anim Pract*. 1989 Mar; 5(1):21–26. https://doi.org/10.1016/s0749-0720(15)31000-8. PMID: 2647234.

Janis C, Theodor J, Boisvert B. 2002. Evolution of pacing locomotion in camelids. *J Vertebr Paleontol*; 22(1):110–121.

47

Regional Intravenous Drug Perfusion

Meredyth L. Jones

Purpose or Indication for Procedure

Regional intravenous (RIV) drug perfusion is used for injection of local anesthetics to provide total analgesia for surgical procedures of the distal limb and for the injection of concentration-dependent antimicrobials for management of septic conditions of the distal limb. Injections are typically made into the dorsal common digital vein, the lateral saphenous vein, or the cephalic vein.

Equipment Needed

The following equipment is needed: clippers with #40 blade, gauze, iodine or chlorhexidine preparatory solutions, isopropyl alcohol, exam gloves, tourniquet (or medical rubber tubing), 19- or 20-gauge × 3/4-inch (1.9-cm) butterfly catheter, and 4 units (U)/mL heparin flush solution. For prolonged catheter use, an 18- to 22-gauge × 1.5- to 2-inch (3.8- to 5.1-cm) over-the-needle catheter may be placed and maintained.

Restraint/Position

Lateral or sternal recumbency is preferred with sedation.

Technical Description of Procedure/Method

The choice of vein to be catheterized follows:

- Dorsal Common Digital Vein: The dorsal surface of the limb is clipped and prepared from the metacarpal/metatarsal region distally to the fetlock. A tourniquet is placed proximal or distal to the carpus (Figure 47.1), and a butterfly catheter is inserted just proximal to the fetlock into the dorsal common digital vein, which lies on midline (Figure 47.2). Alternatively, any visible or palpable vein distal to the tourniquet may be catheterized.
- Lateral Saphenous Vein: The lateral saphenous vein is catheterized proximal to the hock, on the lateral aspect of the tibia (Figure 47.3). The area is clipped and aseptically prepared, and a tourniquet is placed around the distal muscle belly of the gastrocnemius muscle, occluding the vein. A butterfly or over-the-needle catheter is used and is secured using adhesive tape.
- Cephalic Vein: The cephalic vein may be catheterized in camelids as in small animals through use of a tourniquet occluding the vein at the level of the elbow. The region over the antebrachium is clipped and aseptically prepared, and a butterfly catheter or over-the-needle catheter is placed (Figure 47.4). An extension set is attached, and the catheter is secured with adhesive tape.

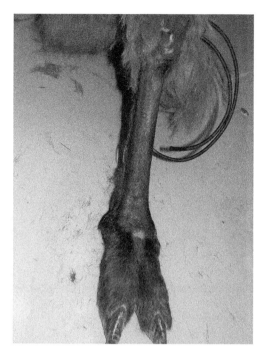

Figure 47.1 Preparation of the dorsal forelimb for RIV perfusion. A tourniquet has been placed proximal to the carpus, and the limb has been clipped and aseptically prepared.

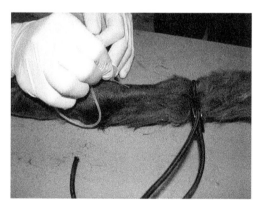

Figure 47.2 Placement of a butterfly catheter into the dorsal common digital vein. The vein lies on the midline, and the catheter is initially inserted at about a 30-degree angle. Any visible and accessible vein in this region may be used for perfusion.

For distal limb anesthesia, 5 mL of 2% lidocaine HCl may be administered through the catheter, which will be distributed and result in anesthesia of the limb distal to the tourniquet. This allows

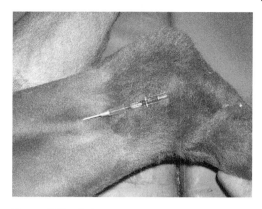

Figure 47.3 Catheterization of the lateral saphenous vein of a llama. A tourniquet is being used to occlude the vein at the level of the gastrocnemius muscle at the proximal tibia.

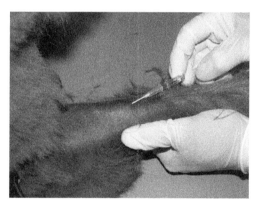

Figure 47.4 An over-the-needle catheter is placed into the cephalic vein.

for the performance of painful procedures of the soft tissues and bone. The tourniquet should not remain in place for longer than 1 hour.

For local perfusion of antimicrobials, the goal is to achieve high concentrations of antimicrobials locally to increase bactericidal activity. Aminoglycosides exhibit concentration-dependent bactericidal effect, meaning that they simply need to reach high concentrations to achieve lethal effect, and are commonly used for RIV perfusion in horses. Beta-lactam antimicrobials are time-dependent antimicrobials, meaning that their concentrations must remain above MIC for a prolonged period of time. There is some evidence, however, that concentration may play a role in the activity of beta lactams and, therefore, they are often selected for RIV perfusion. RIV perfusion may also result in prolonged, higher concentrations of drug in the tissues as compared to systemic administration. Ceftiofur sodium is the most commonly used of the beta-lactams for RIV because, unlike other ceftiofur preparations, it is safe to give IV. RIV dosing often differs by individual, but based on the literature in other species, the author has calculated that ceftiofur sodium is generally administered at approximately 1/2 to 1 times the systemic dose for cattle (RIV dose of 1 mg/kg), while gentamycin is administered at 1/3 (RIV/dose 2 mg/kg) and amikacin at 1/10 (RIV dose 2 mg/kg) the systemic doses for horses.

Practice Tip to Facilitate Procedure

Procedures should be expedited to minimize the time of tourniquet placement on the limb to 30 minutes to 1 hour. The tourniquet may be left in place longer, but it should be a tourniquet that distributes pressure over a wide area. It is not recommended to allow animal to walk with the tourniquet in place, because this may result in tendon damage. Tourniquet pressure should not exceed that required to achieve obstruction of venous outflow and minimize arterial inflow. This is estimated as systemic arterial pressure + 100 mm Hg. A towel or other padding may be placed between the limb and the tourniquet to distribute pressure over a larger surface area. Extremely high or focal pressure can cause significant damage to the nerves, vessels, or muscle at that site.

Potential Complications

Lidocaine toxicity can occur when the dosage of anesthetic exceeds tolerance limits. The safe dose of lidocaine for llamas and alpacas is not specifically known, but it is considered to be approximately 5 mg/kg of body weight. Thus, when using 2% lidocaine HCl (20 mg/mL), the total volume of lidocaine used for any procedure should not exceed 1 mL per 4 kg (9 pounds) or 11 mL per 45 kg (100 pounds) of body weight. Other complications may include hematoma formation, myopathy, and peripheral nerve damage from prolonged tourniquet placement.

Patient Monitoring/Aftercare

Animals should be monitored for complications at the injection site including hematoma or abscess formation. Ambulation should also be monitored closely for tendon or neurological complications of the procedure and for positive progress in their disease condition.

Recommended Reading

Butt TD, Bailey JV, Dowling PM, Fretz PB. 2001. Comparison of 2 techniques for regional antibiotic delivery to the equine forelimb: intraosseous perfusion vs. intravenous perfusion. Can Vet J; 42(8):617–622.

Navarre CB, Zhang L, Sunkara G, et al. 1999. Ceftiofur distribution in plasma and joint fluid following regional limb injection in cattle. J Vt Pharmacol Ther; 22:13–19.

Pille F, de Baere S, Ceelen L, et al. 2005. Synovial fluid and plasma concentrations of ceftiofur after regional intravenous perfusion in the horse. Vet Surg; 34:610–617.

Werner LA, Hardy J, Bertone AL. 2005. Bone gentamicin concentration after intra-articular injection or regional intravenous perfusion in the horse. Vet Surg; 32(6):559–565.

Section X

Urinary System

48

Urinary Tract Examination and Anatomy

Meredyth L. Jones

Anatomic Review

The kidneys of camelids are nonlobulated, with the right kidney more cranially located and typically found ventral to the transverse processes of the fourth to sixth lumbar vertebra. The ureter and urinary bladder are structurally similar to those of other species. The urethra of male camelids is long and sigmoid in shape, with a urethral diverticulum present at the level of the ischial arch, preventing retrograde catheterization of the urinary bladder. The glans penis has a cartilaginous corkscrew appendage, and the external urethral orifice lies beneath this structure (Figure 48.1). The prepuce of camelid males is directed caudally at rest, and males urinate caudally, between the back legs (Figure 48.2). The urethra in females lies at the junction of the vagina and vestibule (Figure 48.3a and 48.3b), where a suburethral diverticulum is present and must be bypassed to catheterize the dorsally located external urethral orifice.

Urinary Tract Evaluation

Animals with urinary tract disease may present with an owner complaint of gastrointestinal or reproductive tract disease (e.g., straining, abdominal distension), making early, accurate interpretation of these signs at the time of initial examination imperative to providing adequate treatment. A thorough health and husbandry history is useful in the management of all cases presented for veterinary care. For animals with signs referable to the urinary tract, owners should be questioned regarding dietary history, duration and progression of clinical signs, treatments administered, response to therapy, and the quality of the last observed urination. For females, pregnancy status, parturition history, and history of dystocia may provide diagnostic direction.

Evaluation should begin with a thorough, systematic physical examination, with the presence of signs of systemic illness, including apparent depression, dehydration, fever, abdominal distension, and first-compartment hypomotility noted and used to localize urinary tract disease. It is common for camelids to delay urination during transport and examination, but the animal should be observed for urination behaviors, with classification of these as normal micturition, dysuria, pollakiuria, or polyuria as well as observation for urine scalding.

Abdominal viscera are not readily palpable in camelids, but ballottement and succussion can provide characterization of the abdominal contents. In males, the urethra can be indirectly observed as it exits the pelvis and traces the body wall to the external urethral orifice. Nonproductive pulsations and generalized or

Veterinary Techniques in Llamas and Alpacas, Second Edition. Edited by David E. Anderson, Matt Miesner, and Meredyth Jones.

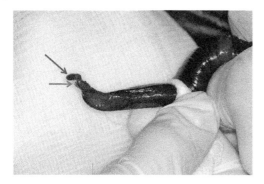

Figure 48.1 The exteriorized penis of a mature alpaca. The cartilaginous corkscrew appendage (*red arrow*) overlies the external urethral orifice (*blue arrow*).

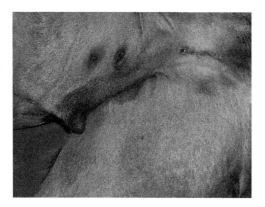

Figure 48.2 The normal prepucial conformation of an alpaca.

focal swellings along this length are suggestive of obstruction, urethral rupture, hematoma, or abscess formation. The vulvar and preputial hairs should be examined for the presence of grit, blood, purulent matter, or urine.

The penis should be exteriorized and the prepuce and free portion of the penis examined. The penis is adhered to the prepuce in prepubertal males, making exteriorization of the penis for examination or catheterization difficult. This can be rarely accomplished in nonsedated animals, usually requiring at least some sedation with or without lumbosacral epidural anesthesia. The use of xylazine should be avoided in animals with potential obstruction due to its diuretic effects.

Urinalysis should be performed in any animal with suspected urinary tract disease or any other systemic disease for which the disease or treatment may impact urinary health (Table 48.1). Free catch urine may be obtained spontaneously during housing or physical examination. Animals that do not voluntarily provide a urine sample and have a patent urinary tract may be catheterized (females) or have cystocentesis performed.

Values for fractional excretion and electrolytes in urine in llamas fed hay-based diets have been published (Lackey et al. 1995).

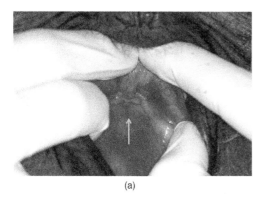

(a)

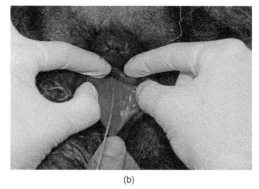

(b)

Figure 48.3a and 48.3b Location of the external urethral orifice in a female alpaca (**3a**). A polypropylene catheter is placed into the urethra (**3b**).

Table 48.1   Urinalysis reference ranges for llamas at sea level (Adapted from Fowler 1998).

Color	Clear, light yellow-amber	
Specific Gravity	1.013–1.048 (mean 1.023)	
pH	7–8.5	
Protein	Negative	Some 1 +
Glucose	Negative	Some 1–3 +
Ketones	Negative	Some 1 +
Urobilinogen	Negative	Some 2–3 +
Bilirubin	Negative	
Blood	Negative	
Sediments	Calcium Oxalate common Uric Acid rare	

Based on results of historical, physical examination and urinalysis findings, complete blood count with fibrinogen determination, serum biochemistry, ultrasound exam, abdominocentesis, excretory urogram, urinary endoscopy, or renal biopsy may be indicated to guide case management.

Recommended Reading

Anderson DE, Constable PD, Yvorchuk KE, et al. 1994. Hyperlipidemia and ketonuria in an alpaca and a llama. *J Vet Intern Med*; 8(3):207–211.

Cardwell JM, Thorne MH. 1999. Hydronephrosis and ureteral duplication in a young alpaca. *Vet Red*; 145(4):104–107.

Dart AJ, Dart CM, Hodgson DR. 1997. Surgical management of a ruptured urinary bladder secondary to a urethral obstruction in an alpaca. *Aust Vet J*; 75(11):793–795.

DeWitt SF, Bedenice D, Mazan MR. 2004. Hemolysis and Heinz body formation associated with ingestion of red maple leaves in two alpacas. *J Am Vet Med Assoc*; 225(4):578–583.

Fowler ME. 1998. *Medicine and Surgery of South American Camelids*, 2nd Edition. Ames:Blackwell.

Gerros TC. 1998. Recognizing and treating urolithiasis in llamas. *Vet Med*; 93(6):583–590.

Gerspach C, Hull BL, Rings DM, et al. 2008. Hematuria and transitional cell papilloma of the renal pelvis treated via unilateral nephrectomy in an alpaca. *J Am Vet Med Assoc*; 232(8):1206–1209.

Kingston JK, Staempfli HR. 1995. Silica urolithiasis in a male llama. *Can Vet J*; 181:1411.

Lackey MN, Belknap EB, Salman MD, et al. 1995. Urinary indices in llamas fed different diets. *Am J Vet Res*; 56(7):859–865.

McClanahan SL, Malone ED, Anderson KL. 2005. Bladder outlet obstruction in a 6-month-old alpaca secondary to pelvic displacement of the urinary bladder. *Can Vet J*; 46:247–249.

McLaughlin BG, Evans NC. 1989. Urethral obstruction in a male llama. *J Am Vet Med Assoc*; 195(11):1601–1602.

Peauroi JR, Mohr FC, Fisher DJ, et al. 1995. Anemia, hematuria, and multicentric urinary neoplasia in a llama (Lama glama) exposed to bracken fern. *J Zoo Wildl Med*; 26(2):315–320.

Poulson KP, Gerard MP, Spaulding KA, et al. 2006. Bilateral renal agenesis in an alpaca cria. *Can Vet J*; 47(2):159–161.

49

Urethral Catheterization
Meredyth L. Jones

Purpose or Indication for Procedure

This procedure is used for collecting a urine sample for urinalysis or microbial culture, emptying the urinary bladder, treating urinary blockage, providing urinary drainage in animals with neurologic disease, performing urinary bladder lavage, quantifying urine output, providing access to the urinary bladder for diagnostic tests, and performing radiographic studies.

Equipment Needed

The following equipment is needed: iodine or chlorhexidine preparation scrub, sterile or exam gloves, water-soluble lubricant, 3.5 to 8 French polypropylene catheter, sterile collection syringe, sterile collection containers (red top evacuated tube or specimen cup), ± sedation.

Restraint/Position

Females may be catheterized while standing or in sternal recumbency in a chute. Males are placed in lateral recumbency and restrained using sedation. NOTE: The urinary bladder of males cannot be catheterized using standard procedures because of the urethral recess at the level of the ischial arch. Special catheters (e.g., curved cardiac vascular catheters) are often required to bypass this structure.

Technical Description of Procedure/Method

In females, the vulva should be cleansed thoroughly after wrapping the tail. The external urethral orifice is visualized or palpated on the vaginal floor (Figure 49.1). A catheter is directed into the dorsal shelf of the urethral orifice to avoid placement in the suburethral diverticulum (Figure 49.2). If the catheter does not advance, the catheter is most likely contained within the suburethral diverticulum and should be redirected. The catheter is then advanced until urine flows. If urine does not flow easily, a syringe should be attached and light suction applied to determine if the catheter is positioned within the bladder. Urine samples are collected by aspiration (Figure 49.3) and placed in the appropriate sampling containers. The syringe may be used to suction, reinject the urine, and repeat these steps several times to create turbulence in the bladder. This method may increase the value of cytological examination by causing sediment to become intermixed with urine.

In males, the prepuce should be cleansed, and the penis exteriorized, which can be difficult,

Veterinary Techniques in Llamas and Alpacas, Second Edition. Edited by David E. Anderson, Matt Miesner, and Meredyth Jones.

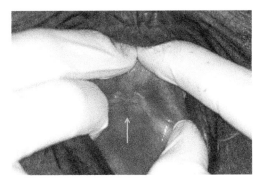

Figure 49.1 Urethral diverticulum and external urethral orifice location in female camelids. The external urethral orifice is located at the dorsum of this orifice.

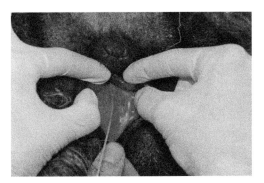

Figure 49.2 An 8Fr polypropylene catheter passed retrograde into the external urethral orifice.

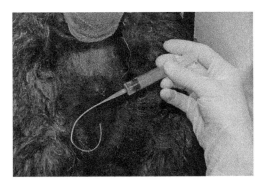

Figure 49.3 As the catheter is passed into the urinary bladder, urine will spontaneously flow and can be aspirated for sampling.

particularly in juveniles. In prepubertal males, adhesions are present between the penis and the prepuce. Sedation is highly recommended. An assistant should be available to grasp the penis with gauze, which has been unfolded and made linear. The penis and prepuce are manipulated

and the penis extended beyond the prepuce (Figure 49.4). The glans penis is grasped with the gauze. (See Figure 49.5). Camelids have a corkscrew cartilaginous process extending from the glans. The urethral orifice is located below the cartilaginous appendage at the end of the penis. (See Figure 49.6). Unlike sheep and goats, this

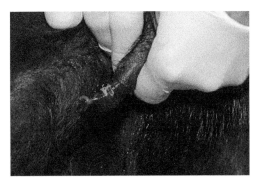

Figure 49.4 Manipulation of the penis and prepuce to exteriorize the glans penis in a mature alpaca.

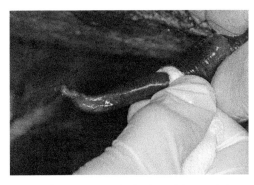

Figure 49.5 Full exteriorization of the penis in a mature alpaca. A 4 × 4 gauze sponge has been unfolded and made linear to encircle the penis for a secure grip.

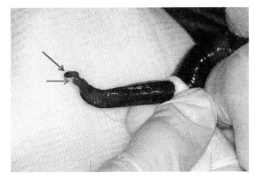

Figure 49.6 The corkscrew cartilaginous process (*red arrow*) and the external urethral orifice (*blue arrow*).

cartilaginous appendage is not a continuation of the urethra. A 3.5 French catheter may then be passed into the urethra. (See Figure 49.7). The distal urethral orifice can be quite small and it can be helpful to use a soft guide wire (as for intravenous catheters) to facilitate catheterization. (See Figure 49.8).

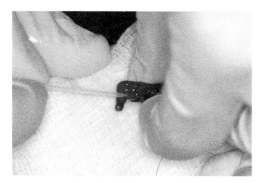

Figure 49.7 A 3.5Fr polypropylene catheter being placed retrograde into the urethra.

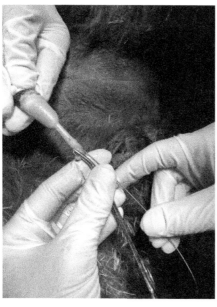

Figure 49.8 An intravenous catheter guide wire being used to facilitate urethral catheterization.

The urinary bladder is rarely successfully catheterized due to the presence of a urethral diverticulum at the level of the ischial arch. This diverticulum readily accepts a catheter, diverting it away from the urinary bladder.

> **Practice Tip to Facilitate Procedure**
>
> Lumbosacral epidural anesthesia, sedation, or short-term general anesthesia can be useful in aiding in the exteriorization of the penis. The technique for lumbosacral epidural anesthesia is covered elsewhere in this text. These should be used with caution depending on the disease condition of concern.

Potential Complications

Potential complications include urinary tract trauma, ascending infection, hemorrhage, and irritation leading to dysuria. Catheterized samples may contain increased red blood cells (RBC), protein, epithelial cells, and contamination from the genital tract and urethra.

Patient Monitoring/Aftercare

Animals should be monitored after catheterization for signs of dysuria or hematuria. Animals with indwelling urinary catheters should be monitored for regular urine production and flow, hematuria, and evidence of cystitis.

Urinalysis should be conducted within 20 minutes after urine collection or may be kept in a sealed container and refrigerated for up to 2 days (Table 49.1).

Values for fractional excretion and electrolytes in urine in llamas fed hay-based diets have been published (Lackey et al. 1995).

Table 49.1 Urinalysis reference ranges for llamas at sea level (Adapted from Fowler 1998).

Color	Clear, light yellow-amber	
Specific Gravity	1.013–1.048 (mean 1.023)	
pH	7–8.5	
Protein	Negative	Some 1+
Glucose	Negative	Some 1–3+
Ketones	Negative	Some 1+
Urobilinogen	Negative	Some 2–3+
Bilirubin	Negative	
Blood	Negative	
Sediments	Calcium Oxalate common Uric Acid rare	

Recommended Reading

Fowler ME. 1998. *Medicine and Surgery of South American Camelids*, 2nd Edition. Ames: Blackwell.

Kingston JL, Staempfli HR. 1995. Silica urolithiasis in a male llama. *Can Vet J*; 36(12):767–768.

Lackey MN, Belknap EB, Salman MD, et al. 1995. Urinary indices in llamas fed different diets. *Am J Vet Res*; 56(7):859–865.

McLaughlin BG, Evans NC. 1989. Urethral obstruction in a male llama. *J Am Vet Med Assoc*; 195(11):1601–1602.

50

Ultrasound of the Urinary System
Matt D. Miesner

Purpose or Indication for Procedure

Stranguria is a common presenting complaint with camelids. Ultrasound, performed percutaneously and transrectally, is a noninvasive and effective way to evaluate potential problems associated with the urinary system. We can use ultrasound to better classify cases of dysuria, trauma, obstruction, and infection. A very complete study can easily be performed due to patient size and anatomical locations of the structures of the urinary system.

Equipment Needed

Ultrasound machine and 3.5- to 7.5-MHz sector and linear probes, clippers, isopropyl alcohol, ultrasound gel, and reproductive lubricant are needed.

Clippers

It is not absolutely necessary to clip the hair from the patient. By parting the hair and applying isopropyl alcohol over the areas of interest, sufficient imaging can be provided. More detailed images will be achieved by clipping the hair. The natural relatively hairless regions of the groin and caudoventral abdomen provide excellent transabdominal ultrasound windows.

Ultrasound Probes

Most structures of the urinary system can be imaged effectively with a 5- to 7.5-MHz linear probe both transrectal and transabdominal. For rectal ultrasound, first infuse the rectum with lubricant for better imaging. For better resolution and deeper focal depth with transabdominal methods, a 3.5-MHz curvilinear probe is suggested.

Restraint/Position

Standing or cushed (sternal) positions are used. It is easiest to evaluate the urinary bladder, ureters, and kidneys with the animal standing when viewing transabdominally. Camelids often object to touching the abdomen and will preferentially cush into sternal position. A camelid restraint chute with suspended support straps may be helpful to keep the patient standing or suspended for imaging, but the straps can obstruct image windows. Additional imaging of the urinary bladder and pelvic urethra will need to be done transrectal.

Technical Description of Procedure/Method

Both kidneys may be imaged through the respective paralumbar fossa., Neonates and juveniles may be imaged through the caudal-ventral abdomen with the probe directed dorsally. The kidneys are located in close association with the dorsal midline of the abdomen, the left kidney being positioned slightly caudal to the right kidney. The author prefers to begin by performing ultrasound on the right kidney through the right paralumbar fossa about the level of the fifth to seventh lumbar transverse processes. (See Figures 50.1 and 50.2.) Camelid kidneys are not lobulated, but an otherwise smooth capsule

incorporates the renal pelvis, medulla, and cortical parenchyma. (See Figure 50.2.) The capsule may appear hyperechoic normally but should not be surrounded by fluid or gas. Normally, the renal pelvis can appear somewhat hyperechoic, and sometimes clear anechoic saccules radiate from the renal pelvis into the medulla. By placing the probe ventral to the left lumbar transverse processes, the left kidney can be imaged. It will be more caudal than the right kidney. (See Figure 50.3.) The spleen will be seen cranial to the left kidney. (See Figure 50.4.) Estimate or measure the size of the kidneys. Both are of equal size ranging from about 5 to 7 cm. Note any changes consistent with obstruction (hydronephrosis), toxicity (echogenic disparity or cortical fluid),

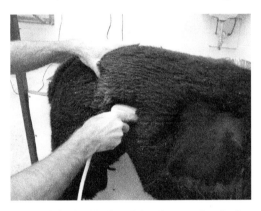

Figure 50.1 Positioning of the ultrasound probe for imaging the right kidney. The clinician's left thumb is at the level of the tuber coxae, and the probe is ventral to the transverse processes of the lumbar vertebrae.

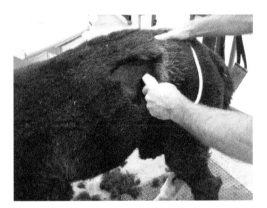

Figure 50.3 Approximate probe positioning for imaging the left kidney is more caudal than the right. By positioning the probe face cranial to the left kidney, the spleen can be located.

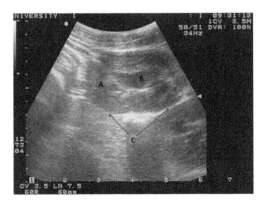

Figure 50.2 Image of the right kidney showing the smooth capsular appearance (**C**), the renal cortical parenchyma (**A**), and pelvis (**B**).

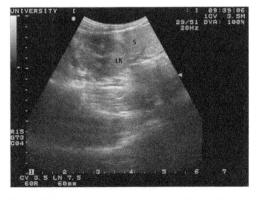

Figure 50.4 An ultrasound image of the left kidney (**LK**), showing the close approximation to the spleen (**S**). Splenic vasculature can be seen coursing through the parenchyma.

infection (fluid density), nephroliths, or neoplasia. Normal ureters are difficult to image, but pathology can usually be recognized (Cardwell and Thorne 1999).

Place the probe in the caudoventral flank and direct it caudodorsally to the pelvis, to allow visualization of the urinary bladder. If the bladder is empty, it will likely not be visualized. Severe distention is easily recognized in cases of urethral obstruction as might be seen with urolithiasis. (See Figure 50.5.) The normal bladder should not be more than 6 to 8 cm in diameter in the adult camelid or appear very tense. Hyperechoic irregularities may be seen suspended in the bladder lumen of normal patients and are not pathognomonic of uroliths or mucosal debris. However, with overdistention and a compatible history of urethral obstruction or cystitis, these refractile bodies may be pathologic.

Rectal ultrasound provides detailed images of the bladder wall, trigone, pelvic urethra, and accessory sex glands in males (Figure 50.6). A form of prostatic hyperplasia and prostatic cysts causing stranguria has been noted by this author in young males, and the occurrence has

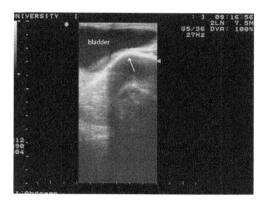

Figure 50.6 An ultrasound image of a normal urinary bladder as seen per the rectum at the level of the pubic eminence (*arrow*).

been briefly mentioned by others (Figure 50.7) (Tibary and Vaughan 2006). Another problem seen in camelids is a form of idiopathic polypoid cystitis (Figure 50.8). To date, biopsy of these lesions has only reported chronic inflammation without specific causes. Some cases resolve with medical management, where others require surgery (Anderson et al. 2010). Bladder wall masses may involve both the serosal and mucosal surfaces and vary in size and

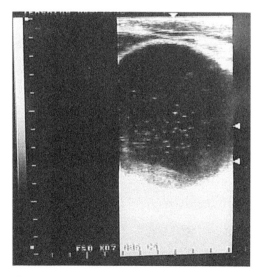

Figure 50.5 Transabdominal ultrasound image showing an overdistended urinary bladder. The measurement scale to the left is in centimeters. Note the refractile bodies within the lumen.

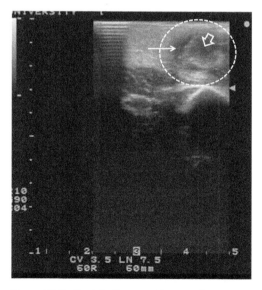

Figure 50.7 Rectal ultrasound image of an enlarged prostate gland (*dashed line*) in a young male alpaca, showing fluid within the parenchyma of the gland (*block arrow*) and well as periglandular fluid (*solid arrow*).

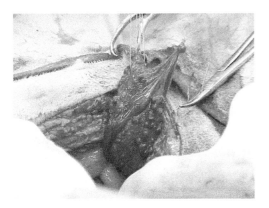

Figure 50.8 Intraoperative photo of a urinary bladder with idiopathic polypoid cystitis.

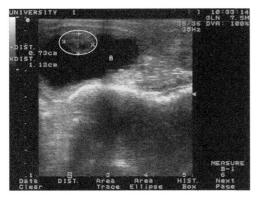

Figure 50.9 Rectal ultrasound image of a large mucosal polyp (*solid circle line*) protruding from the dorsal wall. The bladder lumen toward the trigone is labeled (**B**).

number (Figure 50.9). Although neoplasia from suspected bracken fern toxicosis has been reported in a llama, lesions were isolated to the kidneys and ureters. Gross bladder lesions were not evident as would be expected in cattle (Peauroi et al. 1995).

Practice Tip to Facilitate Procedure

The right and left kidneys are located immediately ventral and medial to the transverse processes on the respective sides of the abdomen. The left kidney is located caudal to the dorsal sac of the first forestomach compartment and caudal and medial to the hilus of the spleen. Transrectal examination of the kidneys

---

provides superior image clarity, but this procedure must be performed cautiously so as not to tear the rectum during manipulation of the ultrasound probe.

Potential Complications

Use caution when utilizing the linear probe per rectum. Image quality is improved by first infusing lubricant into the rectum with a syringe.

Patient Monitoring/ Aftercare

Patient monitoring and aftercare are not necessary assuming no injuries occurred during the procedure.

Recommended Reading

Anderson DE, Schulz KM., Rousseau M. 2010. Laparoscopic cystotomy for removal of a large bladder polyp in a juvenile alpaca with polypoid cystitis. *Vet Surg*; 39(6):661–783.

Cardwell JM, Thorne MH. 1999. Hydronephrosis and ureteral duplication in a young alpaca. *Vet Rec*; 245(4):104–107.

Eibl C, Franz S. 2021. Ultrasonography of kidney and spleen in clinically healthy llamas and alpacas. *Act Vet Scand*; 63(1):49.

Gerspach C, Bateman S, Sherding R, et al. 2010. Acute renal failure and anuria associated with vitamin D intoxication in two alpaca (Vicugna pacos) cria. *J Vet Intern Med*; 24(2):443–449.

Gerspach C, Hull BL, Rings DM, et al. 2008. Hematuria and transitional cell papilloma of the renal pelvis treated via unilateral nephrectomy in an alpaca. *J Am Vet Med Assoc*; 232(8):1206–1209.

Hardefeldt LY, Textor JA, Dart AJ. 2007. Renal agenesis in an alpaca cria. *Aust Vet J*; 85(5):185–187.

Kingston JK, Stäempfli HR. 1995. Silica urolithiasis in a male llama. *Can Vet J*; 36(12):767–768.

McClanahan SL, Malone ED, Anderson KL. 2005. Bladder outlet obstruction in a 6-month-old alpaca secondary to pelvic displacement of the urinary bladder. *Can Vet J*; 46(3):247–249.

Patel JH, Kosheluk C, Nation PN. 2004. Renal teratoma in a llama. *Can Vet J*; 45(11):938–940.

Peauroi JR, Mohr CF, Fisher DJ, et al. 1995. Anemia, hematuria, and multicentric urinary neoplasia in a Llama (Lama glama) exposed to bracken fern. *J Zoo and Wildlife Med*; 26(2):315–320.

Raffaele M, Parry NMA, Gruntman. 2010. Urinary bladder agenesis in an alpaca (Vicugna pacos) cria. *J Vet Diagn Invest*; 22(3):473–475.

Tibary A, Vaughan J. 2006. Reproductive physiology and infertility in male South American Camelids: a review and clinical observations. *Sm Rum Res*; 61:283–298.

51

Cystocentesis

Meredyth L. Jones

Purpose or Indication for Procedure

The cystocentesis procedure provides a sterile urine sample suitable for urinalysis, bacterial culture and sensitivity, and may be used to reduce pressure in an overdistended urinary bladder prior to surgery.

Equipment Needed

The following equipment is needed: clippers, gauze, iodine or chlorhexidine preparation solution, isopropyl alcohol, 18- or 20-gauge × 2- to 5-inch (5.1- to 12.7-cm) needle with or without stylet, 10–20-mL syringe, sterile vial, and ± ultrasound and probe.

Restraint/Position

Standing or lateral recumbency may be used.

Technical Description of Procedure/Method

The lower right abdomen is clipped, and the caudal abdomen is scanned with an ultrasound probe. (See Figure 51.1.) In camelids with significant distension of the urinary bladder, transabdominal palpation may be successful in some animals. Palpation of the urinary bladder in camelids is more difficult than in sheep, goats, or small animals. With ultrasound imaging, the target site for cystocentesis is the location where the urinary bladder lies immediately adjacent to the body wall, absent of other viscera (Figure 51.2). After the urinary bladder is located, the selected site of insertion is aseptically prepared. The operator's hand (with or without ultrasound guidance) is used to stabilize the bladder, and the needle is thrust into the bladder lumen through the body wall (Figure 51.3). It is ideal to enter the urinary bladder at a 45-degree angle to better allow for sealing of the bladder after puncture, but this can be difficult to achieve with body wall motion and position. The syringe is connected to the needle and most or all of the urine is removed from the urinary bladder, to reduce urine leakage from the pressure of the remaining urine. Negative pressure on the syringe and needle apparatus should be released before the needle is withdrawn.

Practice Tip to Facilitate Procedure

If a large volume of urine is to be removed, thus necessitating prolonged needle placement, it is recommended that an extension set be used between the

(Continued)

Veterinary Techniques in Llamas and Alpacas, Second Edition. Edited by David E. Anderson, Matt Miesner, and Meredyth Jones.
© 2023 John Wiley & Sons, Inc. Published 2023 by John Wiley & Sons, Inc.

(Continued)

needle and syringe to allow for repeated aspiration. Additionally, an over-the-needle intravenous catheter may be used and the stylet removed to reduce trauma to the urinary bladder wall.

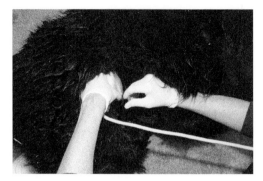

Figure 51.3 Use of an 18-gauge spinal needle, with concurrent ultrasound guidance, to perform cystocentesis.

Values for fractional excretion and electrolytes in urine in llamas fed hay-based diets have been published (Lackey et al. 1995).

Potential Complications

Risks include urinary bladder laceration, rupture, laceration of bowel with subsequent peritonitis. In general, cystocentesis is discouraged in camelids. The urinary bladder is intra-pelvic in location unless distended, and thus, risk of bowel perforation is higher. Ultrasound-guided cystocentesis is always preferred. In cases of urinary outflow obstruction, bladder pressure is sufficient to cause persistent leakage after cystocentesis in some camelids. Thus, this procedure is not suited for transient alleviation of bladder distension unless surgery or other means of clearing the urinary obstruction are performed soon afterward.

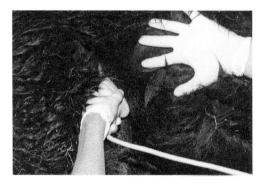

Figure 51.1 Transabdominal ultrasound imaging of the caudal abdomen of a male alpaca.

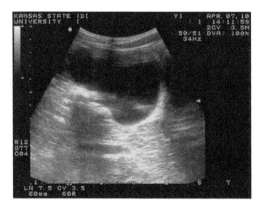

Figure 51.2 Transabdominal ultrasound image of the urinary bladder in an alpaca. The ideal site for needle insertion is the curvature of the urinary bladder as it contacts the body wall.

Patient Monitoring/ Aftercare

The patient should be monitored for normal urination and the development of uroperitoneum. Caution should be exercised for patients with bacterial cystitis or other urinary bladder wall compromise because of increased risk of urine leakage and septic peritonitis.

If xylazine is used alone or in combination to facilitate this procedure, glucosuria should be expected and must be considered when interpreting results.

Urinalysis should be performed within 20 minutes of sample collection or refrigerated/shipped on ice for laboratory testing within 2 days. Reference information for urinalysis can be found in Table 51.1.

Table 51.1   Urinalysis reference ranges for llamas at sea level (adapted from Fowler 1998).

Color	Clear, light yellow-amber	
Specific gravity	1.013–1.048 (mean 1.023)	
pH	7–8.5	
Protein	Negative	Some 1+
Glucose	Negative	Some 1–3+
Ketones	Negative	Some 1+
Urobilinogen	Negative	Some 2–3+
Bilirubin	Negative	
Blood	Negative	
Sediments	Calcium oxalate common uric acid rare	

Recommended Reading

Fowler ME 1998. *Medicine and Surgery of South American Camelids*, 2nd edition. Ames: Blackwell.

Lackey MN, Belknap EB, Salman MD, et al. 1995. Urinary indices in llamas fed different diets. *Am J Vet Res*; 56(7):859–865.

McLaughlin BG, Evans NC 1989. Urethral obstruction in a male llama. *J Am Vet Med Assoc*; 195(11):1601–1602.

Section XI

Female Genital Anatomy

52

Comments Regarding Female Genital Anatomy

David E. Anderson

Llamas and alpacas are expected to live for 15 to 25 years. Females (also known as hembras) reach sexual maturity at around 24 months of age. Sexually mature females are non-seasonal, polyestrous breeders when ample nutrition resources are available. They are receptive to the male all year round with appropriate nutrition and a favorable environment. The average gestation length is 335 to 353 days, and females give birth to their offspring (crias) most often during the morning and early afternoon.

External genitalia of female camelids include the vulva and clitoris. Internal genitalia include the vestibule, cervix, a bicornuate uterus, oviduct, fimbria, and ovaries. The vestibule is approximately 15 to 18 cm long in alpacas and 20 to 25 cm long in llamas. The cervix is composed of fibrocartilage arranged with a spiral ridge that makes three revolutions along the length of the cervix. These are often referred to as cervical "rings." The uterine body is short, and the uterine horns terminate in the oviductal papillae. The oviductal papilla is a muscular mound of tissue composed partly of circular smooth muscle. The muscular papilla prevents retrograde flow of fluids from the uterus into the oviducts. The oviduct is firm and convoluted and terminates in the fimbria, which envelops the ovary. Follicles ovulate on the surface of the ovary.

Alpacas and llamas are induced ovulators, and the female needs to be bred by the male to stimulate the LH surge in the female and cause the follicle to ovulate (Figure 52.1). If the female accepts the male and breeding takes place, then ovulation may occur within 24–48 hours after copulation. Ovulation is expected to occur in approximately 80% of pasture-mated females and 90% of hand-mated females when the animals are bred in the presence of a mature follicle (mature follicles are defined as > 6-mm diameter). After ovulation, the follicle luteinizes to form a corpus luteum (CL). Progesterone concentration increases within 3 to 4 days after copulation, increases rapidly for 6 to 7 days after mating, and peaks 8 to 10 days after copulation. If the female fails to conceive, then the CL will regress after day 10 to 12 post-mating, and the progesterone levels will decline back to base line (<0.2 ng/mL).

During copulation the stud will "orgle." Orgling is a low, humming sound with an occasional grunt. Once the stud has adequately positioned himself, he will then begin to insert his penis and thrust. These thrusts are named "ejaculating thrusts" or "pelvic thrusts." The penis will physically penetrate all the way through the hembra's cervix; llamas and alpacas are intra-uterine ejaculators. Semen is deposited in both the left and right uterine horns. The semen is viscous and needs to liquefy prior to entering the oviducts. Within 6 hours of deposition, semen can be found near the utero-tubal junction. These cells can

Veterinary Techniques in Llamas and Alpacas, Second Edition. Edited by David E. Anderson, Matt Miesner, and Meredyth Jones.

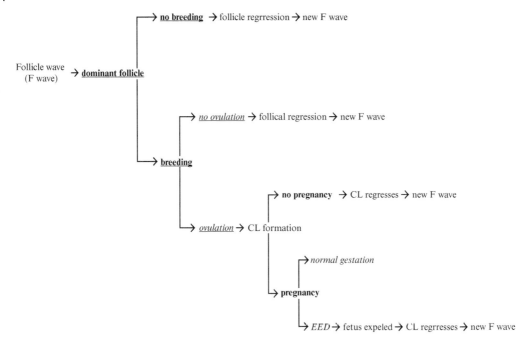

Figure 52.1 Diagram illustrating the various possible sequences of follicle development in alpacas and llamas. Alpacas and llamas are induced ovulators. As such, the follicle should not ovulate without copulation. When no breeding occurs, the mature follicle will regress. With breeding, the follicle will either fail to ovulate or ovulate. If the follicle fails to ovulate, it should regress. If the follicle ovulates, it will be maintained for approximately 10 to 12 days if no pregnancy occurs, or it will persist throughout pregnancy (10 to 11.5 months' gestation).

remain in the oviduct for up to 30 hours to fertilize an ovum. It is believed that the act of orgling, mounting, and positioning of the stud on the female's back act as auditory and neurohormonal stimuli for ovulation. These neurohormonal stimuli initiate a cascade of events that culminate in the ovulation of a follicle. Copulation is expected to occur over a 15- to 20-minute period but can range from 10 to 60 minutes.

In llamas and alpacas, embryos predominantly implant in the endometrium of the left uterine horn (llamas establish approximately 90% left horn pregnancies and 10% right horn pregnancies; alpacas may have slightly increased prevalence of right horn pregnancies). These pregnancies occur from ovulations from either the left or right ovary. Embryotaxis to the left horn occurs for unknown reasons. Placental development in llamas and alpacas occurs with diffuse epitheliochorial placentation. Pregnancy is CL dependent throughout gestation.

Congenital defects are relatively common among camelids. Congenital refers to a trait with which the animal is born (existing at the time of birth). These defects are not necessarily genetically programmed and may have resulted from problems encountered during organogenesis or fetal development *in utero*. Heritable defects are genetically programmed in that animal and can be passed on from the affected animal. A common misconception is that a trait may not be heritable because the dam or sire has produced multiple progeny that were normal. Heritable defects are complex and usually do not result in a high frequency of abnormal neonates. These defects may be passed on to progeny and may surface generations distant from the affected dam or sire. The most common body systems to be affected by congenital defects are the reproductive, musculoskeletal, and cardiovascular.

The most common congenital defects affecting the reproductive tract are segmental aplasia, cryptorchidism, and pseudohermaphroditism. Affected camelids should be removed from the breeding pool by neutering. Segmental aplasia has been seen in many forms including uterus unicornous, cervix aplasia, aplasia of the uterine body, aplasia of the oviduct, and ovarian hypoplasia. Little information is available regarding heritability from the dam or sire, but the breeding combination should not be repeated. Cryptorchidism is uncommon in camelids, and few cases have been reported. Based on breeding studies from other livestock species, cryptorchidism should be considered heritable and affected males gelded. The mode of inheritance is unknown, but the breeding combination should not be repeated. Pseudohermaphroditism also is uncommon. Most affected camelids have female external genitalia but with an enlarged clitoris. Histopathology of the ovaries reveals the presence of ovotestis.

53

Pregnancy Diagnosis
David E. Anderson

Purpose or Indication for Procedure

Pregnancy diagnosis is done most often to determine the results of scheduled matings. However, pregnancy diagnosis also is done to evaluate females that have been exposed to a breeding male, females that have been unintentionally bred, and females prior to being sold to determine if pregnancy is present.

Equipment Needed

The following equipment is needed: camelid restraint chute, lubricant, rectal sleeves, ultrasound machine, 3.5-MHz sector probe for transabdominal scan, 5.0-MHz linear probe for transrectal ultrasound, rigid probe extender for the linear probe, and sedation (e.g., butorphanol at 0.1 mg/kg IV).

Restraint/Position

Standing or sternal recumbency (cushed posture) may be used.

Technical Description of Procedure/Method

Behavior

Camelids are induced ovulators and should only ovulate if they have been bred. Thus, females that are not pregnant and have not been bred recently should accept the male or be "receptive." A percentage of pregnant females will develop dominant follicles on the ovary sufficient to stimulate receptive behavior. Thus, accepting a male for breeding does not, in and of itself, indicate that the female is not pregnant. Females that have been bred recently (within the previous 10 days) and females that are pregnant should have ovulated and have a functioning CL or corpus luteum. This structure produces progesterone hormone and causes suppression of ovarian cyclicity. Thus, the female should reject or "spit-off" the male. Females that have not been bred within the previous 10 days and reject the male >14 days after breeding are consistent with pregnancy. Females with inactive ovaries, ovarian cysts such as luteinized follicular cysts or cystic CLs, or behavioral derangements, may "spit off" the male despite not being pregnant. Thus, rejection of the male, in and of itself, does not mean the female is pregnant.

Typical behaviors of females:

Normal female bred but did <u>not</u> conceive a pregnancy:

Activity	Behavior
Day 0	Receptive to be bred
Day 5 to 10	Spit-off with CL and high progesterone
Day 14	Receptive to be bred

Normal female bred and did conceive a pregnancy:

Activity	Behavior
Day 0	receptive to be bred
Day 5 to 10	Spit-off with CL and high progesterone
Day 14	Spit off
Day 21	Spit off
Day 28	Spit off →cria born 11 months

Rectal Examination: This author does not routinely perform rectal examination for pregnancy diagnosis in alpacas because of concern for damage to the rectum. The rectum and anus are small and difficult to accommodate a hand and arm in nonpregnant or early pregnant females. However, many veterinarians can and do perform this examination successfully. Pregnancy can be determined as early as 30 days after conception. This procedure is more easily performed in females that have had at least one cria and is easier in llamas as compared with alpacas. False negative diagnosis of pregnancy can occur if the pregnancy is too early to detect. False positives can occur by palpation of the bladder, ingesta within a bowel segment, or other masses in the abdomen.

Progesterone: Progesterone hormone concentration in the blood is widely used for "diagnosis" of pregnancy in camelids.

Camelids are induced ovulators, and, therefore, a female that has not been bred should have minimal (<0.2 ng/mL) progesterone in the bloodstream. Females that have been bred will have increased progesterone within 3 to 5 days, and these concentrations usually will remain increased (>2.0 ng/mL) throughout pregnancy. If the female fails to conceive a pregnancy, progesterone will fall back to low concentrations approximately 12 days after breeding. Timing of measurement of progesterone concentration determines the interpretation.

Expected progesterone concentrations:

Day 0 breeding
  Low: <0.2 ng/mL
Day 4 to 8
Increase =<u>ovulation</u> (>2.0 ng/mL)
Low =failure to ovulate
Day 14 to 21
  Increase =<u>conception</u>
  Low =failure to conceive
Day > 21
  High = pregnancy
  Low = early embryonic death

If the female is bred on day 0 and has a progesterone level >2.0 ng/mL on day 7, the interpretation is that she ovulated. If the progesterone remains increased at day 14, the interpretation is that she conceived a pregnancy. Alternatively, she may have not conceived but rather developed a retained CL. Increased progesterone on day 21 is interpreted as successful implantation of the pregnancy into the uterus. Alternatively, the female could have a retained CL, luteinized follicle, or other progesterone-secreting tissue.

Possible causes of hyperprogesteronemia:

- Inappropriate increase in progesterone
  - Persistent CL
  - Cystic CL
  - Ovarian tumors
- Granulosa cell tumor
- Granulosa theca cell tumor

Ultrasonography: Ultrasonography is the preferred method of diagnosis of pregnancy in llamas and alpacas. Transrectal ultrasonography in early pregnancy is done most commonly via rectal examination. The small size of camelids limits the examiner's ability to perform rectal palpation for control of the linear probe. A rigid extender can be manufactured from PVC pipe that is molded to the contour of a linear probe to facilitate control of the probe during the examination (Figures 53.1 and 53.2). This must be done with extreme care so

as not to injure or tear the rectum. Ideally, the camelid is restrained in a chute so that movements are restricted. Sedation is advisable to prevent or minimize unwanted activity during the examination. A lubricant (60 to 120 mL) should be instilled into the rectum prior to insertion of the probe. The nongravid uterus is recognized as a homogeneous gray to white tissue approximately 1 cm in diameter (Figure 53.3). The uterine horns are often curled in a "C" shape, and the ovaries can be found cranial and lateral to the tip of the nongravid uterus (Figure 53.4). The gravid horns straighten and extend cranially with advancement of the pregnancy. Pregnancies <45 days

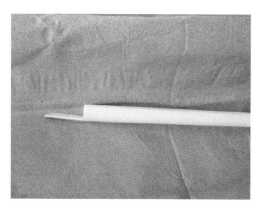

Figure 53.1 A rigid extension can be made from rigid plastic or polymer tubing to facilitate transrectal ultrasonography when transrectal palpation is not possible. Extreme care must be exercised to prevent tearing or other damage to the rectum.

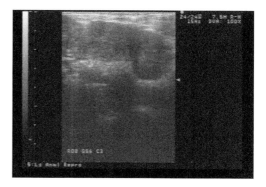

Figure 53.3 The nonpregnant uterus is recognized as having a homogeneous echogenicity with well-defined margins. (Image courtesy of Dr. Maria Ferrer, Kansas State University).

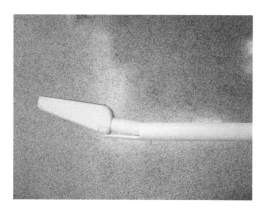

Figure 53.2 The rigid extender must be closely fitted to the rectolinear probe and the exposed edges covered with smooth tape to minimize the risk of injury.

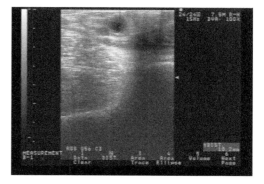

Figure 53.4 A mature follicle is present on the ovary of a female alpaca. The size of the follicle (10 mm) is consistent with a mature follicle ready for breeding. (Image courtesy of Dr. Maria Ferrer, Kansas State University).

are most easily examined via transrectal ultrasonography (Figures 53.5 to 53.7). Pregnancies >60 days but <180 days are most easily found via transabdominal ultrasound on the left side of the abdomen approximately 10-cm cranial to the brim of the pelvis and medial to the stifle (Figures 53.7 and 53.8). Pregnancies >180 days are difficult to find by ultrasound examination. At this stage, the cria resides cranial, ventral, and to the right side of midline in the abdomen. The cria thorax is most consistently found 10- to 20-cm caudal to the xyphoid and 10- to 15-cm to the right of ventral midline (Figures 53.9 to 53.12).

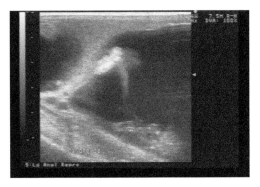

Figure 53.7 By day 60 of pregnancy, the head, neck, thorax, and abdomen can be recognized. (Image courtesy of Dr. Maria Ferrer, Kansas State University).

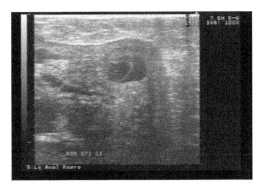

Figure 53.5 A 25-day pregnancy is recognized by focal accumulation of fluid, fine membranes, and a small fetal bud. (Image courtesy of Dr. Maria Ferrer, Kansas State University).

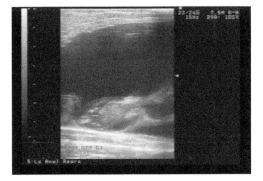

Figure 53.8 At 120 days of pregnancy, the abdominal and thoracic viscera are easily discernible. (Image courtesy of Dr. Maria Ferrer, Kansas State University).

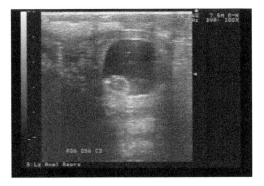

Figure 53.6 A more well-defined fetus is recognized by 37 days of pregnancy. (Image courtesy of Dr. Maria Ferrer, Kansas State University).

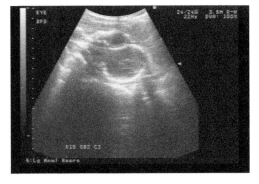

Figure 53.9 The skull and eyes are visible in this 292-day pregnancy image. (Image courtesy of Dr. Maria Ferrer, Kansas State University).

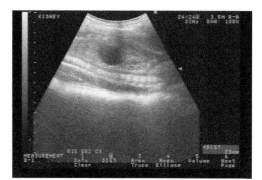

Figure 53.10 At 292 days, individual viscera can be examined such as this kidney (*measure bar*) and stomach (*hypoechoic circular area*). (Image courtesy of Dr. Maria Ferrer, Kansas State University).

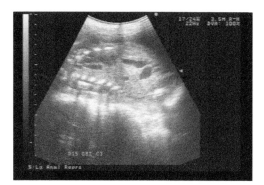

Figure 53.11 The thorax is easily recognized by the presence of ribs, vertebrae, and heart. The lungs are difficult to recognize in this 292-day fetus. (Image courtesy of Dr. Maria Ferrer, Kansas State University).

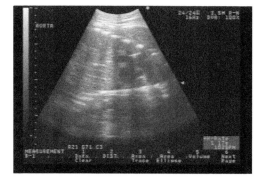

Figure 53.12 Heartbeat can be used to assess fetal viability and stress as is being imaged in this 318-day alpaca pregnancy. (Image courtesy of Dr. Maria Ferrer, Kansas State University).

- Transrectal
  - <45 days
  - Up to 90 days
- Transabdominal
  - Left flank
  - 60 to 180 days
  - Right paramedian
  - >180 days

In llamas, the gestational age of the cria can be estimated by the biparietal diameter using the formula:

$$y = 3.79 * x + 18.8$$

where y = gestational age and x = biparietal diameter (in mm) (Haibel and Fung 1991).

Practice Tip to Facilitate Procedure

A 5-MHz linear transducer can be used for evaluation of all stages of pregnancy (approximately 12 to 15 cm penetration of adequate resolution images). A 3.5-MHz transducer can be used for deeper penetration of the abdomen (up to 20 to 23 cm), but significant loss of image resolution occurs at these depths. Most modern ultrasound machines are equipped for simultaneous B- and M-Mode ultrasonography. This allows assessment of fetal heart rate (FHR) and some quantitative estimates of cardiac contractility. If the uterine fluid appears normal, then we would assume that the fetus-placenta-dam unit is normal. The placenta can be evaluated to a certain extent and premature separation of the placenta or placental edema may be found in females having had a uterine torsion. These findings suggest that a C-section may be necessary to save the life of the cria. If the FHR is normal, we would assume that the fetus is normal (adequate oxygen supply and waste removal). In our fetal stress research, we have determined that normal fetal heart

(Continued)

(Continued)

rate range for alpacas and llamas is 80 to 120 (fetal heart rate ranges from 1.5 to 2.0 × maternal heart rate [MHR]). The late gestation fetus (>6 to 7 months) is positioned in the uterus with the fetal head and thorax located near the maternal xiphoid bone just to the right of midline. Thus, the hair may need to be clipped to allow ultrasonography of the fetal heart. Most owners do not object to having this done because this region of hair removal is not seen and is not economically important. Occasionally the fetal heart cannot be found because of fetal positioning (fetal backbone or maternal viscera obstruction of ultrasound waves, positioning too deep in the abdomen for viewing, etc.).

Potential Complications

Rectal tear or perforation is the most serious complication of transrectal ultrasound. Although rare, death has occurred following full thickness tears into the abdomen. These catastrophic events most commonly occur when using a rigid probe extender in a fractious female that violently resists restraint and examination.

Patient Monitoring/Aftercare

The females should be monitored for 24 hours after ultrasound examinations, especially when transrectal ultrasound has been performed. Immediate attention is warranted if the females demonstrate clinical signs of abdominal pain, depression, lethargy, or anorexia.

Recommended Reading

Adams R, Garry F. 1994 Jul. Llama neonatology. *Vet Clin North Am Food Anim Pract*; 10(2):209–227. https://doi.org/10.1016/s0749-0720(15)30556-9. PMID: 7953955.

Haibel GK, Fung ED. 1991. Real-time ultrasonic biparietal diameter measurement for the prediction of gestational age in llamas. *Theriogenology*; 35(4):683–687.

Johnson LW. 1989 Mar. Llama reproduction. *Vet Clin North Am Food Anim Pract*; 5(1):159–182. https://doi.org/10.1016/s0749-0720(15)31008-2. PMID: 2647232.

Parraguez VH, Cortéz S, Gazitúa FJ, Ferrando G, MacNiven V, Raggi LA. 1997 May. Early pregnancy diagnosis in alpaca (Lama pacos) and llama (Lama glama) by ultrasound. *Anim Reprod Sci*; 47(1–2):113–121. doi: 10.1016/s0378-4320(96)01630-2. PMID: 9233511.

54

Procedure: Vaginoscopy and Uterine Culture
David E. Anderson

Purpose or Indication for Procedure

Vaginoscopy is performed for the purpose of assessment of the vestibule, vagina, and cervix. This can be done as a pre-breeding examination to verify that a female is ready for entry into a breeding program. Most often, vaginoscopy is done during a breeding soundness examination of females that have failed to become pregnant or have failed to maintain a pregnancy. In these cases, uterine culture also is performed.

Equipment Needed

The following equipment is needed: restraint chute; sedation (e.g., butorphanol at 0.1 mg/kg IV; xylazine at 0.2 to 0.4 mg/kg IV); soap and water with gauze pads for cleansing of the perineum, tail wrap, vaginoscope, light source, and guarded uterine swab.

Restraint/Position

Standing or in sternal recumbency in the chute positions are used.

Technical Description of Procedure/Method

The female is restrained in the camelid chute and the tail wrap applied. Roll gauze or non-adhesive bandage material is useful for wrapping the tail. With these materials, the free end is used to tie the tail forward to the halter or around the base of the neck. This tie should be firm enough to keep the tail out of the procedure field of the perineum. Then, the vulva is cleaned thoroughly with soap and warm water. Vaginoscopy can be performed using any tubular material, but commercially available human sigmoidoscopes are ideal for vaginoscopy of camelids (Figures 54.1 and 54.2). Flashlights and extended light sources can be placed into the lumen of the tube to illuminate the vagina, but a circular light source that will attach to the human rigid sigmoidoscope is ideal because it does not obscure the examiner's view (Figures 54.3 and 54.4). These attachments include a magnifying lens to facilitate the examination (Figure 54.5).

Insertion of the vaginoscope is done by applying sterile lubricant to the exterior of one end of the scope. Then, the scope is inserted through the vulva at a 60-degree ventral angle to the spine (the scope will be partially vertically oriented). At this angle, the scope is pushed dorsal

Veterinary Techniques in Llamas and Alpacas, Second Edition. Edited by David E. Anderson, Matt Miesner, and Meredyth Jones.

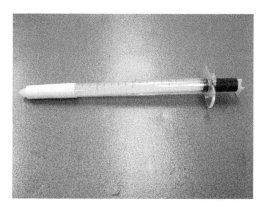

Figure 54.1 Rigid sigmoidoscope, available from WelchAllyn, designed for use in people has useful diameter and length for vaginoscopy of alpacas. The length may be too short for many llamas.

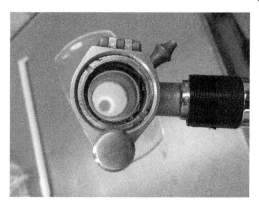

Figure 54.4 The sigmoidoscope light adaptor provides a magnification lens and circumferential light to facilitate examination without light source interference.

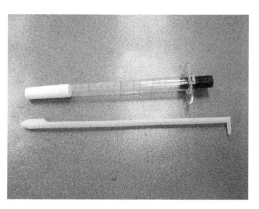

Figure 54.2 The rigid sigmoidoscope has an obturator that is blunt ended making easier entry through the vulva and into the vagina.

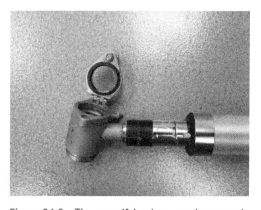

Figure 54.5 The magnifying lens may be opened to allow for sample collection when cytology or cultures are desired.

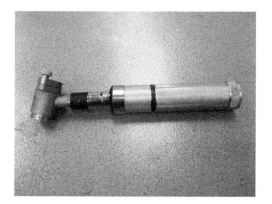

Figure 54.3 The sigmoidoscope light adaptor from WelchAllyn can be attached to most standard hand-held power supplies used for otoscopic and ophthalmic examinations.

and cranial for 5 to 6 cm until slight resistance is felt. When resistance is felt, the free end of the vaginoscope is elevated until advancement is possible. The final position of the vaginoscope is approximately horizontal. The light source is attached or inserted and the cervix identified and inspected (Figure 54.6). The cervix is recognized by the spiral form of the external os. The cranial vagina and cervix normally have a pink color and smooth surface with an absence of fluid. In the presence of a dominant follicle, the cervix is relaxed ("open") and can be recognized by the presence of a noticeable lumen. In the presence of a CL, the cervix is "closed," and the lumen is difficult to detect.

If fluid is present, samples should be obtained for cytology and culture. Guarded

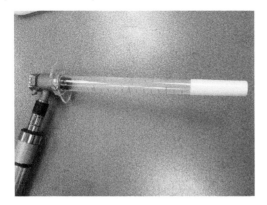

Figure 54.6 The light source adaptor is attached to the sigmoidoscope by threads. This allows the unit to be held and manipulated as one piece with one hand.

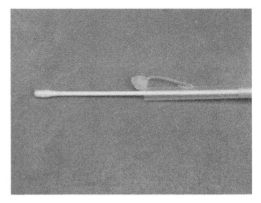

Figure 54.7 Guarded uterine culture swab minimizes contamination during sample collection.

uterine culture swabs are needed to minimize the risk of contamination (Figures 54.7 and 54.8). Uterine cultures are most easily obtained when a mature follicle is present and the cervix is relaxed. The culture swab is inserted through the vaginoscope and directed through the cervix under direct viewing.

Practice Tip to Facilitate Procedure

Llamas will nearly always remain standing for these procedures. Alpacas often lay down in sternal recumbency (cush) during these events. Restraint chutes that are specific to llamas and alpacas may include slings to facilitate maintaining a standing posture (Figure 54.9). Most often, one sling is placed under the sternum and one in front of the rear limbs along the caudal abdomen. These suspension slings can cause increased resistance from the patient. Therefore, many examiners prefer to work with alpacas in a recumbent position. This can be made easier by placing knee pads behind the female for the examiner to kneel onto or the examiner can wear knee pads designed for industrial and mechanical work. Another option is to mount the alpaca restraint chute onto a mechanical (hydraulic or electrical) lift so that the entire chute can be elevated (Figure 54.10). This allows the examiner to position the alpaca in such a way that kneeling is not required.

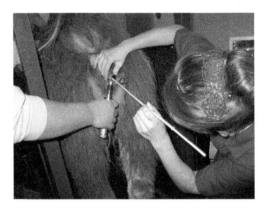

Figure 54.8 When the swab is in position to obtain the sample, the cotton swab is extended beyond the sheath. After sample collection, the swab is retracted within the sheath prior to removal of the unit.

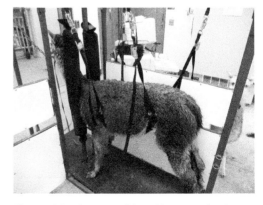

Figure 54.9 Alpaca positioned in a restraint chute with suspension slings in place to prevent lying down.

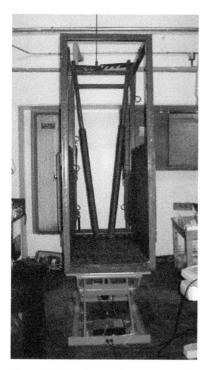

Figure 54.10 Alpaca chute mounted on a hydraulic lift to facilitate examination in sternal recumbency (cushed position).

Potential Complications

Sudden, severe, and agitated movements by the patient can cause injuries from the chute, slings, vaginoscope, or guarded culture swab. Adequate restraint, either manual or chemical, is imperative to prevent such injuries.

Patient Monitoring/Aftercare

No specific aftercare is required. Follow-up examination is indicated in females diagnosed as having uterine infection.

Recommended Reading

Anne Kutzler M, Ing M. 2021 Mar. Use of Hysteroscopy for Diagnosing Causes of Infertility in Camelids. *Vet Clin North Am Food Anim Pract*; 37(1):139-147. doi: 10.1016/j.cvfa.2020.12.004. PMID: 33541695.

55

Teat and Udder Examination

David E. Anderson

Purpose or Indication for Procedure

Diseases of the teat and udder of llamas and alpacas have received little attention. Perhaps the most common problem is poor milk production. However, mastitis (bacterial infection of the mammary gland) can be a significant problem for llamas and alpacas and is a cause of poor milk production and low weaning weights among crias. Nutrition is one of the most critical components of adequate milk production and quality. Poor milk production is one of the most common problems encountered in breeding females. Poor milk production is common among first lactation females, females giving birth to premature neonates, and females that have suffered illness, malnutrition, or severe stress. Poor milk production is most commonly recognized by poor growth of the cria or failure of the cria to gain weight. The female's udder should be immediately examined for swelling, obstruction of the teat to milk flow, pain, heat, and edema. The color and texture of the milk should be assessed. The most common diseases of the udder include mastitis, mammary abscess, and trauma.

Equipment Needed

The following equipment is needed: camelid chute for standing restraint and ultrasound with 7.5 to 10.0-MHz sector probe.

Technical Description of Procedure/Method

Anatomy

The mammary system of llamas and alpacas includes four glands, each of which has one teat (Figure 55.1). The principal supports for the udder are the medial and lateral suspensory ligaments. The medial suspensory ligament is elastic in nature, and although each half of the udder has a medial suspensory ligament, they are tightly adhered to each other. Secondary laminae arise from the medial and lateral laminae to support lobes or quarters of the udder. The indentation formed between the two halves of the udder is associated with the medial laminae and is referred to as the intermammary groove. The two halves of the udder are distinctly separate from each other and are supplied by separate arteries, veins, and nerves. The teat wall is composed of five layers: the inner most layer is a very thin mucosal layer followed by the submucosa; the next layer is the connective tissue layer, which is rich in blood supply; then the muscular layer, which is composed of both circular and longitudinal muscle fibers; and finally, the teat is covered by skin. The teat mucosa surrounds a teat cistern (teat sinus, lactiferous sinus), which, during lactation, is filled with milk. The teat cistern is continuous proximally with

Veterinary Techniques in Llamas and Alpacas, Second Edition. Edited by David E. Anderson, Matt Miesner, and Meredyth Jones.
© 2023 John Wiley & Sons, Inc. Published 2023 by John Wiley & Sons, Inc.

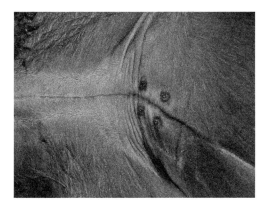

Figure 55.1 Teat and udder conformation in a nonpregnant, nonlactating adult female alpaca.

the gland cistern. Located at the bottom of the teat and connecting the teat cistern to the outside is the streak canal (teat canal, papillary duct). The main purpose of the streak canal is to protect the gland from bacterial infection.

Milk and Mastitis

Llama milk differs from that of other traditional livestock species, having more protein, sugar, and calcium, and less fat, sodium, potassium, and chloride than other ruminants. Acute mastitis may be recognized by the presence of heat, pain, and swelling of the udder. Palpation of the udder may reveal edema, firmness of the gland, and enlargement of the supramammary lymph nodes. Expulsion of milk from the gland may reveal altered color, the presence of flakes or clots, and either a thinner (e.g., serous) or thicker character. Some bacteria may cause septicemia or toxemia as recognized by increased rectal temperature, elevated heart rate, decreased appetite, and marked reduction in milk production.

Subclinical mastitis is the most common form of mastitis. Subclinical mastitis may be recognized by reduced cria growth, neonatal malnutrition, and neonatal death caused by starvation. Subclinical mastitis may be caused by a variety of bacteria. Chronic subclinical mastitis causes progressive fibrosis and decreased ability to produce milk. Diagnosis

of subclinical mastitis is done by palpation of the udder, milk culture, or use of animal side milk tests (e.g., black plate, strip cup, CMT). Occasionally, udder abscesses are recognized by swelling, edema, or rupture of the abscess to the exterior. Herd managers should be encouraged to perform routine udder palpation and milk tests when animals freshen and at appropriate intervals given the management system to evaluate for heat, pain, and edema.

A variety of treatment regimens have been used for treatment of mastitis. Response to treatment varies with the type of pathogen causing disease. Response to parenteral (IV, IM, SC) treatment of mastitis during lactation is highly variable with some pathogens being poorly responsive (e.g., *Staphylococcus aureus*) and some pathogens being highly responsive (coagulase negative *Staphylococcus, streptococci*) to treatment. Supportive care is the most important component of the treatment regimen. Supportive care includes anti-inflammatory medication, optimal feed intake, hydrotherapy or hot packing of the udder, and "stripping" milk out of the udder. Intramammary infusions are an accepted practice, but little research has been published evaluating this procedure. In our experience, a combination of anti-inflammatory drugs, antibiotics, and hot packing results in a high cure rate in camelids. The cria should be allowed to "strip" the milk out of the udder as part of normal nursing because "stripping" by hand causes excessive soreness to the teats, and this may cause the female not to allow the cria to nurse. Prevention of mastitis is best accomplished by close attention to hygiene, optimal nutrition, and excellent animal care and housing.

Poor Milkability

Camelid milk should be white, free of clots or debris, and should be able to be expressed. The body condition score (BCS) of the female should be assessed to determine adequacy of nutrition. Lactating females having a BCS of 3 or less out of 10 should be examined to determine if malnutrition, disease, or parasitism is present. Lactating females with BCS > 7 out of 10 may have hypogalactia of obesity either because of adipose tissue invasion in the udder or because of fat interference with hormone receptors within the mammary cells. Domperidone and herbal supplements have been used to improve lactation in some females. Domperidone has been used in horses to combat the negative effects of fescue endophyte toxins on milk production. However, the drug may be used to stimulate milk production in a variety of situations because the effect is to increase endogenous levels of prolactin hormone. Prolactin is responsible for stimulating the mammary tissues to produce milk. We have observed beneficial effects of both of these products and routinely use them to stimulate lactation in poor milking females when no cause can be found for the poor milk production.

Practice Tip to Facilitate Procedure

Sedation and restraint in lateral recumbency greatly facilitates examination. Milk samples may be more easily obtained by using a homemade "breast pump." This is made from a 20-cc syringe. The plunger is removed and the needle end of the syringe cut off flush with the barrel of the syringe. Then, the plunger is replaced into the syringe from the cut end. The flanged end of the syringe is placed over the teat and held gently but firmly against the udder. A small amount of petroleum jelly can be placed on the contact surface of the flanged end of the syringe to improve the seal. The plunger is withdrawn repeatedly so as to form a pulsating vacuum within the lumen of the syringe.

Potential Complications

Examination and milk collection can cause discomfort to the patient. This may cause resistance to restraint and the risk of self-trauma.

56

Mastectomy (Udder Amputation)

Matt D. Miesner

Purpose or Indication for Procedure

Mastectomy is indicated in cases of chronic udder disease, where local and systemic manifestations result in poor quality of life. Acute or toxic mastitis may render the patient a high anesthetic risk, and should be resolved medically prior to deciding on mastectomy. Fortunately, severe mastitis is a rare problem in camelids and neoplasia is rare., If selected, alternative arrangements for colostrum and nutritional support of offspring must be made in advance of future parturition.

Equipment Needed

A general surgical pack, absorbable and non-absorbable suture material, Penrose drain (optional), and general anesthesia are needed.

Restraint/Position

The patient is preferably intubated and anesthetized under general inhalant anesthesia. They should be positioned in dorsal recumbency, with assisted ventilation and monitoring equipment available. Injectable anesthesia and a high-volume epidural may be sufficient in situations where the surgeon is familiar with the procedure and patient health status allows.

Technical Description of Procedure/Method

The mastectomy procedure is also called udder amputation. Camelids have four mammary quarters and teats and a relatively nonpendulous udder. (See Figure 56.1.) An elliptical incision is made around the udder at a level at which sufficient skin remains to allow suture closure of the wound. (See Figure 56.2.) An alternative "inverted clover leaf" method recently reported in small ruminants may also be useful. (Hermida et al. 2021) The udder is removed while systematically ligating the major vasculature (Figure 56.3) and followed by closure of the skin. Infected or necrotic wounds on the udder or teats should be covered or sutured closed before beginning the mastectomy. A wide surgical margin should be clipped, surgically scrubbed, and draped.A skin incision is made surrounding the udder. Preserve about 2 cm of the dorsal mammary skin to facilitate primary closure. The incision will eventually be an ellipse, alternatively inverted cloverleaf, surrounding the udder and enough tissue must be retained for appositional closure (Figure 56.4). The external pudendal arteries and veins exiting the inguinal rings and coursing along the lateral aspect of both sides of the udder should be isolated and ligated during the early phases of the procedure to limit blood flow into the udder and reduce intraoperative hemorrhage.

Veterinary Techniques in Llamas and Alpacas, Second Edition. Edited by David E. Anderson, Matt Miesner, and Meredyth Jones.

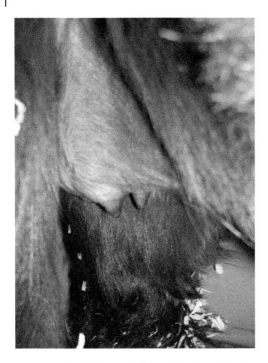

Figure 56.1 A right craniolateral photograph of a llama udder showing the relatively nonpendulous orientation of the gland and teats.

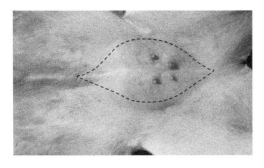

Figure 56.2 Approximate location (*dashed line*) of the elliptical incision for mastectomy in an alpaca. Note that the lateral portions of the incision will preserve approximately 2 cm of dorsal mammary skin for closure after the gland in removed.

Approach carefully through the subcutaneous fat and lateral suspensory ligament toward the inguinal ring. Frequently palpate for the pulse of the external pudendal artery to avoid inadvertent cutting trauma of the artery and vein which lie just deep to the suspensory ligament and in close approximation with one another. (See Figure 56.5.)

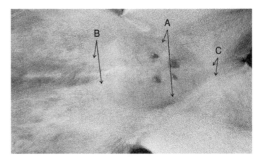

Figure 56.3 Approximate locations of the major blood vessels of the mammary gland. Paired pudendal arteries and veins (**A**) arise from the inguinal rings dorsal to the gland. Subcutaneous abdominal veins and branches (**B**) cranial to the udder and perineal arteries and veins (**C**) caudally.

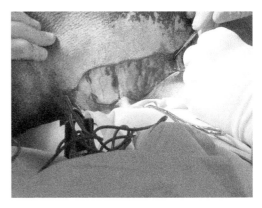

Figure 56.4 Initial incision is made on the lateral side of the udder preserving a portion of dorsal skin for closure. Continue approach through the lateral suspensory ligament to the inguinal ring.

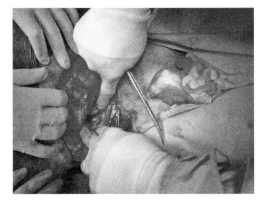

Figure 56.5 The pudendal artery and vein can be seen coursing from the inguinal ring.

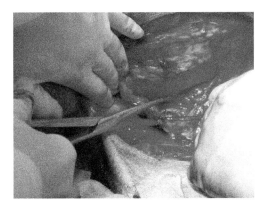

Figure 56.6 Ligate and transect the pudendal and artery on each side before continuing amputation. Attempts should be made to ligate the pudendal artery before ligation of the vein.

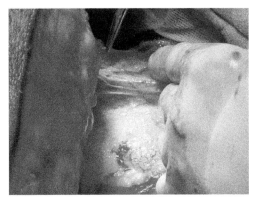

Figure 56.7 Continue lateral incisions cranial and caudal to isolate and ligate the subcutaneous abdominal vein(s) and large branches as well as the perineal artery and vein.

Isolate and ligate the external pudendal artery first, followed by the vein near the inguinal ring. (Figure 56.6). By ligating the artery first, circulatory blood volume is preserved by allowing the udder to drain into circulation. Use of absorbable suture material is indicated. Braided suture are preferred to ensure holding power on tissues while tightening. Double ligation of the arteries using No. 2 chromic gut or No. 1 braided suture such as PGA-910 are desirable. Transect the vessels and check for bleeding. Repeat these first steps on the opposite side.

After ligating and transecting the external pudendal arteries and veins, continue the skin incisions cranially in an elliptical fashion to meet at the cranial midline. Isolate and ligate the subcutaneous abdominal veins (cranial superficial epigastric veins) and large branches at the craniolateral aspect of the udder. (See Figure 56.7.) Next, continue the skin incisions caudal to meet at the caudal midline of the udder. Isolate and ligate the perineal vessels (ventral perineal veins).

At this point, all major blood vessels should have been ligated and transected. Begin lifting the udder at the cranial aspect and cutting the median suspensory ligament about 1 cm from its attachment to the abdominal wall. Continue lifting the udder and cutting the suspensory

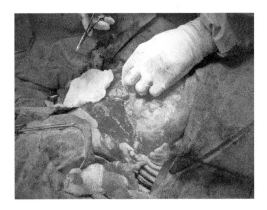

Figure 56.8 Undermine the udder from its abdominal attachments and transect the median suspensory ligament about 1 cm distal to the abdomen to incorporate into skin closure. Recheck ligatures for security.

ligament caudally until the udder is removed. (See Figure 56.8.)

Check the security of the remaining vessel ligatures and begin skin closure. Multiple simple interrupted sutures (also known as walking sutures) can be used to close dead space. Skin is closed using a single layer closure. Added suture line security can be gained by anchoring the skin sutures to the remaining median suspensory ligament along the skin edges. A few interrupted tension-relieving sutures are placed first, followed by an intermittent continuous closure in a forward (FORD) interlocking pattern.

Postoperative seroma formation is common and occasionally may pose a problem. Depending on the case and size of the wound, a Penrose drain may be placed in the tissue defect remaining after udder removal. These drains are typically placed deep to the incision from caudal to cranial during closure and maintained for 3 to 4 days after surgery. In addition, soft leg hobbles are made and placed on the metatarsal region of the pelvic limbs to prevent splaying of limbs during recovery and for several days after surgery.

Practice Tip to Facilitate Procedure

Separation of the external pudendal artery and vein before ligating individually may be difficult to impossible in some cases. The author has ligated them simultaneously on occasion without complications such as arteriovenous fistula.

Potential Complications

Excessive hemorrhage is possible both intra and postoperatively. Consider having a blood donor available or precollected whole blood to address hemorrhage. Assume a total blood volume of 8% and adjust accordingly with the size of the patient and estimated blood loss volume. A safe volume of blood to collect from a donor is equivalent to 10 mL per kilogram body weight. (e.g., a healthy 70-kg alpaca would be able to safely donate 700 mL of whole blood).

Patient Monitoring/Aftercare

Monitor the patient closely for evidence of excessive hemorrhage for 48 hours. Maintain vigilance against infection for 2 weeks after surgery. Stall confinement for 2 weeks and broad-spectrum antimicrobial therapy are indicated. Remove skin sutures 18 to 21 days after surgery. If a drain was placed, it should be removed within 3 to 5 days after surgery, depending on the nature and amount of discharge.

Recommended Reading

Braga WU, Chavera A, Gonzalez A. 2006. Corynebacterium pseudotuberculosis infection in highland alpacas (Lama pacos) in Peru. *Vet Rec*; 159(1):23–24.

Cable CS, Peery K, Fubini SL. 2004. Radical mastectomy in 20 ruminants. *Vet Surg*; 33(3):263–266.

Fubini SL. 2004. Surgery of the mammary gland. In: *Farm Animal Surgery*, Fubini and Ducharme Ed., Elsevier Saunders, Philadelphia, PA, pp. 403–407.

Hermida JA, Baird AN, Hawkins JF, et al. 2021. Mastectomy in 25 small ruminants (2002-2019). *Vet Surg*; 50(1):104–110.

Hull BL. 1995. Teat and udder surgery. *Vet Clin N Am Food Animal Pract*; 11(1):14–16.

Leichner TL, Turner O, Mason GL, et al. 2001. Cutaneous metastases of a mammary carcinoma in a llama. *Can Vet J*; 42(3):204–206.

Riek A, Gerken M. 2006. Changes in Llama (Lama glama) milk composition during lactation. *J Dairy Sci*; 89(9):3484–3493.

57

Cesarean Section

(also known as Hysterotomy)

David E. Anderson

Purpose or Indication for Procedure

Dystocia is relatively uncommon in llamas and alpacas with fewer than 5% of birthings expected to require assistance. Elective C-sections are discouraged because of the risk of fetal death. The most common causes of dystocia in llamas and alpacas are fetal malpositioning, uterine torsion, and poor cervical dilation. Dystocia may be relieved without surgery if the following criterion can be achieved: (1) the cervix is adequately dilated and the pelvis is of adequate size to extract the fetus, (2) the pelvic dimension allows introduction of a hand into the uterus for fetal manipulation, and (3) the uterus has sufficient room to grasp and manipulate the fetus. If these criteria cannot be met, the decision to perform a C-section should be made without delay. If the dam is stable or after supportive therapy has been initiated in the dam, the presentation, position, and posture of the fetus and presence and extent of vaginal and uterine injury should be determined. If the size of the dam precludes evaluation of the uterus or fetus, then ultrasonography may be done to assess the fetus. Immediate exploratory surgery and C-section may be the most prudent action if labor has been prolonged, fetal heart rate cannot be assessed, or the condition of the fetus or birth canal precludes transvaginal delivery.

Equipment Needed

The following equipment is needed: clippers, preparation for aseptic surgery (povidone iodine scrub, alcohol rinse, gauze pads), surgery cap and mask, sterile drapes, sterile gloves, sterile gowns, suction apparatus, sterile saline or lactated Ringer's solution (LRS) rinse, soft tissue surgery instruments, suture materials, and bandaging material (cotton sheets, brown roll gauze, elastic non-adhesive tape, adhesive tape). Additional needs include anesthesia supplies, IV fluid supplies, and antibiotics and nonsteroidal anti-inflammatory drugs.

Restraint/Position

Patient assessment is critical to successful alleviation of dystocia. Cardiovascular shock must be treated prior to correction of dystocia. Females having clinical signs of dehydration, hypotension, and shock should have an IV catheter placed and crystalloid fluids administered as needed. Nonsteroidal anti-inflammatory drugs (e.g., flunixin meglumine, 1 mg/kg IV) and/or antibiotics (e.g., ceftiofur sodium, 2 mg/kg body weight IV) may be used when appropriate. In dystocia, if the uterus or fetus is not accessible or the cervix is closed, immediate C-section is indicated. Damage to the cervix or uterus is more likely when trying

Veterinary Techniques in Llamas and Alpacas, Second Edition. Edited by David E. Anderson, Matt Miesner, and Meredyth Jones.
© 2023 John Wiley & Sons, Inc. Published 2023 by John Wiley & Sons, Inc.

to force manipulation of the fetus despite inadequate space or cervical dilation. If the size of the dam precludes transvaginal palpation, immediate C-section should be chosen. Delay in the decision to perform surgery may result in morbidity or death of the fetus and/or dam.

Technical Description of Procedure/Method

Cesarean section is most easily performed via paralumbar fossa or ventral midline laparotomy. Ventral midline laparotomy for C-section has been recommended but is best performed with the dam under general anesthesia. This author prefers to perform C-section via a left paralumbar approach. This allows C-section to be performed with the dam sedated and restrained in right lateral recumbency but not anesthetized. In this author's experience, this approach results in crias that are more vital and maternal-neonate bonding occurs more readily. Also, milk let-down and early lactation are expected to be more rapid. General anesthesia is discussed elsewhere in this text. A useful sedative for left laparotomy is butorphanol (0.1 mg/kg IV). If necessary based on maternal activity, xylazine (0.1 mg/kg IV) may be used. Clinical depression of the fetus is minimal, and xylazine may be reversed using yohimbine or tolazoline if needed. The female is haltered, placed in right lateral recumbency, and the head and limbs are tied to prevent excessive movement. Then, lidocaine HCl 2% is used to establish a line block at the site of the incision. Caution should be used not to exceed 4 mg/kg body weight total dose of lidocaine so as not to induce lidocaine toxicity. Lidocaine toxicity is recognized by lethargy, ataxia, slow and labored breathing, weakness, hypotension, and diminished response to stimuli.

For flank laparotomy, the skin incision is begun approximately 8 to 10 cm cranial and ventral to the tuber coxae and is extended cranially and ventrally approximately 15 cm in length toward the costochondral junction.

Care must be taken when incising the external abdominal oblique muscle, internal abdominal oblique muscle, and the transverses abdominus muscle so as not to invade the peritoneal cavity prematurely. With the left side approach, the C1, spleen, and left kidney lay positioned against the abdominal wall and can be inadvertently lacerated during entry. On the right side of the abdomen, the C3, duodenum, right kidney, and small intestine lay positioned close to the abdominal wall.

The uterus should be exteriorized from the abdomen if possible to prevent leakage of uterine fluids into the abdomen. This is critical if extensive attempts at manual correction of dystocia have been tried or if the fetus is dead or emphysematous. The uterus is remarkably thin, and care should be exercised when opening the uterus in order to not cause injury to the fetus. In most cases, the placenta is left *in situ* after extraction of the fetus. If the placenta can be easily separated from the endometrial wall, it may be removed at the time of hysterotomy.

In most llamas and alpacas, the healthy uterus can be closed in a single layer with No. 0 polydioxanone or poliglecaprone. When uterine laceration or compromise to the uterine wall is present (e.g. edema, mural hematoma), a double layer closure should be done to ensure that an adequate serosal seal is achieved. The uterus should be thoroughly lavaged clean of all blood clots prior to being replaced into the abdomen. However, the surgeon should not use gauze pads or other abrasive materials to remove blood or fibrin because this will increase the likelihood of postoperative adhesions.

Ventral midline celiotomy incisions can be closed in interrupted or simple continuous suture patterns. This author uses No. 1 polydioxanone or PGA910 suture material in the linea alba. In camelids, paralumbar incisions have a greater risk of postoperative incisional hernia as compared with ventral midline incisions. The muscle layers should be precisely reconstructed in simple continuous suture patterns. The author prefers No. 1 PG-910 or PGA because of the supple nature of the suture and tissue-holding characteristics in muscle. The skin can be apposed using No. 1 nylon or polypropylene suture in an interrupted or Ford interlocking suture pattern. After surgery and when the dam is standing, an abdominal support bandage can be used to minimize incision strain for 10 to 14 days. This may minimize the risk of incisional hernia. A three-layer bandage composed of a thick layer of cotton padding, a conforming layer using non-adhesive bandaging tape or roll gauze, and an outer layer of adhesive tape provide support for the abdomen during the first 2 weeks after surgery.

Practice Tip to Facilitate Procedure

Infiltration of lidocaine for local anesthesia can easily accumulate dosages approaching toxicity. The total body dosage of lidocaine should not exceed 4 mg/kg body weight (1 mL per 5 kg body weight). Lidocaine toxicity can be treated by administration of IV fluids and supportive care.

CAUTION: Dinoprost, a PGF2-alpha drug, is not recommended for use in llamas and alpacas because of the risk of hyper-tension and death.

Potential Complications

Complications of laparotomy include peritonitis, hemorrhage, incisional seroma or hematoma, incisional infection, incisional dehiscence, and incisional hernia. These complications are infrequent when aseptic technique, careful tissue handling, and accurate reconstruction of tissues using appropriate materials and techniques are used. Interestingly, incisional hernias appear to be more common in llamas and alpacas with paralumbar incisions as compared with other ruminant species. An abdominal support bandage is recommended to be used for 10 to 14 days after surgery to support the incision in an attempt to minimize this risk.

Complications of hysterotomy include peritonitis, uterine adhesions, paraovarian adhesions, retained placenta, metritis, endometritis, and infertility. Early decision for C-section will optimize the condition of the dam, fetus, and tissues and therefore minimize the risk of complications. Retention of the placenta is not uncommon, but the placenta is expected to pass within 24 hours after surgery with minimal to no treatment. Closprostenol (250 μg total dose, IM) has been used to encourage lysis of the CL and continuation of placental separation from the endometrium. Caution should be observed with the use of oxytocin. Oxytocin should only be used in the presence of an open cervix. Oxytocin has been associated with abdominal pain in llamas and alpacas, and the dosage and response to therapy should be closely monitored.

Patient Monitoring/Aftercare

Antibiotics and nonsteroidal anti-inflammatory drugs are administered routinely before surgery and continuing for 3 days after surgery. Therapy may be prolonged if uterine laceration, abdominal contamination, or emphysematous fetus were present. Close attention should be paid to the dam for 5 to 7 days after surgery to monitor for the onset of peritonitis. Antimicrobial therapy should include both Gram-positive and Gram-negative spectrum. When C-section is performed early in dystocia and sterile technique is used, the re-breeding success rate is expected to be good.

Recommended Reading

Anderson DE. 1999. Common surgical procedures in camelids. *J Camel Pract Res*; 6(2):191–201.

Anderson DE. 2009, Jul. Uterine torsion and cesarean section in llamas and alpacas. *Vet Clin North Am Food Anim Pract*;

25(2):523–538. doi: 10.1016/j.cvfa.2009.02.002. PMID: 19460653.

Bravo PW. 2002. Female Reproduction. In: *The Reproductive Process of South American Camelids*, Bravo PW, Seagull Printing, Salt Lake City, pp. 1–31.

Cebra CK, Cebra ML, Garry FB, Johnson LW. 1997. Surgical and nonsurgical correction of uterine torsion in New World camelids: 20 cases (1990–1996). *J Amer Vet Med Assoc*; 211:600–602.

Miller BA, Brounts SH, Anderson DE, Devine E. 2013, Mar 1. Cesarean section in alpacas and llamas: 34 cases (1997-2010). *J Am Vet Med Assoc*; 242(5):670–674. doi: 10.2460/javma.242.5.670. PMID: 23402415.

Saltet J, Dart AJ, Dart CM, Hodgson DR. 2000, May. Ventral midline caesarean section for dystocia secondary to failure to dilate the cervix in three alpacas. *Aust Vet J*; 78(5): 326–328. doi: 10.1111/j.1751-0813.2000. tb11782.x. PMID: 10904816.

58

Diagnosis and Management of Uterine Torsion

David E. Anderson

Purpose or Indication for Procedure

The term uterine torsion refers to a condition where the pregnant uterine horn rotates along the long axis of the uterus from the normal position. Uterine torsions are most often diagnosed because of abnormal clinical signs in the dam. Uterine torsions likely occur at some stages of pregnancy without our knowledge and without causing harm. However, uterine torsion associated with clinical signs should be addressed as an emergency in order to save the viability of the fetus and the life of the dam. Fatalities of the fetus and dam have been observed because of delays in treatment, and deaths have been caused by ischemia to the uterus, rupture of the uterus, and fatal hemorrhage into the abdomen.

Uterine torsion most commonly occurs in late gestation in llamas and alpacas with clinical cases most often occurring after the ninth month of gestation and most often 2 weeks or more before the due date for parturition (Cebra et al. 1990–1996). When possible, the author leaves the gestating cria in utero to continue until the natural birthing process because of the poor survival rate of crias born prematurely.

The ability to diagnose the direction of uterine torsion is critical to non-surgical correction. Failure to correctly diagnose the direction of torsion before attempting correction by rolling can cause exacerbation of the torsion, loss of blood flow to the fetus, or ischemia to the uterus. The direction of the rotation of the uterine horns can be described as either clockwise (torsion of the left horn rotating dorsally and then to the right side) or counter-clockwise (torsion of the right horn dorsally and then to the left side). This refers to the direction of rotation of the gravid uterine horn about the long axis of the uterus and the nongravid horn similar to the direction of the rotation of the hands of a clock. This terminology assumes that the observer is standing behind the animal and looking at the rear end of the llama or alpaca. The rear quarters are used to visualize a clock face with the vulva at the center. In a normal, nongravid uterus, the uterine horns are positioned at 3 o'clock (right horn) and 9 o'clock (left horn) on the clock face. During pregnancy, the gravid horn of the uterus normally rotates ventrally and toward midline because of volume displacement and gravity. This shifting of the gravid horn creates a 90-degree rotation ipsilateral to the gravid horn. Although the uterus is rotated, the broad ligaments of the uterus are relatively straight and course from the caudal dorsal attachments to a cranial ventral position. The broad ligaments remain relatively parallel to each other and become more obvious as the pregnancy advances and the uterus becomes laden with fluid. Uterine

Veterinary Techniques in Llamas and Alpacas, Second Edition. Edited by David E. Anderson, Matt Miesner, and Meredyth Jones.
© 2023 John Wiley & Sons, Inc. Published 2023 by John Wiley & Sons, Inc.

torsions are based (maximum point of gravity) on the gravid horn. Thus, clockwise torsions occur when a left horn pregnancy (90%) is present, and counter-clockwise torsions occur when a right horn pregnancy (10%) is present. In the situation when the left horn rotates dorsal and lateral to the right horn, then the horn is described as having moved clockwise similar to the hands of the clock. In the situation of a counter-clockwise uterine torsion, a right horn pregnancy is present, and the gravid right horn rotates dorsal and lateral to the left horn of the uterus. The torsion can be anywhere from 180 to 360 degrees and beyond. The caudal extent of the torsion is normally near the cervix, but it may be based in the uterine body cranial to the cervix or in the vagina caudal to the cervix. In term pregnancies, the torsion often prevents the cervix from dilating fully and will prevent birth if it is not corrected.

Equipment Needed

A restraint chute for standing or sternal recumbency examination, lubricant, examination gloves, rectal palpation sleeves, and an ultrasound machine with 3.5- to 5.0-MHz sector probe are needed.

Restraint/Position

Standing, sternal recumbency, and lateral recumbency positions may be used.

Technical Description of Procedure/Method

Vaginal speculum examination or transvaginal palpation can be used to diagnose the presence of a uterine torsion in many cases. A vaginal speculum is placed into the vagina, and the vestibule is inspected for deviations, compression, or twisting of the walls of the vagina or vestibule. The author prefers to use a human rigid

sigmoidoscope for vaginoscopic examinations, but any suitably sized and cleansed tube and light source may be used. Diagnosis of uterine torsion is made when the vaginal vault is twisted and narrowed and the direction of the torsion is inferred by the direction of the twisting or distortion of the vaginal vault. However, the examiner must understand that distortion of the vagina is consistently observed only with post-cervical uterine torsion. In many cases of uterine torsion in llamas and alpacas, the vaginal examination is nondiagnostic, and a definitive diagnosis requires either rectal palpation or exploratory laparotomy.

Careful rectal palpation can be used to identify the uterus and broad ligaments (Figure 58.1). The broad ligaments are thinner, more pliable, and less easily defined compared with that of cattle and horses. Thus, some experience is required to accurately identify the uterus and broad ligaments. Rectal examination must be performed carefully so as not to tear or perforate the rectum. Techniques used to increase the safety of rectal palpation include restraint in a camelid stocks, sedation with drugs having analgesic properties (e.g., narcotics are preferred because alpha-2 agonists can cause decreased uterine perfusion), use of large quantities of obstetrical lubricant, epidural anesthesia (e.g., 2% lidocaine HCl), and application of lidocaine jelly directly on the anal sphincter and in the rectal lumen. When needed, butorphanol tartrate (0.1 mg/kg IV) provides excellent sedation with minimal to no untoward effects on the fetus. Clinical signs of uterine

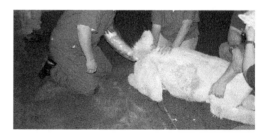

Figure 58.1 Rectal palpation for diagnosis of uterine torsion in an adult female alpaca. In this case, a left-horn-over-right, or "clockwise," uterine torsion is present.

torsion are variable and range from mild, including depression, lethargy, reluctance to rise, and anorexia, to more severe signs of colic including increased heart rate and respiratory rate, rolling, thrashing, vocalizing, and straining without effect. Uterine torsion should be suspected when a dam is in late gestation and shows signs of abnormal behavior, distress, abnormal labor, or labor without progression.

Diagnosis of uterine torsion is based on palpation of deviation of the broad ligaments. In the gravid uterus, both broad ligaments course from caudal and dorsal in the pelvic canal to cranial and ventral in the abdomen. In the presence of a uterine torsion, the broad ligament associated with the gravid uterine horn courses from caudal and dorsal to the horn, across the pelvic canal dorsal to the uterine body, and cranial and ventral to the contralateral side of the abdomen. The broad ligament associated with the nongravid horn courses from caudal and dorsal in the pelvic canal, can be felt continuing ventral to the cervix and uterine body, but cannot be palpated because it continues cranial and ventral in the abdomen. The examiner should make the owner aware that a small amount of bleeding from the anal sphincter is common when rectal palpation is performed. The bleeding is caused by over-stretching of the mucous membrane and sphincter muscle. This procedure is unlikely to pose a risk to the animal but does cause swelling and discomfort.

Nonsurgical Correction of Uterine Torsion

Uterine torsion can be corrected either with medical or surgical intervention. Medical intervention generally entails rolling the female while stabilizing the uterus to "untwist" the torsion. Transvaginal correction can be done if cervical dilation is sufficient for entry of a hand into the uterus alongside of the fetus, but this is possible only in a minority of cases. If sedation is needed to roll the dam, a mixed agonist-antagonist narcotic (e.g., butorphanol, 0.05 to 0.1 mg/kg IV) is recommended to minimize cardiopulmonary effects on the dam and fetus. The rolling

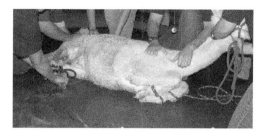

Figure 58.2 A halter and leg ropes are applied after attaining recumbency.

procedure is done by placing the dam on the same side as the direction of the torsion. A halter is placed on the patient, and ropes are placed on the front and hind limbs to aid in control of the limbs during the procedure (Figure 58.2). For example, if an alpaca has a clockwise uterine torsion, then the alpaca would be placed on her right side to begin the procedure (Figure 58.3). Then, transabdominal palpation is used to identify and stabilize the gravid horn of the uterus by feeling the fetus (Figure 58.4). Most often, the backbone of the fetus is present along the abdominal wall. While maintaining pressure on the gravid horn, the female is rolled over her back to her other side (Figures 58.5 to 58.7).

This procedure may need to be repeated. A rectal examination is done after each attempt to determine the extent of correction (Figure 58.8). Correction of the torsion is confirmed by palpating the broad ligaments, uterine body, and fetus.

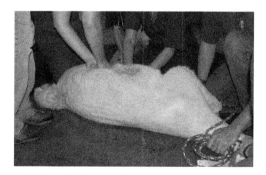

Figure 58.3 The female is initially placed into right lateral recumbency (90 degrees to sternal) to begin rolling correction of a clockwise uterine torsion. The examiner palpates the fetus and provides manual stabilization of the uterus during rolling of the dam.

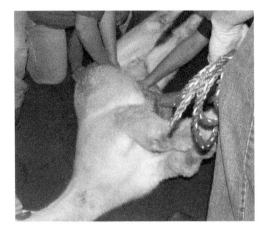

Figure 58.4   The female is rolled to right lateral oblique position (135 degrees from sternal) while the examiner maintains the position of the uterus.

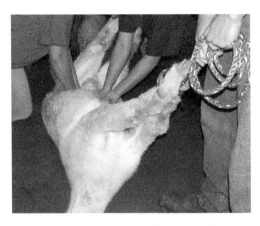

Figure 58.5   The female is rolled to right lateral to dorsal oblique (approximately 155 degrees from sternal) while the examiner maintains the position of the uterus.

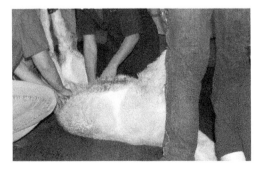

Figure 58.6   The female is rolled into dorsal recumbency (180 degrees from sternal) while the examiner maintains the position of the uterus.

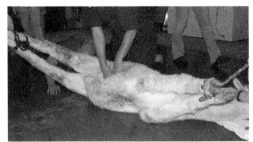

Figure 58.7   The female is rolled to left lateral oblique position (225 degrees from sternal) while the examiner maintains the position of the uterus.

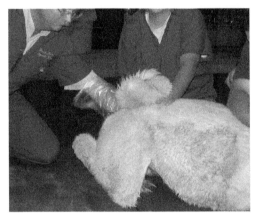

Figure 58.8   After completion of the corrective rolling procedure, the female is positioned either in a cushed (sternal) position (picture here) or standing and rectal palpation repeated to confirm correction of the torsion.

If rolling is successful, the dam should be walked but not allowed to roll for up to 30 minutes and then reexamined. Uterine torsion often reoccurs within a short period of time in up to 20% of females. This may be associated with incomplete correction during the rolling procedure. If rolling is not successful, a decision should be made quickly regarding surgical correction.

Practice Tip to Facilitate Procedure

Rectal palpation can be facilitated by sedation (butorphanol tartrate, 0.1 mg/kg IV) and by instillation of a mixture of lidocaine and lubricant into the rectum (55 mL OB lubricant mixed with 5 mL lidocaine 2%).

Potential Complications

Uterine torsion presents a significant risk to the life of the dam and cria. Possible complications of uterine torsion can include fetal death or compromise, premature birth, death of the dam, uterine compromise by ischemia, rupture of the uterine or ovarian artery with hemorrhage, uterine rupture and subsequent peritonitis, and, if surgical correction is necessary, all of the complications associated with laparotomy and C-section such as retained placenta, metritis, and adhesions. Return to breeding soundness is of concern to breeders, but females without significant complications are expected to return to the breeding program successfully.

Patient Monitoring/Aftercare

The cause of uterine torsion is unknown. Studies in other species have documented risk factors including large fetal size, having a male fetus, breed predispositions, and maternal illness. Dam behaviors such as rolling excessively, right horn pregnancies, and prolonged gestation may be associated with increased risk of uterine torsions. Excessive rolling is often seen when females are moved to a new area during late gestation. This situation occurs when females are moved to a new pasture or to maternity pens or barns. Ideally, dams should not be stressed in the last several months of gestation. When relocation of females to a maternity area is required or desired, this should ideally be done at least 60 days before birthing to minimize the risk of excessive rolling (e.g., dusting behavior) by the dam. Close observation of late-term dams can help to detect uterine torsion before harm occurs to the fetus or dam. Any dam that shows signs of colic or has prolongation of Stage 2 labor should be evaluated as soon as possible.

Recommended Reading

Anderson DE. 2009 Jul. Uterine torsion and cesarean section in llamas and alpacas. *Vet Clin North Am Food Anim Pract*; 25(2):523–38. doi:10.1016/j.cvfa.2009.02.002. PMID: 19460653.

Cebra CK, Cebra ML, Garry FB, Johnson LW. 1990–1996. Surgical and nonsurgical correction of uterine torsion in New World camelids: 20 cases. *J Amer Vet Med Assoc* 1997; 211:600–602.

Miller BA, Brounts SH, Anderson DE, Devine E. 2013. Cesarean section in alpacas and llamas: 34 cases (1997–2010). *J Amer Vet Med Assoc*; 242(5):670–674.

Pearson LK, Rodriguez JS, Tibary A. 2012. Uterine torsion in late gestation alpacas and llamas: 60 cases (2000–2009). *Small Rumin Res*; 105(1–3):268–272.

Purohit G. 2012. Dystocia in camelids: the causes and approaches of management. *Open J Anim Sci*; 2:99–105. doi:10.4236/ojas.2012.22013.

Section XII

Male Genital Anatomy

59

Male Genitalia Anatomical Comments and Breeding Behavior and Soundness

David E. Anderson

Purpose or Indication for Procedure

Male llamas and alpacas (also known as studs or machos) have important similarities and differences from other livestock. Anatomical examination of males is most often done immediately after birth to establish viability and normalcy; males also are routinely examined when potential future sires are being selected and when males are being used for breeding services. Breeding soundness examinations are most often performed immediately prior to or following sire sales. Male alpacas are frequently presented to the veterinarian for evaluation after they have failed to successfully breed multiple females or females fail to achieve a pregnancy after breeding.

Equipment Needed

Sedation and restraint chute are needed.

Restraint/Position

Standing, sternal recumbency, and lateral recumbency positions may be used.

Technical Description of Procedure/Method

Male llama and alpaca genital anatomy is most similar to ruminants. The scrotum of camelids is not pendulous, but rather is positioned horizontally in the perineal region and has a broad base of attachment to the perineal skin. The testicles can be oriented vertically or horizontally depending on ambient temperature. During summer months, the scrotum becomes more pendulous in an attempt to improve thermoregulation of the testicles. The penis is covered by a sheath and prepuce, which is attached to the penis at the fornix (Figure 59.1). The penis is fibrovascular in structure, and therefore, the diameter and length of the penis does not change. The position of the penis is dictated by its rigidity, which changes with engorgement of the vascular channels of the corpus cavernosus penis (CCP) and corpus spongiosus penis (CSP). When the penis is not engorged, it is withdrawn within the sheath by the retractor penis muscles resulting in an S-shaped sigmoid flexure (Figure 59.2). The sigmoid flexure is positioned cranial to the scrotum and medial to the limbs. The sigmoid flexure most often lies horizontally or diagonally. Engorgement of the CCP and CSP results in straightening of the penis and rigid erection for

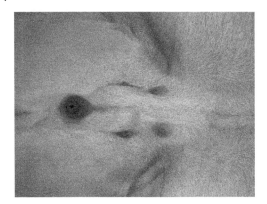

Figure 59.1 The penis and prepuce are retracted and entirely covered by the sheath when not breeding.

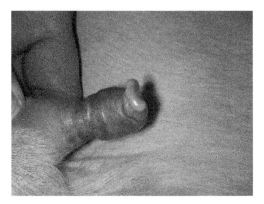

Figure 59.3 Extension of the penis and prepuce from the sheath in an alpaca. The glans penis (*diamond*) and cartilagenous process (*solid arrow*), prepuce (*star*), and sheath with preputial orifice (*circle*) are seen.

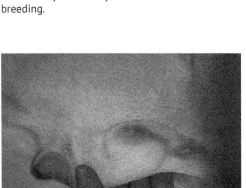

Figure 59.2 Retraction of the flaccid fibrovascular penis results in the formation of a sigmoid flexure in the penis. This is located along the ventral midline ventral to the pelvis.

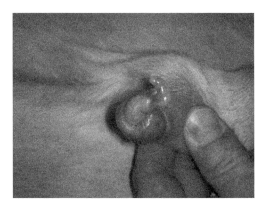

Figure 59.4 The cartilaginous process (*solid arrow*) serves to facilitate intromission of the penis through the cervix during breeding. The urethral opening (*open arrow*) is located at the base of this process.

breeding activity. The tip of the penis in composed of the glans penis, cartilagenous process, and urethral opening (Figure 59.3). In camelids, the urethra opens on the glans penis near the base of the cartilaginous process, unlike sheep and goats in which the urethra is contained within the vermiform process and opens at the tip of that process (Figure 59.4).

Llamas and alpacas have two prominent, paired accessory sex glands: bulbourethral and prostate. The bulbourethral glands are spherical structures located dorsal and lateral to the pelvic urethra at the level of the ischial arch. These glands are found immediately cranial to the anus and bulbospongiosus muscles. The bulbourethral gland has a duct that empties the secretions into the urethral diverticulum during ejaculation. The urethral diverticulum is a blind pouch extension of the urethra and is located caudal to the ischial arch and extends from the caudal margin of the urethra. A "flap" of urethral mucosa prevents retrograde flow of secretions, semen, and urine. For this reason, the bladder cannot be catheterized retrograde from the tip of the penis in the vast majority of males. The bilobed prostate glands are located immediately caudal to the vas deferens and trigone region of the bladder. These glands are oval in shape and extend dorsal and lateral from the dorsal surface of the pelvic urethra. These glands should be symmetrical and ultrasound measurements of their dimensions should be within 10% of the contralateral gland.

Libido (Breeding Behavior and Aggressiveness)

Many factors can adversely affect breeding behavior, and these often make evaluation of libido difficult. Breeder data on duration of breeding is useful for evaluation of changes in libido. Overuse of males decreases semen quality and may decrease conception rates. Breeding studs may show different behaviors in a pasture breeding setting as opposed to those males that are housed separately from females. Studs that are cohabitated with the herd may exhibit more seasonality in breeding activities. Through the use of pasture breeding, studs will be less aggressive and may be more selective of the females that they breed. Breeding studs that are exclusively used in hand-mating scenarios will often demonstrate more aggressive libido. During breeding, the male will sit down behind the female with the hind limbs completely flexed and resting on the surface of the foot pads and hocks. As the stud sits behind the female, he will "clasp" her around the neck with his front limbs. This action provides a neural stimulus to the female, which helps induce ovulation of a mature follicle. The macho will emit variable sounds during breeding termed orgling. As the male inserts his penis through the cervix, he will begin to thrust the rear quarters, termed "ejaculatory thrusts." Duration of copulation in llamas and alpacas typically ranges from 10 to 60 minutes. Short duration breeding times may decrease the probability of conception.

Practice Tip to Facilitate Procedure

Few texts are available for study of detailed anatomy of the male genitalia. The examiner can develop familiarity with normal structures and examination procedures of the male alpaca by studying normal males at commercial breeding farms.

Potential Complications

Overuse of breeding males may cause transient subfertility. Also, males may suffer debilitating musculoskeletal problems such as vertebral spondylitis/arthritis.

Patient Monitoring/Aftercare

No patient monitoring or aftercare is required except for sedation protocols.

Recommended Reading

Bravo PW, Solis P, Ordonez C, Alarcon V. 1997. Fertility of the male alpaca: effect of daily consecutive breeding. *Animal Reproduction Science*; 46:305–312.

Johnson LW. 1989 Mar. Llama reproduction. *Vet Clin North Am Food Anim Pract*; 5(1):159–82. doi: 10.1016/s0749-0720(15)31008-2. PMID: 2647232.

Lichtenwalner AB, Woods GL, Weber JA. 1998. Male llama choice between receptive and nonreceptive females. *Applied Animal Behavior Science*; 59:349–356.

Sumar J. 1994. Effects of various ovulation induction stimuli in alpacas and llamas. *Journal of Arid Environments*; 26:39–45.

Tibary A, Campbell A, Rodriguez JS, Ruiz AJ, Patino C, Ciccarelli M. 2021. Investigation of male and female infertility in llamas and alpacas. *Reproduction, Fertility and Development*; 33(2):20–30.

Tibary A, Ruiz A. 2018. "Investigation of male infertility in llamas and alpacas." *Spermova*.

Tibary A, Vaughan J. 2006. Reproductive physiology and infertility in male South American camelids: a review and clinical observations. *Small Ruminant Research*; 61(2–3):283–298.

60

Examination of the Penis and Prepuce
David E. Anderson

Purpose or Indication for Procedure

Examination of the penis and prepuce may be done as part of a pre-breeding examination or because of subfertility. This examination is also performed as part of a diagnostic examination in response to changes in urination (e.g., dysuria, stranguria). Although uncommon, preputial and penile trauma has been observed to occur.

Equipment Needed

The following equipment is needed: gloves, gauze pads, sedation, and a 3.5, 5, and 8 French red rubber catheter.

Restraint/Position

Lateral recumbency with sedation or general anesthesia is used.

Technical Description of Procedure/Method

A complete examination of external genitalia should include palpation of the sheath, examination of the prepuce and penis, and palpation of the scrotum, testicles, epididymis, and spermatic cords (Figure 60.1). Full extension of the penis and prepuce is required to confirm normalcy. This can be done during breeding of a female or after heavy sedation and with the male in lateral recumbency. Some males require general anesthesia in order to allow complete examination of the penis and prepuce (Figure 60.2). The preputial epithelium and frenulum should be fully separated from the penis by 36 months old in llamas and alpacas. In most males, this separation has occurred by 18 to 24 months (about 70% of males), and in some males this has occurred at 12 months age (about 10% of males).

Camelids have a fibrovascular penis that is retained within the sheath by the retractor penis muscles (Figure 60.3). This is accomplished by the formation of a sigmoid flexure when the non-engorged penis is retracted. The urethra courses along the ventral margin of the penis and can be identified by careful palpation of a groove, or depression, in the fibrous sheath of the corpus spongiosum penis. The tip of the free end of the penis includes the glans penis and a cartilaginous projection (Figure 60.4). This cartilaginous projection has a spiral curve to it, and the urethral opening is found on the tip of the glans penis close to the base of this cartilage (Figure 60.5). Note: the urethra in llamas and alpacas opens at the tip of the glans penis as these species do not have a urethral process

Veterinary Techniques in Llamas and Alpacas, Second Edition. Edited by David E. Anderson, Matt Miesner, and Meredyth Jones.
© 2023 John Wiley & Sons, Inc. Published 2023 by John Wiley & Sons, Inc.

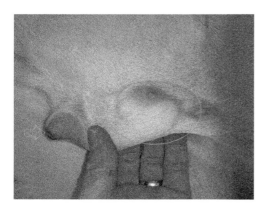

Figure 60.1 The penis and prepuce are retracted and entirely covered by the sheath when not breeding. The preputial orifice (*arrow*) is closed and represents the junction of the external sheath and the prepuce. Retraction of the flaccid fibrovascular penis results in the formation of a sigmoid flexure (*circle*) in the penis. This is located along the ventral midline ventral to the pelvis.

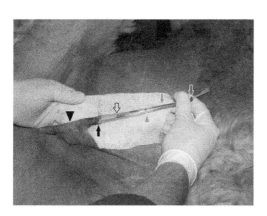

Figure 60.2 Complete extension of the penis and prepuce from the sheath in an alpaca. The glans penis and cartilaginous process (*open yellow arrow*), prepuce (*solid orange arrow*), fornix (preputial attachment to the penis; *solid orange triangle*), prepuce (*open black arrow*), preputial orifice (*solid black arrow*), and sheath (*solid black triangle*) are seen. A polyurethane catheter is in place to demonstrate the location of the urethral opening.

as is seen in sheep and goats. The prepuce is attached to the penis at the fornix.

When the penis is retracted within the sheath, the examiner can clearly evaluate the preputial orifice and sheath and can palpate the penis, sigmoid flexure, and retractor penis

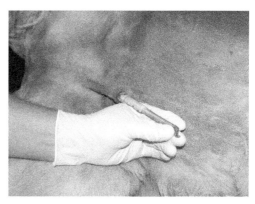

Figure 60.3 The fibrovascular penis is flaccid when not engorged and tightly erect during engorgement for breeding.

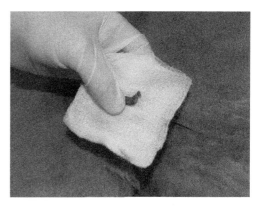

Figure 60.4 The cartilagenous process serves to guide the penis through the cervix and into the uterine body. Ejaculation takes place within the uterine horns of the female during breeding.

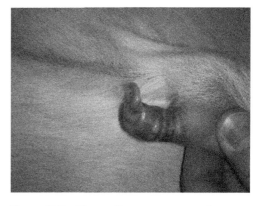

Figure 60.5 The cartilagenous process of the penis in llamas and alpacas is spiral in shape.

muscles. When the penis is fully extended, the examiner can clearly identify the glans penis and free portion of the penis, the fornix, the prepuce, the preputial orifice, and the sheath. Careful palpation of the penis allows identification of the paired retractor penis muscles attached to the penis at the level of the distal sigmoid flexure and coursing caudal and dorsal to their attachment at the ischial arches of the pelvis. The penis, prepuce, and sheath should be freely movable.

Practice Tip to Facilitate Procedure

Palpation of the penis and prepuce can be performed during mounting and breeding of a receptive female. However, this approach allows only a limited view and access and therefore does not provide a thorough examination. When concerns arise regarding injury or disease of the penis or prepuce, sedation or general anesthesia is recommended to facilitate the exam. In cases where the penis cannot be extended, preputial endoscopy can be used to examine the interior of the preputial cavity and the free portion of the penis. Ultrasonography is useful to examine the penis and associated tissues caudal to the fornix and when extension cannot be achieved. Air within the preputial cavity limits ultrasound examination of the prepuce and free portion of the penis when retracted.

Potential Complications

Damage to the penis or prepuce during forced extension may occur.

Patient Monitoring/Aftercare

Males should be monitored for straining to urinate, swelling in the area surrounding the sheath, and discharge from the prepuce for 24 hours after completion of the examination.

Recommended Reading

Gariépy A, Desrochers A, Guarnieri E, Torabi A, Francoz D. 2022 Sep. Surgical treatment of a paraphimosis in a castrated alpaca secondary to a preputial avulsion. *Can Vet J*; 63(9):943-946. PMID: 36060489; PMCID: PMC9377188.

Timm KI, Watrous BJ. 1988 Apr 1. Urethral recess in two male llamas. *J Am Vet Med Assoc*; 192(7):937-938. PMID: 3366683.

61

Examination of Accessory Sex Glands

David E. Anderson

Purpose or Indication for Procedure

Accessory glands most often are examined as part of a breeding soundness examination of sub-fertile males. These glands may also be examined as part of a prepurchase exam or, in the case of the prostate glands, as part of workup for dysuria. Although uncommon, idiopathic prostatomegaly, prostatic abscess, prostatic cysts, and prostatitis have been observed in alpacas and llamas.

Equipment Needed

Examination gloves, lubricant, sedation, and ultrasound with rectolinear probe (7.5 to 10 MHz) are needed.

Restraint/Position

Standing or sternal recumbency positions, restraint in a chute, and sedation, if needed, may be used.

Technical Description of Procedure/Method

Llamas and alpacas have two prominent and paired accessory sex glands: bulbourethral and prostate. Seminal vesicles are not present in camelids.

Bulbourethral Glands

The bulbourethral glands are spherical structures located dorsal and lateral to the pelvic urethra at the level of the ischial arch. These glands are found immediately cranial to the anus and bulbospongiosus muscles and can be palpated using the fingers of a gloved and lubricated hand. The bulbourethral gland has a duct that empties its secretions into the urethral diverticulum during ejaculation. The urethral diverticulum is a blind pouch extension of the urethra and is located caudal to the ischial arch and extends from the caudal margin of the urethra. A "flap" of urethral mucosa prevents retrograde flow of secretions, semen, and urine. For this reason, the bladder normally cannot be catheterized retrograde from the tip of the penis. High frequency ultrasound probes (7.5 to 10 MHz) are desirable for evaluation of these glands so that higher resolution images can be obtained. During ultrasound examination, the bulbourethral glands appear to have a homogenous soft tissue density (Figure 61.1). The bulbospongiosus muscle encircles the caudal half of the gland and appears hypoechoic in comparison. This creates the appearance of a crescent moon shape around that portion of the glands. The glands are symmetrical spheres and measure approximately 1 cm in diameter (Table 61.1). Size asymmetry of up to 10% is acceptable for each gland if the echotexture is normal. Although rare, bulbourethral

Veterinary Techniques in Llamas and Alpacas, Second Edition. Edited by David E. Anderson, Matt Miesner, and Meredyth Jones.
© 2023 John Wiley & Sons, Inc. Published 2023 by John Wiley & Sons, Inc.

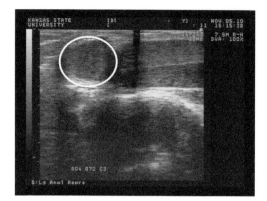

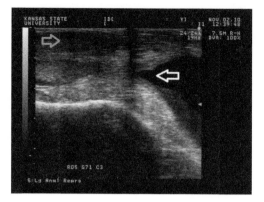

Figure 61.1 The bulbourethral glands are located immediately dorsal to the ischial arch and cranial to the anal sphincter. The glands are recognized by their spherical shape and homogeneous echotexture.

Figure 61.2 The prostate glands are located within the pelvic canal and caudal to the trigone of the bladder and attachment of the vas deferens. The trigone (*open white arrow*) is most easily recognized when the bladder contains a sufficient volume urine. The prostate is homogeneous in echotexture and caudal to the trigone.

cysts and focal mineralized lesions have been observed in the gland parenchyma. The clinical significance of these lesions is unknown.

Prostate Glands

The bilobed prostate glands are located immediately caudal to the attachment of the vas deferens to the pelvic urethra caudal to the trigone region of the bladder (Figure 61.2). These glands are oval in shape and extend dorsal and lateral from the dorsal surface of the pelvic urethra. These glands have a broad base and can be difficult to measure accurately, but the prostate glands should be symmetrical and ultrasound

measurements of their dimensions within 10% of the contralateral gland (Table 61.1). The prostate can, occasionally, be evaluated by palpation. More often, ultrasound examination via the rectum is required. High frequency ultrasound probes (7.5 to 10 MHz) are desirable for this evaluation so that higher resolution images can be obtained. In alpacas, a rectal linear ultrasound probe can usually be inserted through the anal sphincter far enough to visualize the glands. In llamas, the probe may need to be controlled via rectal palpation or fitted to a rigid extender (50-cm long), such as a molded PVC

Table 61.1 Mean bulbourethral (BU) gland and prostate gland size in the alpaca.

Age (years)	BU length (cm)	BU width (cm)	Prostate length (cm)	Prostate width (cm)
1	0.8	0.5	1.5	1
2	1.1	0.8	2.1	1.4
3	1.5	0.9	2.7	1.9
4	1.6	0.9	2.6	2.1
5	1.9	0.9	2.7	2.1

Adapted from Bravo 2002, Chapter 4, page 51.

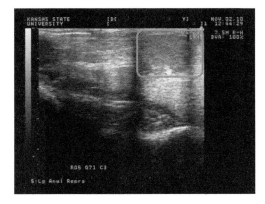

Figure 61.3 The bilobed prostate should be symmetrical with minimal (<10%) difference in width or length between the right and left lobes. The prostate glands have a homogenous echotexture and collecting ducts often can be detected during ultrasonography.

tube, so that the probe can be inserted through the rectum far enough for complete examination. These glands should be assessed for symmetry, size, and tissue echotexture. The glands should be homogeneous in nature, and the prostatic duct can often be visualized coursing through the center of the gland and connecting to the pelvic urethra (Figure 61.3). The pelvic urethra and bladder also are examined at this time. Camelids, especially alpacas, can suffer prostatitis, prostatic abscesses, prostatic cysts, and idiopathic prostatomegaly.

Practice Tip to Facilitate Procedure

Sedation is suggested for transrectal examination of males. This will minimize the risk of inadvertent damage to the rectum during palpation or rigid probe insertion. Ample lubricant should be utilized to increase the safety of this procedure.

A combination of lidocaine and obstetrical lubricant (50 mL lubricant + 5 mL lidocaine HCl 2%) has been used to improve the comfort and safety of transrectal ultrasonography in camelids. Infusing the mixture into the rectum with a syringe prior to probe insertion enhances clinical visualization and patient comfort.

Potential Complications

Rectal trauma may occur.

Patient Monitoring/Aftercare

The patient should be monitored for abdominal discomfort (e.g., colic), rectal bleeding, or straining to urinate.

Recommended Reading

Bravo PW 2002. *The reproductive process of South American Camelids*. Salt Lake City, Utah. Seagull Printing, pp. 57–61.

Gray GA, Dascanio JJ, Kasimanickam R, Sponenberg DP. 2007. Bilateral epidiymal cysts in an alpaca male used for breeding. *The Canadian Veterinary Journal*; 48(7):741.

TIBARY A, 2022. Applied Animal Andrology: camelids. *Manual of Animal Andrology*, p.120.

Tibary A, Campbell A, Rodriguez JS, Ruiz AJ, Patino C, Ciccarelli M. 2021. Investigation of male and female infertility in llamas and alpacas. Reproduction. *Fertility and Development*; 33(2):20–30.

62

Examination of the Scrotum and Testicles

David E. Anderson

Purpose or Indication for Procedure

Examination of the scrotum, testicles, and epididymides is most commonly performed during sire selection, pre-breeding examination, and around the time of sale of herd sires. The size, symmetry, texture, and mobility of these structures are important components of the examination. Diseases of the scrotum and testicles can include inguinal hernia, cryptorchidism, orchitis, epididymitis, paradidymal cysts, testicular neoplasia, hematoma, hypoplasia, and testicular degeneration.

Equipment Needed

Gloves, lubricant, alcohol, ultrasound machine, and transducer are needed.

Restraint/Position

Standing, sternal recumbency, and lateral recumbency positions may be used.

Technical Description of Procedure/Method

The male to be examined is placed into a camelid chute or contained between solid barriers. The tail is lifted and the scrotum and each individual structure palpated. Sedation may be required for thorough examination in uncooperative males or when a disease condition is painful to palpation.

Llama and alpaca males should have both testicles descended into the scrotum at the time of birth. Although failure to be present at birth could be considered a form of cryptorchidism, the testicles are extremely small and may be difficult to distinguish at this time. Identification is easily performed by weaning age (4 to 6 months) at which time a presumptive diagnosis of cryptorchidism can be made.

Mature (3 years old or older) male alpacas should have testicles that are approximately 3.0-cm long and 2.5-cm wide, each (Table 62.1). Male llamas should have testicular dimensions of approximately 5-cm long and 3-cm wide. Males having smaller testicles may be at increased risk of having reduced testicular volume; smaller testicles have been associated with low daily sperm output in multiple species. The testicles and epididymides should be equal in size and firmness. In cool weather, the testicles are held upright along the vertical perineum. In warmer weather, the scrotum elongates to aid in thermoregulation, and this causes ventral displacement of the testicles, which then rest in a more horizontal plane. In the vertically positioned testicle, the epididymides are found on the cranial and medial aspect of the testes. The head of the epididymis is located at the ventral end of the

Veterinary Techniques in Llamas and Alpacas, Second Edition. Edited by David E. Anderson, Matt Miesner, and Meredyth Jones.

Table 62.1 Mean testicular size and testosterone concentrations by age in llamas and alpacas.

Age (months)	Llama size (cm)	Testosterone (pg/mL)	Alpaca size (cm)	Testosterone (pg/mL)
6	2.1 × 1.4	120	1.0 × 0.4	67
12	3.4 × 2.3	150	2.3 × 1.5	213
18	3.5 × 2.6	140	2.8 × 1.9	1156
24	3.9 × 2.3	500	3.3 × 2.2	2163
30	4.4 × 2.5	600	3.6 × 2.4	2835
36	4.5 × 2.7	800	2.6 × 2.4	5385
Sires	5.4 × 3.3	1000	3.7 × 2.5	5247

Adapted from Bravo 2002, Chapter 4, page 49.

testes, the body courses along the median aspect of the testes, and the tail of the epididymis is positioned at the dorsal aspect of the testis. In the horizontal testicle, the epididymides are found on the dorsal and medial aspect of the testes. The head of the epididymis is located at the cranial end of the testes, the body courses along the median aspect of the testes, and the tail of the epididymis is positioned at the caudal aspect of the testes.

Ultrasonography of the scrotum can be done using a sector scan probe or a linear array probe. High MHz probes are desired to increase the resolution of the tissues being imaged. Care should be taken to identify and assess each structure. The testicles should reveal a homogenous tissue texture on ultrasound. Hyperechoic (brighter on the image) or hypoechoic (darker on the image) lesions in the testicles or epididymides may indicate trauma, infection, cysts, or other abnormal conditions that may affect fertility. A diseased testicle may cause suppression of the normal testicle so that the fertility of the male is impaired. The head and tail region of the epididymis can be identified by the cluster of tubules. The tubules are recognized as multiple hypoechoic foci arranged in a concentric area at each end of the testicle. The body of the epididymis is difficult to follow and assess.

Testicular biopsy or fine needle aspiration can be performed to assess ultrastructure and determine prognosis for fertility. The procedures are not recommended to be done on the epididmi because of the risk of fibrosis and obstruction of the tubules. However, these procedures can be successfully done on the testicles with minimal risk. Biopsy of the testicle allows for histopathologic examination of the tissue architecture. This aids in establishment of prognosis by examination of the germinal epithelium. Fine needle aspirates provide samples sufficient to establish if active spermatogenesis is occurring and to allow for culture of the tissues when orchitis is suspected.

Practice Tip to Facilitate Procedure

Alcohol is used to soak the skin of the scrotum before lubricant is applied to facilitate ultrasound probe contact and eliminate artifacts.

Potential Complications

Injury to testicle from aggressive handling in uncooperative males may occur.

Patient Monitoring/Aftercare

No patient monitoring or aftercare is required.

Recommended Reading

Abraham MC, Puhakka J, Ruete A, Al-Essawe EM, De Verdier K, Morrell JM, Båge R. 2015. Testicular length as an indicator of the onset of sperm production in alpacas under Swedish conditions. *Acta Veterinaria Scandinavica*; 58(1):1–8.

Bravo PW 2002. *The reproductive process of South American Camelids*. Salt Lake City, Utah. Seagull Printing, 57–61.

Stelletta C, Juyena NS, Salazar DP, Ruiz J, Gutierrez G. 2011. Testicular cytology of alpaca: comparison between impressed and smeared slides. *Animal Reproduction Science*; 125(1–4):133–137.

Tibary A, Vaughan J. 2006. Reproductive physiology and infertility in male South American camelids: a review and clinical observations. *Small Ruminant Research*; 61(2–3):283–298.

63

Semen Collection and Evaluation

David E. Anderson

Purpose or Indication for Procedure

Semen is most often collected as part of a breeding soundness examination. As alternative reproductive technologies such as artificial insemination and *in vitro* fertilization become accepted in the industry, semen collection may be requested to fulfill these needs. Semen collection in alpacas and llamas is far more challenging than similar procedures in cattle, sheep, or goats. However, this is a vital component of the breeding soundness examination of males. Collection and evaluation of semen in young male camelids is usually not done until normal penile extension is achieved. Young male alpacas should reach full mating ability by the time they are 3 years old. The frenulum connecting the penis to the prepuce begins to break down starting at around 12 months old and is completely disrupted by 18 to 24 months old. The frenulum may be retained up to 36 months in some males. Although breeding maturity is most often attained by 36 months old, some males do not become active breeders until they are 4 to 5 years old. The significance of late onset sexual maturity is not known.

Artificial breeding technologies offer the advantages of improved herd biosecurity. Also, artificial breeding technologies offer the advantage of dissemination of superior genetics. Provided that appropriate, consistent, and reliable genetic or phenotypic standards are identified, these genetics may be marketed without the risks associated with animal transportation and with fewer obstacles for importation and exportation of genetics. Frozen semen or embryos may be able to be stored indefinitely for preservation of genetic materials.

Equipment Needed

The following equipment is needed: vaginal speculum, vaginal speculum illumination source, glass slides, slide warmer, microscope, AI pipette or polyurethane catheter (10 F), syringe (20-mL Luer tip; 60-mL catheter tip), live/dead stain, receptive female or artificial vagina system, electroejaculator, sperm morphology counter, semen collection and processing tubes, general anesthesia for electroejaculation.

Restraint/Position

Natural service breeding posture (mounting followed by cushing) and lateral recumbency for electroejaculation may be used.

Veterinary Techniques in Llamas and Alpacas, Second Edition. Edited by David E. Anderson, Matt Miesner, and Meredyth Jones.

Technical Description of Procedure/Method

A variety of methods have been employed to collect semen from llamas and alpacas including the use of live, receptive females, mannequin females housing artificial vaginas, and electro-ejaculation under general anesthesia. Semen samples have been recovered from receptive females by aspiration of seminal fluids from the cranial vagina and cervix, vaginal inserts, vaginal sponges, and hand held artificial vaginas. The most reliable method yielding the highest quality samples have been collected via a mannequin female with an artificial vagina warmed to the appropriate temperature and equipped with a stricture that is made to resemble a natural cervix. However, aspiration of seminal fluids from receptive females immediately after coitus is the most common technique used because these devices are not readily available.

Aspiration of seminal fluids from the cranial vaginal vault and cervix is the most common method for semen collection when performing breeding soundness examination (Figures 63.1 and 63.2, Video 63.1: Llama semen collection). This method of collection yields a mixed sample

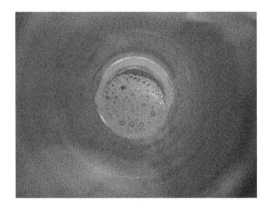

Figure 63.2 Seminal fluids pooled in the cranial vagina of a llama female 5 minutes after copulation with a male llama.

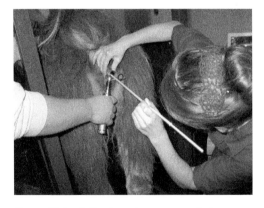

Figure 63.1 Collection of semen sample by aspiration of seminal fluids from the cranial vagina immediately caudal to the cervix. Vaginoscopy is performed to identify sample pool; AI pipette is used to aspirate the sample for examination.

of seminal fluids, vaginal debris, and blood. Blood is often present in the female's vagina after copulation and is associated with bruising of the vagina and cervix. Thus, the semen sample obtained is usually of low volume, low sperm cell concentration, and of inconsistent quality. In this method, the male to be examined is allowed to breed a receptive female llama or alpaca. A vaginal examination of the female should be done before the male is allowed to breed so that the vagina can be verified to be free of discharge or other contaminants. The male is allowed to breed until he voluntarily dismounts the female. In most cases, breeding can be disrupted after 30 minutes. The female is allowed to stand and is prepared for vaginal speculum examination. During this time (5 to 10 minutes), post-coitus uterine contractions will expel some of the seminal fluids that the male has deposited in the uterus. Seminal fluids can be harvested by the vaginal speculum if a sufficient volume of fluid is present (>1 mL) or aspirated by passing an AI pipette through the speculum and applying suction with a 20-mL syringe. A single drop of semen is placed directly on a warmed slide for immediate assessment of viability and motility. If there is sufficient volume, the sample is placed in a warmed vial and agitated to attempt to separate sperm cells from the highly viscous gel fraction of the semen.

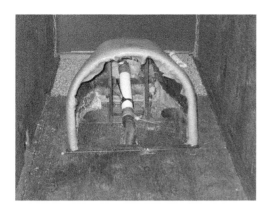

Figure 63.3 Artificial vagina (AV) designed to be placed on top of the rear quarters of a cushed female during breeding. The male's penis is diverted into the AV unit after mounting the female and achieving sternal recumbency.

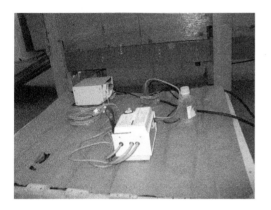

Figure 63.4 A warm water blanket or similar heating system is used to prevent cold-shock of the semen samples during the collection period.

Video available online

[[img]]Go to www.wiley.com/go/anderson veterinary to view videos of these procedures.

Artificial vaginas (AV) have been used to attempt semen collection in llamas and alpacas (Figures 63.3, 63.4, and 63.5). Llamas and alpacas do not readily accept AVs, and considerable effort has been expended to design systems that can be used reliably (Video 63.1). Various types of mannequins have been used, and these devices are most often covered with a tanned hide from a female llama or alpaca. These designs include various types of artificial vaginas mounted within the mannequin.

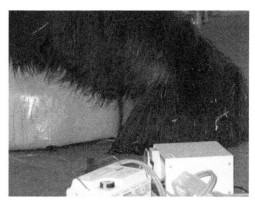

Figure 63.5 Male llama mounted unto AV unit with adjacent warm water system.

These AVs often include an artificial cervix to provide penile stimulation (camelids are intrauterine ejaculators) and appropriate heating pads or warm water systems to keep the AV warm through the extended copulation period. Artificial vaginas provide the most representative semen sample, and these samples have the greatest sperm cell concentration and are of the highest quality compared with all other semen collection techniques. Unfortunately, the significant time and expense as well as the poor mobility of these systems have limited their adoption among veterinarians and breeders.

Electroejaculation (EEJ) is often used as a method of last resort for semen collection. EEJ must be done with the male anesthetized and does not consistently yield a sufficient sample to allow thorough assessment of potential fertility. Further, EEJ often causes concomitant dilution and contamination of the semen with urine. This procedure is performed after induction of general anesthesia using a short duration injectable regimen. The male is laid in lateral recumbency and 120 mL obstetrical lubricant is inserted into the rectum. Then, a small ruminant electroejaculator (ram probe) is inserted into the rectum with the electrical conducting elements positioned ventrally overlying the pelvic urethra (Figure 63.6). The stimulation pulses (rate, duration, rhythm) can be applied using a predetermined program

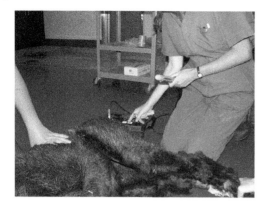

Figure 63.6   Ram electroejaculator ready for use to collect semen from an alpaca. The alpaca is anesthetized using short duration injectable anesthesia for the procedure.

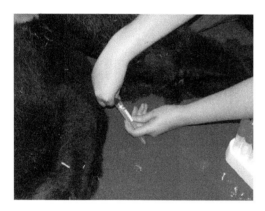

Figure 63.7   During electroejaculation under general anesthesia, the penis is extended and held during sample collection.

or can be adjusted based on the erection and extension or the penis or the ability to stimulate ejection of seminal fluids. A warmed sample collection vial is held over the glans penis and the sample collected and processed as described above (Figure 63.7).

Semen Evaluation

The semen sample is evaluated for volume, consistency, and color. Then a representative sample is examined microscopically and assessed for motility and morphology of the sperm cells. The motility of semen varies by collection technique. In normal males, samples successfully collected by electroejaculation are expected to yield better motility (>50%) estimates as compared with that typically appreciated after vaginal aspiration (motility often < 50%). Sperm cell motility is best assessed in samples obtained by artificial vagina (usually > 75%). Normal sperm cell morphology in breeding sound males varies considerably in samples collected by vaginal aspiration and by EEJ. Normal sperm morphology would be expected to be > 70% in samples collected by AV, whereas samples harvested via vaginal aspiration or EEJ often have approximately 50% normal sperm cells. These differences are attributed to dilution and contamination of the sample, entrapment of live, normal sperm cells in the gel fraction of the semen, and handling artifacts. Abnormal sperm cell morphology noted upon microscopic examination may include malformed sperm cell heads, midpiece defects, cytoplasmic droplets, detached heads, and a variety of sperm cell tail defects.

Semen characteristics include color, motility, concentration, percent live/dead, and morphology. The color tends to be milky white and very viscous. Motility is difficult to evaluate because of the gel-like consistency of the semen. Motility should be evaluated using a warm slide, and the ejaculate should be spread thin to get a more accurate observation of motility. Concentration can be measured with a hemocytometer, and the percentage of live and dead sperm can be evaluated after staining with a live/dead stain. In this stain, sperm cells that are dead at the time of staining will take up the stain and appear dark microscopically. Live cells resist stain uptake and appear white or clear during microscopic examination. The proportion of sperm cells expected to be alive at the time of staining ranges from 50 to 90% in normal males. Abnormal morphology is classified into primary and secondary defects of the sperm cells. These defects include tail abnormalities, head abnormalities, and cytoplasmic droplet retention. Abnormal sperm cells should not represent more than 40% of the cells examined.

Practice Tip to Facilitate Procedure

Availability of a receptive female greatly facilitates semen collection for evaluation. Motility and morphology must be cautiously interpreted in these samples, but the consistency and ease of collection far exceeds that of electro-ejaculation. For EEJ, depth of anesthesia has an important effect on the success rate of this procedure. Samples are most easily harvested from males that are more deeply anesthetized.

Potential Complications

The most common issue is failure to obtain a diagnostic sample. Caution should be exercised in the performance of EEJ so as not to damage the rectum.

Patient Monitoring/Aftercare

Monitor males for colic, straining to defecate, and straining to urinate.

Recommended Reading

Abraham MC, de Verdier K, Båge R, Morrell JM. 2017. Semen collection methods in alpacas. *Veterinary Record*; 180(25):613–614.

Bravo PW. 1994. Reproductive endocrinology of llamas and alpacas. *Vet. Clin. North Am.: Food Anim. Pract.*; 10:265–279.

Bravo PW 2002. *The reproductive process of South American Camelids*. Salt Lake City, Utah. Seagull Printing, 57–61.

Bravo PW, Flores U, Garnica J, Ordonez C. 1997. Collection of semen and artificial insemination of Alpacas. *Theriogenology*; 47:619.

Brown BW. 2000. A review on reproduction in South American camelids. *Anim. Reproduction Sciences*; 58:169–195.

Del Campo MR, Del Campo CH, Adams GP, Mapletoft RJ 1995. *The application of new reproductive technologies to South American Camelids*. Butterworth Heinemann.

Garnica J, Achata R, Bravo PW. 1993. Physical and biochemical characteristics of alpaca semen. *Animal Reproduction Science*; 32(1–2):85–90.

Morton KM., Thomson PC, Bailey K, Evans G, Maxwell WMC. 2010. Quality parameters for alpaca (Vicugna pacos) semen are affected by semen collection procedure. *Reproduction in Domestic Animals*; 45(4):637–643.

Szymkowicz P, Purdy SR, 2012. Semen collection, evaluation, artificial insemination, and correlation of semen parameters with pregnancies in alpacas. *University of Massachusetts, Amherst, Commonwealth College Honors Research Thesis*.

Vaughan J, Galloway D, Hopkins D. 2003. Artificial insemination in alpacas (Lama pacos). *Rural Industries Research and Development Corporation, Kingston, ACT, Australia*; 1(2):3.

Walter Bravo P, Flores D, Ordoñez C. 1997. Effect of repeated collection on semen characteristics of alpacas. *Biology of Reproduction*; 57(3):520–524.

64

Castration
Meredyth L. Jones

Purpose or Indication for Procedure

Castration is performed to remove non-breeding quality males from the breeding population and prevent aggressive behavior.

Equipment Needed

The following equipment is needed: clippers, gauze, iodine or betadine preparation solution, isopropyl alcohol, sedation, 2% lidocaine, Kelly hemostats, needle driver, thumb forceps, scalpel blade and handle, and absorbable suture (#2–0 to 0). Tetanus prophylaxis and perioperative antimicrobials should be considered. White's emasculators are optional.

Restraint/Position

The first option is chute restraint with standing sedation, and the second option is lateral recumbency with heavy sedation or injectable anesthesia.

Technical Description of Procedure/Method

Preoperative Preparation

If possible, animals should be withheld from feed and/or water for 12 hours if sedation or anesthesia will be used for surgery. Individuals may elect to place animals on antimicrobial therapy, although the author does not routinely administer antibiotics, even in the field setting. If a tetanus toxoid has been administered in the past 6 months to the animal, it is recommended that a tetanus toxoid booster be administered at the time of surgery. If the animal has not received a tetanus toxoid or the vaccination history is unknown, the animal should receive 1,500 units of tetanus antitoxin, with subsequent toxoid administration. Analgesic agents, such as NSAIDs may be administered for perioperative analgesia.

Anesthetic Options

Camelid castration may be performed in the standing or recumbent animal. Sedation and analgesia are covered elsewhere in this text, but a common protocol used is xylazine (0.3 mg/kg IM for llamas; 0.4 mg/kg IM for alpacas) and butorphanol (0.1 mg/kg IM for llamas and alpacas) for standing castration. These drugs may be administered with ketamine (3 mg/kg IM for llamas; 4 mg/kg IM for alpacas) to achieve recumbent anesthesia.

Regardless of the systemic anesthetic protocol used, it is recommended that the scrotum be blocked with local anesthetic by injecting 1–1.5 mL 2% lidocaine into the median raphe, with an additional 1 mL injected into each spermatic cord. Alternatively, caudal epidural

Veterinary Techniques in Llamas and Alpacas, Second Edition. Edited by David E. Anderson, Matt Miesner, and Meredyth Jones.

anesthesia may be utilized, however, lidocaine and lidocaine/xylazine caudal epidurals have been shown to give inadequate analgesia for castration in alpacas (Padula 2005).

Prescrotal Approach

Prescrotal castration should be performed only in recumbent, anesthetized animals (Figure 64.1). The prescrotal region is clipped and aseptically prepared, with asepsis being more of a concern with prescrotal castration than for scrotal castration. One testicle is pushed forward into the prescrotal region. A 3- to 4-cm incision is made over the testicle on midline (Figure 64.2). The incision is continued (Figure 64.3) until the testicle and tunic can be exteriorized together and the cord separated from the scrotum and inguinal fat. (See Figure 64.4.) The spermatic cord is clamped close to the body wall with Kelly hemostats (Figure 64.5). A transfixing or encircling ligature is placed distal to the hemostats on the spermatic cord using absorbable suture material. The suture material of choice should be one that is absorbed over a short time span such as 0 polyglecaprone, 0 chromic gut, or 2–0 polyglactin 910. (See Figure 64.6.) The cord is then transected distal to the suture, grasped with thumb forceps, the hemostat is removed, and

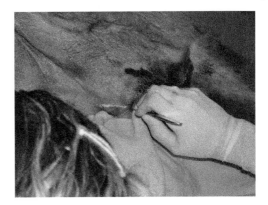

Figure 64.2 Initial midline incision into the prescrotal region. The operator's left thumb is pushing one testicle up and maintaining its position under the incision to protect the penis from accidental incision.

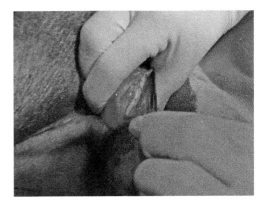

Figure 64.3 Pressure is applied under the testicle into the incision, and the incision is extended until the testicle (with tunic intact) is exteriorized.

the cord is slowly lowered into the body while monitoring for hemorrhage. The second testicle is then advanced to the same incision and exteriorized, ligated, and removed. The single incision (Figure 64.7) is then closed using the same absorbable suture in an intradermal pattern. (See Figures 64.8 and 64.9.)

Scrotal Approach

Scrotal castration may be performed in the standing or recumbent animal. The scrotum is

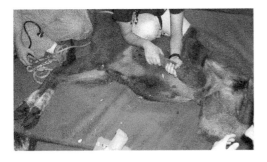

Figure 64.1 Preferred restraint position for animals under injectable field anesthesia for castration. The nose of the animal should be placed lower than the pharynx, accomplished by the placement of a towel under the neck. The upper hind limb is held by an assistant or may lay abducted in animals deeply anesthetized.

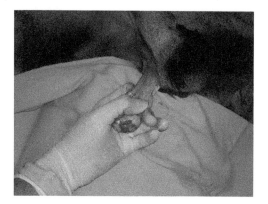

Figure 64.4 The testicle, tunic, and scrotal fat are exteriorized, and the spermatic cord is isolated.

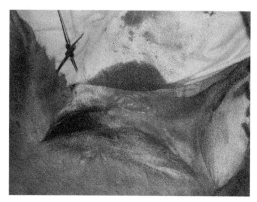

Figure 64.7 Both testicles have been removed, and the single prescrotal incision remains. Some operators will leave this incision open to heal.

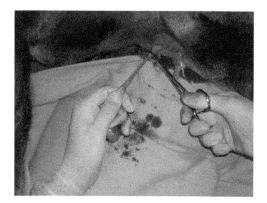

Figure 64.5 The isolated spermatic cord is clamped with Kelly hemostats near the body wall.

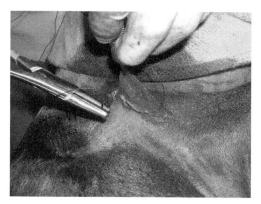

Figure 64.8 The prescrotal incision is closed using absorbable suture in an intradermal pattern.

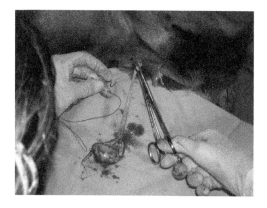

Figure 64.6 Absorbable suture material is used to place a transfixing or encircling ligature around the spermatic cord.

prepared aseptically, and incisions are made over each testicle, parallel to the median raphe along the ventral aspect of the scrotum. The incision should be made only through the scrotal skin, leaving the vaginal tunic intact. The testicle and tunic are exteriorized and freed from scrotal attachment, and the cord is clamped with Kelly hemostats. A transfixing or encircling ligature is placed distal to the hemostats on the spermatic cord using 0 polyglecaprone, 0 chromic gut, or 2–0 polyglactin 910. The cord is then transected distal to the suture, grasped with thumb forceps, the hemostat is removed, and the cord is slowly returned into

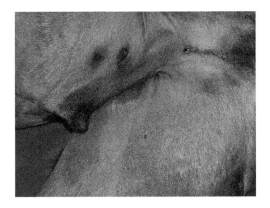

Figure 64.9 The completed, closed prescrotal castration results in an aesthetically pleasing surgical site that is not excessively attractive to flies.

the body while monitoring for hemorrhage. Emasculation with small white emasculators may be performed, but in this author's experience, the small diameter of the camelid spermatic cord does not allow for adequate hemostasis without ligation. After both testicles are removed, the scrotal incisions are left open to heal by second intent.

Comparison of Scrotal and Prescrotal Techniques

A study by Baird and colleagues (1996) compared scrotal and prescrotal techniques in llamas. Prescrotal castration was favorable in requiring less aftercare, less incisional pain, and improved aesthetics, but it did require a significantly longer operative time. Scrotal castration is a faster technique, but it may be less suitable during fly season.

Practice Tip to Facilitate Procedure

If using emasculators, it is recommended that the cords be crushed for at least 3 to 5 minutes to achieve adequate hemostasis.

Cautionary Statements

Castration should not be considered a guarantee in treating behavior in males showing aggression toward humans or other animals. In general, the older the male is at the time of castration, the less likely behavioral modification will occur. Early castration has been associated, by many camelid experts, with musculoskeletal abnormalities. These are likely caused by failure of regulation of the physes of the long bones by androgenic hormones. Clinical manifestations include tall stature, overly straight conformation, patellar luxation, angular limb deformity, and degenerative joint disease. As a precaution, castration is not recommended in llamas younger than 18 to 24 months old and in alpacas younger than 12 to 18 months old.

Potential Complications

Anesthetic complications, hemorrhage, incisional infection, scirrous cord, and tetanus may occur.

Patient Monitoring/Aftercare

Fly spray should be applied during fly season. Animals do not need to be confined, but the incision should be monitored and animals encouraged to walk to minimize swelling.

Recommended Reading

Baird AN, Pugh DG, Wenzel JGW, Lin HC. 1996. Comparison of two castration techniques for castration of llamas. *J Am Vet Med Assoc*; 208(2):261–262.

Barrington GM, Meyer TF, Parish SM. 1993. Standing castration of the llama using butorphanol tartrate and local anesthesia. *Equine Practice*; 15(5):35–39.

Dargatz DA, Johnson LW. 1997. Castrating the llama: a step-by-step guide. *Vet Med*; 625–627. Padula AM. 2005. Clinical evaluation of caudal epidural anaesthesia for the neutering of alpacas. *Vet Rec*; 156:616–617.

Pugh DG, Baird AN, Wolfe DF, Wenzel JGW, Lin HC. 1994. A prescrotal castration technique for llamas. *Equine Practice*; 16(4):26–28.

Section XIII

Nervous System

65

Neurological Examination and Anatomy

Meredyth L. Jones and Matt D. Miesner

Camelids frequently present to veterinarians for ataxia, head tilt, recumbency or other potential neurologic manifestations. In all cases, a systematic neurologic evaluation should be performed and lesion localization used to refine the list of differential diagnoses (Table 65.1).

Information regarding the number of animals involved on the farm, nutrition and water access, exposure to other species, breeding activity, vaccination and anthelmintic use, previous medical issues, and response to any therapies should be obtained. The Sign-Time Graph (Figure 65.1) may be used with the historical information on duration and severity of clinical course and can help delineate possible etiologies.

Neurologic evaluation should begin with a distance examination of posture, balance, ambulation, ability to negotiate obstacles, and behavior. Based on the results of the initial distance evaluation, a thorough neurologic examination may be performed to provide more specific information. Gloves should be worn during examination and handling of all animals with potential neurologic disease. Clinical signs noted may provide lesion localization based on the following criteria:

- Cerebrum: Symptoms may include a depressed mental state, cortical blindness normal pupillary light response (PLR), circling/leaning, yawning, head pressing, opisthotonus, seizures, and bizarre behavior.

 - Vision: Blindness may be from cerebral or brainstem origin (central) or may originate between the optic chiasm and the globe itself (peripheral). The menace response is commonly used to test for vision, but it must be carefully executed and interpreted. First, the examiner must not generate wind currents, which induce blinking due to corneal sensation. Additionally, the menace response is learned and therefore is not present in the early neonatal period. Vision testing is best performed using an obstacle test in ambulatory animals. The PLR is used in blind animals to determine if the blindness is central or peripheral. Centrally blind animals have normal PLR, while peripherally blind animals have an absent PLR.

- Cerebellum: Symptoms may include ataxia without paresis, mental alertness, intention tremors, nystagmus, truncal sway, base-wide stance, hypermetria, picking up feet and slamming them down hard, normal to increased muscle tone, falling over backwards, no conscious proprioceptive deficits, and possible loss of menace response but with normal vision.

- Brainstem and Central Vestibular System: Symptoms may include depression, mania, ataxia and paresis, cranial nerve deficits (Figure 65.2), irregular respiration, head tilt, eyelid droop, circling, hemiparesis, nystagmus,

Veterinary Techniques in Llamas and Alpacas, Second Edition. Edited by David E. Anderson, Matt Miesner, and Meredyth Jones.

Table 65.1 Clinical signs referable to specific regions of the neurologic system and major differential diagnoses for each.

Region	Expected clinical features of diseased region	Primary neurologic diseases affecting region	Diseases with clinical appearance of an affected region	Diseases of nonspecific or multi-region involvement
Cerebrum	<u>Altered mentation:</u> wandering, hyper, depression, head pressing	Listeria, cerebral hypoxia (neonates), rabies, Polioencephalomalacia, viral enceph (EHV-1, EEE, WNV), vascular insult, hydrocephalus, trauma, *P. tenuis*	Hepatic encephalopathy	Metabolic disease—calcium, magnesium
	<u>Cranial nerve deficits:</u> cortical blindness		Uremic encephalopathy,	Nutritional—(weakness/wasting)
	(PLR), head tilt, rotary nystagmus		<u>Acute abdomen:</u> perforated C-3 ulcers (pain and toxemia)	Heat stress Hypothermia
Brainstem	<u>Vestibular:</u> head tilt, tremors, balance, clinical signs may be exacerbated when blindfolded	Neoplasia, *P tenuis,* otitis media/interna,	Ryegrass staggers (lolitrem)	Pregnancy toxemia Septicemia/meningitis Mega-esophagus Neoplasia *Strep. zooepidemicus*
Cord	UMN all limbs	*P tenuis*	Bilateral patellar luxation, coxofemoral disease, congenital musculoskeletal	
C1–C5	LMN (front), UMN (hind)	<u>Toxic:</u> tetanus		
C6–T2	Norm (front), UMN (hind)	<u>Spinal Trauma/ abscess Congenital:</u> kyphosis, scoliosis, other spinal dysraphism		
T3–L3	Norm (front), LMN (hind)			Toxic—Botulism
L4–S2	± LMN (hind), urinary			Tick paralysis
S1–S3	incontinence			Plants (many) Chemical (i.e., OPs)

UMN: upper motor neuron; LMN: lower motor neuron.

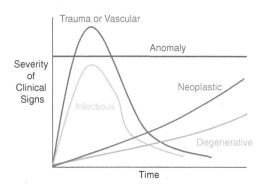

Figure 65.1 The Sign-Time Graph for determining etiologic classification of neurologic disease by severity of onset and progression of clinical signs.

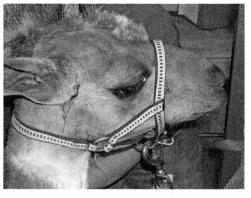

Figure 65.2 Facial paralysis in a llama following otitis media with surgical drainage.

ataxia with weakness, recumbency (lesion side down) with contralateral limbs hyperextended and hyperreflexic, loss of appetite.

The following symptoms may exist:

- Common cranial nerve signs include muscular atrophy, dropped jaw, inability to chew, ptyalism, loss of facial sensation (test ear and nose [V—trigeminal n.])
- Droopy eye, ear, lip, muzzle deviation (VII—facial n.)
- Food retention in mouth (VII—facial n., XII—hypoglossal n.)
- Head tilt (VIII—abducent n.)
- Abnormal tongue tone and movement (XII—hypoglossal n.)
- Abnormal swallowing (IX—glossopharyngeal n., X—vagus n.).

- Peripheral Vestibular System: Though patients are usually not depressed, they may exhibit head tilt, ear droop, leaning, circling all toward lesion, horizontal nystagmus, ataxia without weakness, bright, alert, good appetite.
- Spinal Cord: Symptoms may include paresis, ataxia, dysmetria, recumbency, normal mental status.
- Reflexes: Flexor, patellar, triceps, and crossed extensor reflexes may be tested. When reflexes are exaggerated an upper motor neuron (UMN) lesion is indicated, reduced reflexes indicate a lower motor neuron (LMN) lesion.
  - C1-C5: Altered head and neck movements, CP deficits and ataxia/weakness of all four limbs (Figure 65.3), recumbency, truncal sway, knuckling, stumbling, all four limbs hyperreflexive (UMN)
  - C6-T2: CP deficits and ataxia/weakness to all four limbs, recumbency, hyporeflexive front limbs (LMN), hyperreflexive hind limbs (UMN)
  - T3-L3: CP deficits and ataxia/weakness to hind limbs, hyperreflexive hind limbs (UMN)
  - L4-S2: CP deficits and ataxia/weakness to hind limbs, hyporeflexive to hind limbs (LMN)

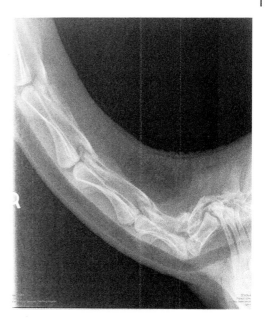

Figure 65.3 C5-C6 subluxation in an alpaca, likely traumatic in origin. This animal presented ambulatory but with ataxia of all four limbs.

- S2-Cd: Loss of anal tone, urinary bladder dribbles (LMN bladder).
- Peripheral Nerves: Symptoms include weakness, paralysis, decreased muscle tone, muscle atrophy.
  - Obturator: the patient cannot adduct hind limbs—splay hind legs
  - Sciatic: extended stifle, flexed hip, flexed or extended hock or fetlock
  - Femoral: flexed stifle, extended hip, crouching stance in young calves
  - Peroneal: extended hock, flexed fetlock
  - Tibial: partially knuckled fetlock, flexed hock
  - Suprascapular: short-strided gait, abduction of the leg and shoulder during weight bearing, atrophy of supraspinatus and infraspinatus mm
  - Radial: dropped elbow to complete forelimb paralysis. Animals with high damage may not be able to bear weight and have a flexed elbow and fetlock
  - Animals with low damage can bear weight with a flexed fetlock.

Recommended Reading

Nagy DW. 2004. *Parelaphostrongylus tenuis* and other parasitic diseases of the ruminant nervous system. *Vet Clin N Am Food Anim Pract*; 20(2):393–412.

Whitehead CE, Bedenice D. 2009. Neurologic diseases in llamas and alpacas. *Vet Clin N Am Food Anim Pract*; 25(2):385–405.

66

Cerebrospinal Fluid Collection and Interpretation
Meredyth L. Jones

Purpose or Indication for Procedure

Indications include recumbency, weakness, and ataxia for further differentiation of neurologic disease in animals after neurologic examination and localization. This procedure provides information regarding inflammatory and traumatic conditions and can demonstrate the etiologic agent of infectious diseases.

Equipment Needed

The following equipment is needed: clippers with #40 blade, sterile gloves, gauze, iodine or chlorhexidine scrub solution, isopropyl alcohol, 20-gauge × 2.5-inch (6.4-cm) spinal needle for atlanto-occipital (AO) tap or 20- to 18-gauge × 3.5-inch (8.9-cm) needle for lumbosacral (LS) tap, 6- or 12-mL syringe, lidocaine HCl 2%, purple (EDTA) × and red top (serum) tubes.

Restraint/Position

Animals undergoing AO tap must be under general anesthesia, and it is typically performed in lateral recumbency. LS taps can be performed in the standing or recumbent animal with good restraint with or without sedation. The llama or alpaca should be positioned in sternal recumbency (cushed posture) to allow for easiest needle insertion and guidance. LS taps can be done in lateral recumbency, but this position contributes to a greater degree of difficulty in maintaining ideal position of the needle.

Technical Description of Procedure/Method

Sampling may occur from two sites: the cisterna magna at the AO joint and the lumbar cistern at the LS junction. The AO site is preferred for suspected intracranial disease, but it has greater risk due to needle placement near the brainstem. AO taps are performed under general anesthesia with the animal in lateral recumbency. The large AO space is palpated, clipped, and prepared aseptically. The head may be flexed ventrally to widen the AO space. A 20-gauge × 2.5-inch (6.4-cm) spinal needle is inserted perpendicular to the skin (Figure 66.1) and advanced through the dura mater and into the subarachnoid space. Two slight "pops," or a sudden change in resistance, may be felt as the needle is passed. The operator may remove the stylet and check for flow of cerebrospinal fluid (CSF) from the hub of the needle. Also, the stylet may be swiped along the back of the operator's sterile gloved hand to detect the presence of moisture, indicating a location in or close to the subarachnoid space. When CSF is detected,

Veterinary Techniques in Llamas and Alpacas, Second Edition. Edited by David E. Anderson, Matt Miesner, and Meredyth Jones.
© 2023 John Wiley & Sons, Inc. Published 2023 by John Wiley & Sons, Inc.

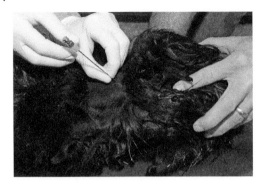

Figure 66.1 Needle placement for an AO CSF tap. The animal's nose is to the right and the head is maintained in a slightly flexed position. Absolute restraint is necessary, preferably with general anesthesia. The needle is introduced at the atlantooccipital joint at the base of the skull.

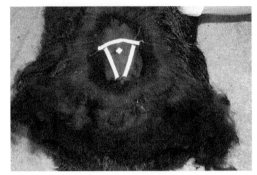

Figure 66.2 Site for lumbosacral CSF tap. The animal is in sternal recumbency and restrained manually or with sedation. Cranial is to the top of the photo. The cranial piece of tape marks the level of the ileal wings. The target site for needle insertion is slightly caudal to the level of the ileal wings, where there is a palpable widening of the intervertebral space.

a syringe is used to aspirate the sample, or the CSF may be allowed to passively drip into the collection tubes.

LS taps are safer than AO taps and may be performed in standing animals, animals in sternal recumbency, or animals in lateral recumbency. The flow of CSF courses from cranial to caudal, and LS taps may be useful for both intracranial and spinal disease. With the animal standing or in the cushed position with the hind limbs flexed to open the space, the operator locates the wide LS space between the ileal wings (Figure 66.2). An easy method to select the site of penetration of the skin is to find the palpable dorsal spinous processes of the lumbar vertebra and continue to move the finger caudally until a large space is identified. The area for CSF tap should be surgically clipped and prepared and 0.5 mL of 2% lidocaine injected subcutaneously to aid in the procedure. A 20- or 18-gauge × 3.5-inch (8.9-cm) needle with stylet is inserted in the LS space, perpendicular to the spine (Figure 66.3). The needle is advanced between the vertebrae until a slight "pop" is felt as the needle passes through the interarcuate ligament (dorsal spinous ligament). As the needle is advanced into the subarachnoid space, a second, more subtle "pop" may be felt. The second "pop" is often associated with a sudden reflex movement activity, and an

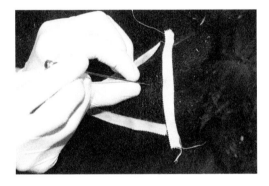

Figure 66.3 Insertion of the spinal needle into the lumbosacral space. The needle is grasped with sterile gloves both at the hub and near the skin in order to stabilize and guide the needle.

assistant should provide effective restraint in anticipation of this reaction. At that time, the stylet is removed (Figure 66.4) and wiped across the operator's sterile gloved hand. If moisture is present on the stylet, CSF may be aspirated (Figure 66.5).

CSF should be collected into red top and purple top tubes for culture and cytology, respectively. Ideally, 5 mL of CSF should be harvested to allow 3 mL to be used for cytologic examination and 2 mL to be used for biochemistry testing. If inadequate sample volume is obtained,

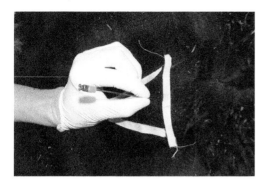

Figure 66.4 Once the needle is suspected to be in the subarachnoid space, the stylet is removed, the needle stabilized, and the hub of the needle is observed for flow of CSF. If none is seen, the stylet may be wiped across the back of the operator's sterile glove to check for moisture, then aspiration is performed. If no fluid is obtained, the stylet is replaced and the needle repositioned.

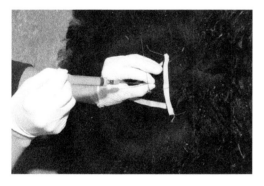

Figure 66.5 A sterile syringe is used to aspirate the CSF sample. Slow, steady aspiration should be performed with the needle stabilized to minimize trauma.

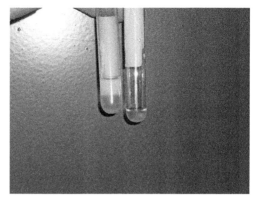

Figure 66.6 Samples of CSF obtained from an animal with meningitis. Note the visible opacity of the sample, indicating a total nucleated cell count of > 400 cells/µL.

hemorrhagic should be interpreted carefully based on the difficulty of obtaining the tap. In the absence of a traumatic tap, hemorrhagic CSF is most consistent with trauma. In trauma cases, cytology would be expected to find erythrophagocytosis. In the event that the CSF must be shipped to a laboratory, a preservative may be added to minimize any cellular changes during transit. See Practice Tip for preservation procedure. Reference ranges for CSF parameters are included in Table 66.1.

The finding of an elevated TNCC and total protein (TP) usually indicates inflammation and should be interpreted according to predominant cell type. The most common

which is common, the author prioritizes the purple top tube for cytology in most cases. In general, there is no need to withdraw more than 1 to 2 mL. If the animal is a rabies suspect, the tubes and shipping container should be marked as such to notify all handling personnel of the safety concern. Gross observation of CSF is useful and is normally clear and colorless, similar to pure water.

CSF that is grossly turbid is consistent with totalnucleated cell counts (TNCC) > 400 cells/µL (See Figure 66.6.) Foamy CSF generally contains > 200 mg/dL of protein. CSF that is grossly

Table 66.1 CSF Reference Ranges for Llamas (Welles et al., 1994/American Veterinary Medical Association).

TNCC = < 3/µL

RBCs = 53.5–458.9/µL

Protein = 38.5–47 mg/dL

Pandy (globulins) = negative

Glucose = 60–80% of blood glucose concentration

Sodium = 151–157 mEq/L

CK = 525–1,862 IU/L

Xanthochromia = negative

findings in camelid CSF include neutrophilic pleocytosis (Figure 66.7), indicating septic meningitis and eosinophilic pleocytosis indicative of meningeal worm infection. A low glucose level is indicative of sepsis and glucose consumption by inflammatory cells and bacteria. The Pandy test detects globulins and may be positive from protein exudates, hemorrhage, or local production. Creatine kinase (CK) is an indicator of axonal degeneration but has been shown to be of limited use diagnostically. In horses, elevated CK in CSF was associated with poor prognosis, regardless of cause.

Practice Tip to Facilitate Procedure

Total protein in CSF is in milligrams per deciliter (mg/dL) and can therefore not be measured on a handheld refractometer, which is only sensitive to grams per deciliter (g/dL).

If CSF is to be submitted to a reference laboratory and immediate analysis is not available, CSF samples may be preserved using the patient's own serum. To do this, place 0.2 mL of CSF into a plastic vial (red top tubes containing silica chips and cannot be used) as a reserved sample for total protein determination. For the cytology and differential count sample, collect the animal's blood and allow it to clot for 30 minutes. Centrifuge the blood for 5 minutes and place 0.250 mL of CSF into a 1- or 2-mL EDTA (purple top) tube and add 0.030 mL (two large drops) of the animal's nonhemolyzed serum into the CSF sample. Be sure to mark this serum-spiked sample as the TP will be significantly altered. Both tubes then may be shipped overnight on cold packs to the laboratory.

Potential Complications

Brain stem damage from improper needle placement at the AO tap may result in acute death or respiratory failure. LS taps can lead to subdural hemorrhage and spinal cord compression. In camelids, the spinal cord ends in

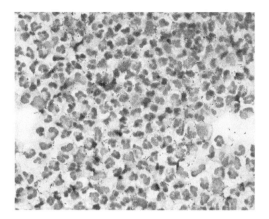

Figure 66.7 Microscopic, stained image of CSF from an alpaca with streptococcal meningitis. Note the severe neutrophilic pleocytosis and intra and extracellular bacteria present.

the midsacral region. Contamination of the needle during collection can result in abscess formation.

Patient Monitoring/Aftercare

The animal's neurologic status should be monitored and managed according to the results of the neurologic exam and ancillary testing.

Recommended Readings

Bohn AA, Callan RJ. 2007. Cytology in Food Animal Practice. *Vet Clin N Am Food Anim Pract*; 23(3):443–479.

Jones M, Miesner M, Grondin T. 2009. Outbreak of *Streptococcus equi* ssp. *zooepidemicus* polyserositis in an alpaca herd. *J Vet Intern Med*; 23(1):220–223.

Nagy DW. 2004. *Parelaphostrongylus tenuis* and other parasitic diseases of the ruminant nervous system. *Vet Clin N Am Food Anim Pract*; 20(2):393–412.

Welles EG, Pugh DG, Wenzel JG, et al. 1994. Composition of cerebrospinal fluid in healthy adult llamas. *Am J Vet Res*; 55(8):1075–1079.

Whitehead CE, Bedenice D. 2009. Neurologic diseases in llamas and alpacas. *Vet Clin N Am Food Anim Pract*; 25(2):385–405.

Section XIV

Ophthalmology

67

Eye Exam

Tracy Miesner and Matt Miesner

Purpose or Indication for Procedure

Eye exams are performed in the following cases: suspected eye problem, pre-purchase exam, routine physical exam, and insurance exam.

Equipment Needed

A bright, focused light source; direct or indirect ophthalmoscope; 2% lidocaine; 25-gauge needle; and 1–3 cc syringe are needed.

Restraint/Position

Standing restraint, sedation, and anesthesia may be used.

Technical Description of Procedure/Method

Initial eye examination should be done on the unsedated animal from a distance sufficient to see both eyes at the same time. First observations should determine facial symmetry, ocular symmetry, any swellings or protrusion of the head, any evidence of head trauma, symmetry of the orbital bones, angle of the eyelashes, and rate of blinking. Pupillary light reflexes are checked,

both direct and consensual. Assessment of sclera for monitoring *Haemonchus contortus* risk with FAMACHA scoring has also been validated. (Storey et al. 2017).

After all of the neurologic and symmetry questions have been answered, then the animal can be sedated, only if needed, and eyelid paresis can be induced. Working from the outside to the inside, eyelid margins, eyelashes, conjunctiva, third eyelid, cornea, anterior chamber, iris, and pupil are all visualized in low light with a bright, focused light, such as a transilluminator. A slit beam and magnification can help define any opacities or floaters found in the anterior chamber and the lens. For further examination, the pupil must be dilated with 1% tropicamide. Atropine should be used judiciously since the mydriasis caused by atropine can last for many days. With the pupil dilated, the iris is evaluated for normal contracture. The lens should be inspected for opacities. The vitreous can be inspected for floating objects, and the retina can be visualized. Direct ophthalmoscopic exams will give a small but magnified view of the retina. Indirect ophthalmoscopy using a transilluminator and a 20- or 25-diopter lens will give a larger field of view with less magnification. Binocular ophthalmoscopy will give the examiner better depth perception. Any of the three techniques are acceptable, and each has strengths and weaknesses.

Topical anesthesia with proparacaine will allow thorough examination of both surfaces of

Veterinary Techniques in Llamas and Alpacas, Second Edition. Edited by David E. Anderson, Matt Miesner, and Meredyth Jones.

the third eyelid and intraocular pressure determination with a TonoPen.5® or a TonoVet.5®. Intraocular pressures measured by rebound tonometry maybe slightly higher than applanation tonometery. (McDonald et al. 2017) Schiotz tonometry is impractical unless in lateral recumbency. Xylazine can affect intra-ocular pressures and, if this parameter is very important, topical anesthesia and pressures should be done prior to sedation. Both topical anesthesia and the act of taking pressures can affect the clarity of the cornea. To control for the pressure alterations caused by medications, both eyes should be tested. Normal ocular pressures have been reported to be between 13–20 in alpacas and 14–20 in llamas (Willis et al. 2000). In cases of suspect tear film abnormalities and other surface diseases, Schirmer tear test values can be compared to normal alpacas (McDonald et al. 2018). Assessment of corneal sensitivity can also be performed utilizing the Cochet-Bonnet anesthesiometer in adults and crias (Rankin et al. 2012).

Nasolacrimal duct patency and corneal integrity can both be checked by instilling fluorescein stain to the eye. Fluorescein solution can be made by placing the fluorescein strip into a 3-cc syringe and adding 1.5 cc of eyewash or sterile saline. Alternatively, the fluorescein strip can be inserted into the lateral canthus of the eye, and some eyewash or sterile saline can be dripped onto the surface of the eye to distribute the stain across the corneal surface and into the nasolacrimal duct. The stain is expected to be present in the nasal passage of an animal with patent ducts within a couple of minutes. However, we have found this to be an inconsistent finding in normal camelids. Nasolacrimal flushing can be achieved retrograde or normograde with a tomcat catheter and warm saline. (This technique is more thoroughly described in a separate location in this manual.) Nasolacrimal duct atresia does occur in camelid species.

Normal Anterior Segment Anatomical Structures

The normal anterior segment is complete bony orbital rim with a large notch palpable dorsally in the frontal bone, pigmented conjunctiva, a large pupillary rough on the dorsal and ventral borders of the iris (Figures 67.1a, 67.1b, and 67.1c), and iris pigmentation varying from very dark to non-pigmented and often mixed colors.

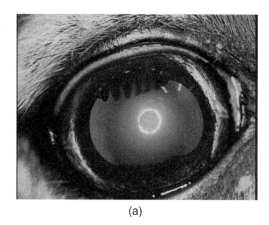

(a)

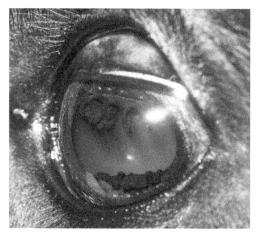

(b)

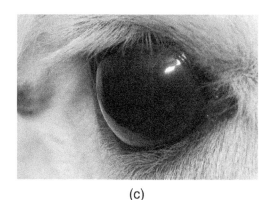

(c)

Figure 67.1 Normal alpaca (**a**) photo courtesy of R. Allbaugh and llama (**b & c**) photo courtesy of A. Metzler.

Normal Posterior Segment Anatomical Structures

The fundus lacks a tapetum but is highly reflective. Fundic pigmentation varies with fiber color and areas of non-pigmented areas can be found in light colored animals with white markings. The retinal vascular pattern is prominent with 3 to 5 pairs of vessels originating from the optic disc (Figures 67.2a, 67.2b, and 67.3).

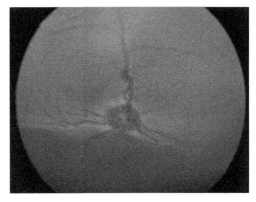

Figure 67.3 Normal 17-year-old grey alpaca with cortical lenticular sclerosis. Photo courtesy of R. Allbaugh.

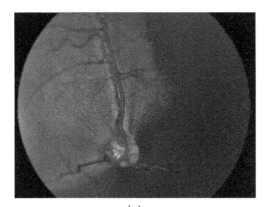

(a)

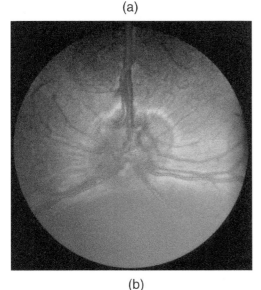

(b)

Figure 67.2 Normal alpaca (**a**) photo courtesy of R. Allbaugh and llama (**b**) fundus photo courtesy of A. Metzler.

Practice Tip to Facilitate Procedure

Sedation and eyelid paresis make the eye exam much easier to perform.

Potential Complications

Extended mydriasis may occur.

Patient Monitoring/Aftercare

Protect the patient from bright light until pupillary response returns to normal.

Recommended Reading and References

Lavach JD. 1990. Large Animal Ophthalmology. In: *Veterinary Ophthalmology*, 4th Edition. Mosby. Gellat K, 2007, Blackwell, pp. 1315–1320.

McDonald JE, Knollinger AM, Dees DD, et al. 2017. Comparison of intraocular pressure measurements using rebound (TonoVet®) and applanation (TonoPen-XL®) tonometry in clinically normal alpacas (Vicugna pacos). *Vet Ophthal*; 20(2):155–159.

McDonald JE, Knollinger AM, Dees DD, et al. 2018. Determination of Schirmer tear test-1 values in clinically normal Alpacas (Vicugna pacos) in North America. *Vet Ophthal*; 21(1):101–103.

Nuhsbaum MT, Gionfriddo JR, Powell CC, Aubin ML. 2000. Intraocular pressure in normal llamas (Lama glama) and alpacas (Lama pacos). *Vet Ophthalmol*; 3:31–34.

Personal Communications and imagery:
Allbaugh, Rachel, DVM, MS, DACVO.
Metzler, Anne, DVM, MS, DACVO.

Rankin AJ, Hosking KG, Roush JK. 2012. Corneal sensitivity in healthy, immature, and adult alpacas. *Vet Ophthal*; 15(1):31–35.

Storey BE, Williamson LH, Howell SB, et al. 2017. Validation of the FAMACHA© system in South American Camelids. *Vet Parasit*; 243:85–91.

Willis AM, Anderson DE, Gemensky AJ, Wilkie DA, Silveira F. 2000. Evaluation of intraocular pressure in eyes of clinically normal llamas and alpacas. *Am J Vet Res*; 61:1542–1544.

68

Nasolacrimal Duct Cannulation
Meredyth L. Jones

Purpose or Indication for Procedure

This procedure is used to establish patency and diagnose conditions of the nasolacrimal (NL) duct. Occlusion of the NL duct may be congenital (atresia of the puncta or duct) or acquired from debris accumulation. The function of the NL duct is to drain tears and debris from the eye out to the nasal passage. Animals with occluded, stenotic, or atretic ducts often present for chronic, acute unilateral, or bilateral ocular discharge that has been refractory to topical therapies. The discharge may be serous, mucoid, or mucopurulent, and conjunctivitis may be present.

Equipment Needed

The following equipment is needed: standing sedation, 3.5- to 5-French polypropylene catheter, syringe, and saline eye flush. For diagnostic imaging, barium or other radiopaque contrast may be used.

Restraint/Position

Standing, cushed, and lateral recumbency ± sedation may be used.

Technical Description of Procedure/Method

Camelids have a nasal punctum and a superior and inferior conjunctival puncta. The simplest method of cannulating the NL duct of camelids is by use of a 5-French (adults) or 3.5-French (cria) polypropylene catheter passed retrograde from the nasal puncta. The nasal puncta is visualized on the floor of the nasal passage (Figure 68.1). The catheter is introduced into the puncta, and the operator's finger is used to occlude the nasal puncta around the catheter (Figure 68.2). A syringe of saline eye flush is attached, and the catheter is advanced as the saline is pulsed through the catheter. In most animals, debris will be expelled through the ocular puncta of the duct, and the saline will flow over the eye. Close attention will verify the presence of both a superior and inferior puncta. Flushing is continued until the duct is thoroughly cleared and the catheter withdrawn.

For animals with suspected atresia or unresolved occlusion of the duct, contrast media may be infused through the catheter and radiographs obtained to determine the extent of the blockage or atresia. In most cria with congenital nasolacrimal duct atresia, the nasal puncta is not present. In these cases, a 3.5-French polypropylene catheter is passed via the inferior conjunctival puncta, and saline is pulsed while

Veterinary Techniques in Llamas and Alpacas, Second Edition. Edited by David E. Anderson, Matt Miesner, and Meredyth Jones.
© 2023 John Wiley & Sons, Inc. Published 2023 by John Wiley & Sons, Inc.

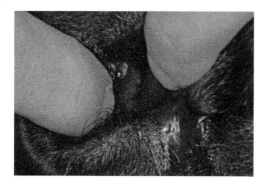

Figure 68.1 The nasal punch of the NL duct present on the ventral surface of the nasal passage.

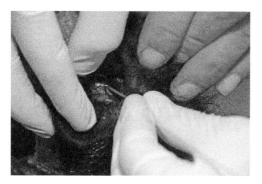

Figure 68.2 The passage of a 5-French polypropylene catheter in a retrograde fashion into the nasal puncta to facilitate flushing of the NL duct.

performing an intranasal examination. In most cases of atresia, a membrane can be seen pulsing over the site of the nasal puncta. In these cases, a #15 scalpel blade or 14-gauge needle can be used to puncture the membrane. Then, a saline flush is continued until the duct is thoroughly cleared and the catheter withdrawn. In atresia cases where no nasal puncta can be observed, surgical conjunctivorhinostomy may be required to establish tear flow.

Practice Tip to Facilitate Procedure

Instilling fluorescein stain into the eye and monitoring for passage into the nares is not diagnostic of an occluded duct. Many animals with patent ducts will not show passage of the stain.

Potential Complications

With gentle manipulation, little or no trauma is expected from catheterization of the NL duct. If an obstruction is met, saline flushing rather than mechanical pressure should be used to relieve the obstruction. The catheter should not be passed in a retrograde fashion completely to the ocular puncta to avoid contact with the cornea.

Patient Monitoring/Aftercare

The animal should be monitored for reoccurrence of the obstruction or continued epiphora. It is not anticipated that topical ophthalmic medications will be necessary in cases of uncomplicated NL duct occlusion.

Recommended Reading

Faulkner J, Williams DL, Mueller K. 2020. Ophthalmology of clinically normal alpacas (Vicugna pacos) in the United Kingdom: a cross-sectional study. Vet Rec; 186(16):e7. https://www.repository.cam.ac.uk/handle/1810/301802.

Mangan BG, Gionfriddo JR, Powell CC. 2008. Bilateral nasolacrimal duct atresia in a cria. Vet Ophthal; 11(1):49–54.

Sandmeyer LS, Bauer BS, Breaux CB, Grahn BH. 2011. Congenital nasolacrimal atresia in 4 alpacas. Can Vet J; 52(3):313–317.

Sapienza JS, Isaza R, Brooks DE, et al. 1996. Atresia of the nasolacrimal duct in a llama. Vet Comp Ophth; 6(1):6–8.

69

Conjunctivorhinostomy for Alleviation of Nasolacrimal Duct Obstruction

David E. Anderson

Purpose or Indication for Procedure

Obstruction of the nasolacrimal duct may occur as a congenital problem (atresia) or be associated with chronic inflammation. Obstruction is suspected when clear to cloudy ocular discharge is noted at the medial canthus of the eye. Obstruction may develop days, weeks, or months after birth in cases of atresia. Acquired obstructions can occur at any age. There are two puncta at the medial canthus that merge and drain to the tear sac, which drains via the nasolacrimal duct at a single nasal opening near the nares. The nasal opening is a faint oval depression seen on the ventral aspect of the rostral nasal passage near the opening of the nares. Acquired obstruction of the nasolacrimal ducts may be caused by chronic infection or trauma. In most cases, acquired obstructions can be resolved by flushing the nasolacrimal duct. In cases of permanent damage to the nasolacrimal duct, conjunctivorhinostomy is indicated. Conjunctivorhinostomy refers to the creation of a permanent tunnel from the conjunctiva to the nasal passageway in such a way that a new nasolacrimal duct is created. This procedure also is indicated in cases of nasolacrimal duct atresia, which may occur unilaterally or bilaterally. In most llamas and alpacas, NL duct atresia occurs at the distal opening. These cases are readily treated by opening the membrane covering the distal opening using sharp dissection. When atresia of either the inferior (lower) puncta or both puncta exists, conjunctivorhinostomy is used to establish efficient drainage. Also, conjunctivorhinostomy is curative in cases where the NL duct atresia is located at the midpoint of the NL duct.

Equipment Needed

The following equipment is needed: sedation or general anesthesia, minor surgery pack, nested trochar set or large bore needle (e.g., 12 to 14 gauge with stylette), No. 8 French long (>15 cm) polyurethane catheter, and No. 2 monofilament suture (e.g., No. 2 PDS).

Restraint/Position

Sternal recumbency (cushed posture) or lateral recumbency with affected eye uppermost may be used.

Technical Description of Procedure/Method

When NL atresia is present at the distal opening, the normal location of the NL duct opening can usually be identified by the presence

Veterinary Techniques in Llamas and Alpacas, Second Edition. Edited by David E. Anderson, Matt Miesner, and Meredyth Jones.

of an opaque, white membrane at the ventral aspect of the nasal passage approximately 5 to 10 mm proximal to the nares. This is easily identified as the junction of pigmented and nonpigmented epithelium. Sedation or general anesthesia is needed to allow for examination and correction of the obstruction. The membrane can be opened using a No. 15 scalpel blade or the beveled edge of a 14-gauge needle to slice the membrane open. This is most easily done by cannulating the ventral puncta at the medial canthus and pressurizing the duct by manual pressure infusion of 0.9% sterile saline. The operator can "pulsate" the pressure to increase the visibility of the obstructing membrane, but excessive pressure should be avoided to prevent inadvertent rupture of the NL duct. Optionally, a stent can be inserted along the length of the NL duct and maintained during the early phases of healing. This can be done by placing a catheter through the NL from the medial canthus, threading it distally through the newly created distal opening, and then threading a monofilament suture through the catheter. The author prefers using a No. 3.5 or 5.0 French polyurethane catheter through which No. 2 monofilament suture (e.g. PDS, polypropylene) material is passed. The catheter is removed and the suture tied in place in such a way as to not cause irritation to the cornea and to maintain patency of the duct. The suture is then removed in 7 to 10 days.

Conjunctivorhinostomy is performed using a 2- to 3-mm-diameter, 8- to 10-cm-long nested trochar. The nested trochar assembly has a cannula with sharp trochar, which is used to puncture a hole from the medial canthus of the orbit to the nasal passage. Alternatively, a bone marrow biopsy needle may be used (e.g. Jamshidi). The cannula is seated deeply in the medial canthus along the margin of the orbital rim and angled ventrally, medially, and rostrally. After puncturing through to the nasal passage, a No. 5 French polyurethane or red rubber catheter is threaded through the cannula until it exits out through the nares. After the cannula is removed, either the catheter

can be maintained as a stent or a No. 2 monofilament suture material (e.g., PDS, polypropylene) can be passed through the catheter as described for obstruction of the distal NL duct opening. When suture is used, the material is grasped and the polyurethane catheter removed. The suture is secured in place for 14 to 21 days to allow epithelialization of the tract. Once mature, this tract will replace the function of the NL duct.

> **Practice Tip to Facilitate Procedure**
>
> A magnification lens with built-in light source facilitates visualization of the distal NL duct opening. This procedure is greatly facilitated by sedation or general anesthesia.

Potential Complications

The principal complications are corneal ulceration and re-obstruction of the duct. If corneal opacity, excessive tearing, or clinical signs of eye pain occur, the eye should immediately be evaluated for the presence of ulcers and the stents removed. Re-obstruction occurs in approximately 10% of cases of membranous obstruction of the distal NL duct opening and an estimated 25% of cases of conjunctivorhinostomy.

Patient Monitoring/Aftercare

Once opened, an ophthalmic antibiotic ointment should be applied two to three times daily for 7 to 10 days or until healed.

Recommended Reading

Czerwinski SL. 2019. Ocular Surface Disease in New World Camelids. *Vet Clin Exot Anim Pract*; 22(1):69–79.

Gionfriddo JR, Friedman DS. 2009. Ophthalmology of South American

Camelids: llamas, Alpacas, Guanacoes, and Vicunas. In: *Current Veterinary Therapy: Food Animal Practice*, 5th Edition. Anderson DE, Rings DMEds. Saunders Elsevier, pp. 430–434.

Ledbetter EC. 2022. Ophthalmology of Tylopoda: camels, Alpacas, Llamas, Vicunas, and Guanacos. In: *Wild and Exotic Animal Ophthalmology*. Cham, Springer, pp. 119–143.

Mangan BG, Gionfriddo JR, Powell CC. 2008. Bilateral nasolacrimal duct atresia in a cria. *Vet Ophthalmol*; 11(1):49–54.

Rubin LF. 1984. Large Animal Ophthalmic Surgery. In: *The Practice of Large Animal Surgery*, Vol. II. Philadelphia, Saunders, pp. 1151–1201.

Sandmeyer LS, Bauer BS, Breaux CB, Grahn BH. 2011. Congenital nasolacrimal atresia in 4 alpacas. *Can Vet J*; 52(3):313.

Sapienza JS, Isaza R, Johnson RD, Miller TR. 1992. Anatomic and radiographic study of the lacrimal apparatus of llamas. *Am J Vet Res*; 53(6):1007–1009.

70

Ocular Extirpation

David E. Anderson

Purpose or Indication for Procedure

Ocular disease and injury occur occasionally in llamas and alpacas. In many instances, medical management is sufficient for resolution and amelioration of clinical signs. In selected cases, surgical intervention is required. Thorough physical examination, proper preparation of the patient, appropriate perioperative management, and precise surgical technique will assure the best results possible. Extirpation of the eye is indicated in cases where the cornea has ruptured, persistent or recurrent panophthalmitis is present, permanent damage to the globe has occurred, or ocular neoplasia is apparent. In most cases, extirpation is recommended as opposed to enucleation. The term enucleation refers to removal of the globe, and ocular extirpation refers to removal of the globe and all orbital structures including muscles, lymph node, and adnexa.

Equipment Needed

Soft tissue surgery pack, general anesthesia, angled forceps, #2–0 or 0 absorbable suture (e.g., poly-glecaprone), and #1 nonabsorbable monofilament suture (e.g., polypropylene, nylon) is needed.

Restraint/Position

Lateral recumbency under general anesthesia is recommended.

Technical Description of Procedure/Method

Surgical Site Preparation

The hair and eyelashes should be clipped using No. 40 clipper blades for a wide zone (e.g., 10 cm) around the orbit. The eye and conjunctiva can be cleansed with a saline solution containing dilute iodine (0.1%). The skin is disinfected with antiseptic scrub solutions such as povidone iodine. Saline rinse rather than alcohol should be used between the disinfectant scrubs to prevent painful irritation.

Ocular Extirpation

A transpalpebral ablation technique is utilized to remove the eye and associated soft tissues. The upper and lower eyelids are sutured closed using No. 0 monofilament suture material (e.g., polypropylene) in a simple continuous suture pattern. This procedure improves sterility by establishing coverage of the cornea, conjunctiva, and associated structures such as the tear ducts. This facilitates *en bloc* removal of the

Veterinary Techniques in Llamas and Alpacas, Second Edition. Edited by David E. Anderson, Matt Miesner, and Meredyth Jones.
© 2023 John Wiley & Sons, Inc. Published 2023 by John Wiley & Sons, Inc.

tissues and minimizes risks of intraoperative contamination. A circumferential skin incision is made approximately 5 -mm from the edges of the eyelids. After the skin incision is completed, the skin is reflected to the level of the orbital rim. Then the scalpel or Metzenbaum scissors are used to dissect the soft tissues along the bony orbit. Dissection should occur adjacent to the bone to ensure excision of all orbital tissues. Using a combination of blunt and sharp dissection, curved Metzenbaum or Mayo scissors are used to dissect through the orbicularis oculi muscle, fascia, and subcutaneous tissues surrounding the eye. Complete excision of orbital tissue is necessary in most cases of eye removal. The retrobulbar musculature and the optic nerve should be transected as far caudally as feasible. Angled forceps are useful to clamp the optic nerve and artery. Care must be taken to prevent excessive tension on the optic nerve so that unwanted parasympathetic response is avoided. Excessive stimulation of optic nerve can cause excessive parasympathetic tone and result in acute, severe hypotension, bradycardia, and cardiovascular collapse ("vasovagal response"). This complication has been observed in camelids during ocular extirpation. Use of an angled vascular clamp can aid in hemostasis and diminish traction placed on the nerve while additional excision of remaining orbital tissue is undertaken. Rapidly absorbable suture materials (e.g., polyglecaprone No. 0) should be utilized for any vascular ligation to limit the period of time the suture foreign body is present.

If skin sutures are applied at this point, an undesirable cosmetic appearance will result from collapse of the skin into the depth of the bony orbit. A more cosmetic result can be achieved by placement of a transorbital suture prior to closure of the skin. This must be done with permanent suture material and therefore is not recommended in cases where there is infection present or the risk of infection is considered significant. Placement of a transorbital suture (a.k.a Trampoline sutures) is done by anchoring nonabsorbable suture material in the periosteum on the dorsal and ventral rim of the orbit. A simple continuous pattern using No. 0 polypropylene or equivalent nonabsorbable suture is placed and the sutures tightened to ensure support of the overlying ocular skin. After postoperative swelling resolves, the skin will adhere to the trampoline suture level to the orbital rim. The skin incision can be closed using a variety of appositional suture patterns including the simple interrupted, continuous interlocking, interrupted cruciate, or simple continuous patterns. Skin suture should be applied using nonabsorbable suture such as No. 0 or 1 nylon or polypropylene. The skin sutures are removed in 14 to 21 days. If present, the transorbital sutures are left in place as a permanent support unless complications are noted.

Practice Tip to Facilitate Procedure

Uncontrolled parasympathetic responses have been observed during enucleation in camelids. Vagal response is noted by acute, severe bradycardia and hypotension. Although rare, the surgeon and anesthetist must be pre- pared to address this life-threatening problem. Treatment is most often successful by administration of atropine (0.02 mg/kg IV) and IV fluids. If hypotension persists, a continuous rate infusion of dopamine or dobutamine may be used to provide cardiovascular support. Application of local anesthesia to the optic nerve is useful to mitigate the risk of this adverse event.

Potential Complications

Postoperative complications can include incisional infection, orbital infection, dehiscence of the incision, infection of the periorbital tissues, or progression of neoplasia. If purulent drainage is noted after extirpation, a portion of the incision may be opened to facilitate drainage and allow for orbital lavage using a dilute wound disinfectant solution. Antibiotic therapy is recommended until no evidence of infection is noted.

Patient Monitoring/Aftercare

The disease and surgical procedure will determine the severity of anti-inflammatory therapy required. Nonsteroidal anti-inflammatory drugs (e.g., flunixin meglumine 1 mg/kg IV) are given immediately before surgery, and the need for further anti-inflammatory drug therapy is based on clinical signs. Broad spectrum systemic antibiotic therapy is indicated, and the disease process will influence the duration of antibiotic therapy. Intra-orbital antibiotic therapy is not recommended because of the local tissue irritation that can be associated with these products. Systemic antibiotics combined with close attention to asepsis during surgery will limit the need for prolonged antibiotic therapy.

The animal should be kept in a confined area for several days after surgery to allow for appropriate hemostasis to occur, pain to resolve, and the patient to adapt to their surroundings. Daily observation of the surgical site and assessment of general well-being is recommended until suture removal.

Recommended Reading

Gionfriddo JR, Friedman DS. 2009. Ophthalmology of South American Camelids: llamas, Alpacas, Guanacoes, and Vicunas. In: *Current Veterinary Therapy: Food Animal Practice*, 5th Edition. Anderson DE, Rings DM Eds., Saunders Elsevier, pp. 430–434.

Rubin LF. 1984. Large Animal Ophthalmic Surgery. In: *The Practice of Large Animal Surgery*, Vol. II. Philadelphia, Saunders, pp. 1151–1201.

71

Subpalpebral Lavage System

Tracy Miesner

Purpose or Indication for Procedure

This procedure is used for frequent application of ophthalmic medications, application of ophthalmic medication in uncooperative animals, and application of ophthalmic medication into unstable or fragile eye conditions.

Equipment Needed

The following equipment is needed: subpalpebral lavage system, local anesthetic 1 mL (2% lidocaine or bupivicaine), 25-gauge needle, clippers, iodine scrub and sterile saline rinse, proparacaine ophthalmic anesthetic, nonabsorbable suture, white tape, and gauze squares (Figure 71.1).

Restraint/Position

Standing sedation with assistant to restrain head. Recumbent anesthesia if needed.

Technical Description of Procedure/Method

The patient must be sedated or anesthetized. The upper eyelid is clipped from just above the eyelashes to 1 inch above the orbital rim (Figure 71.2). Surgical preparation of this skin using alternating iodine scrub and sterile saline wipes (alcohol should be avoided) for a minimum of three repetitions. A local block should be placed at the orbital rim and another at approximately 1 cm cranial to the orbital rim using up to 1 mL of 2% lidocaine (Figure 71.3). Apply a small amount of proparacaine to the cornea for topical anesthesia (Figure 71.4). The trocar needle of the lavage system is loaded with the nondisc end of the lavage tubing. The rest of the tubing is held in the gloved hand. The trocar needle is held along the index or middle finger of the dominant hand. The index or middle finger of the dominant hand is slid up the inside of the upper eyelid with the needle facing bevel out. At the fornix of the upper eyelid, as far proximally as possible the trocar needle is pushed through the upper eyelid at the orbital rim being careful to keep the tubing in the needle (Figure 71.5).

Needle and tubing are advanced and pulled completely through the eyelid being careful to protect the cornea from needle trauma with the gloved finger. When the needle has been passed completely through the eyelid, the needle is removed from the tubing and the tubing is advanced through the eyelid until the disc at the end of the tubing is pulled firmly into the upper eyelid fornix, again, being careful to protect the cornea from damage associated with the plastic disc, using the gloved finger (Figure 71.6).

Veterinary Techniques in Llamas and Alpacas, Second Edition. Edited by David E. Anderson, Matt Miesner, and Meredyth Jones.

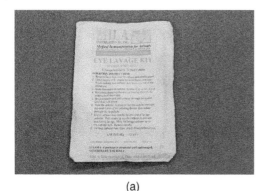

(a)

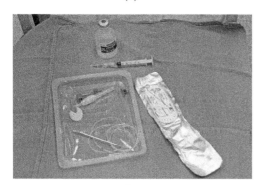

(b)

Figure 71.1 Materials needed.

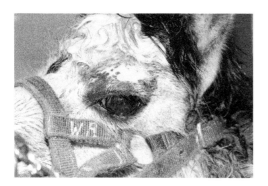

Figure 71.2 Clip hair and prep from eyelashes to 2.54 cm above orbital rim.

When the disc is in place, the tubing is dried, and either the provided plastic rings are used or white tape wings are used to secure the tubing to the upper eyelid. This author's preference is

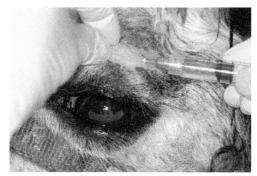

Figure 71.3 Local anesthesia using up to 1 mL of 2% lidocaine at the orbital rim for trocar penetration and another 1 cm proximal for stay suture placement.

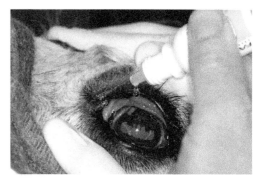

Figure 71.4 Topical anesthesia achieved using a couple drops of proparacaine.

to use white tape to create wings that can be sutured to the skin (Figure 71.7), but the kit comes with a plastic loop that can be used. This plastic securing device must be used correctly; the tubing is passed through the small holes over the top of the large loop, and the suture is placed through the large loop to the head. Additional stay sutures can be placed if security is questionable, at the veterinarian's discretion.

The kit provides a catheter and an end cap to be placed in the distal end of the tubing (which can be cut shorter if desired). The end cap must be placed onto the catheter before placing the catheter into the tubing. Care must be used to avoid puncturing the tubing

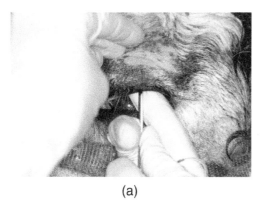

(a)

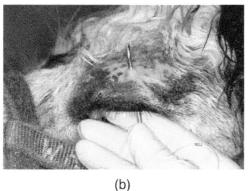

(b)

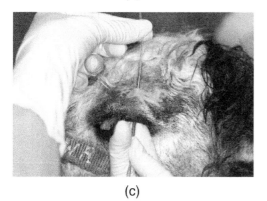

(c)

Figure 71.5 Protecting the cornea with gloved finger, advance trocar to fornix of eyelid and pass through. After trocar is through, advance tubing and then pull trocar completely through the upper eyelid.

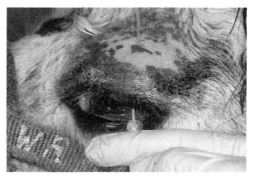

Figure 71.6 Advance tubing and protect cornea from damage from disc by using the gloved finger to position the disc in the fornix of the upper eyelid.

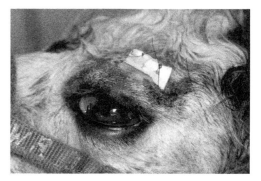

Figure 71.7 Dry tubing and apply white tape wings for suturing.

Practice Tip to Facilitate Procedure

Air is very irritating to the eye, so priming the tubing with saline, applying an ophthalmic ointment directly to the eye while the animal is sedated, or shortening the tubing and filling it with saline while the animal is still sedated and under the influence of corneal anesthetic may make the treatments less irritating to the animal. Ointments cannot be given through the lavage system. Some clinicians prefer to use air to push the medications through the system, but if you have previously determined the volume of the tubing, you could use saline to push the medications to the eye. It does not take a long time for an animal to associate manipulation of the end of the lavage tubing with the application of eye medications, so there will still be some resistance to treatment, but there is less risk of accidental damage to the eye during treatment.

with the introducer needle, pulling the sharp portion into the catheter, after it has been introduced to the tubing is helpful. The catheter is advanced all the way to the hub, the needle is discarded, the end is capped, and the remaining tubing is secured to the animal (Figure 71.8).

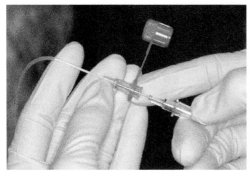

(a)

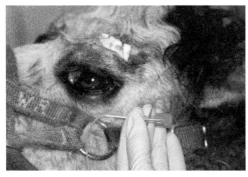

(b)

Figure 71.8 Place blue cap retainer ring onto catheter, then introduce catheter into tubing being careful not to puncture tubing, advance to hub, remove stylette, flush line, and applycap.

Potential Complications

If the stay tape or apparatus slips, the disc could slip down to the cornea and cause further damage. Visual cues can be put in place such as a permanent mark on the tubing, or manually checking the tube can be done by gently pulling on the tubing to ensure that the disc continues to be tightly held in place. Tubing may become blocked or damaged. Upper eyelid swelling can occur and should be investigated. Moist dermatitis of the lower eyelid from ocular discharge or medication overflow may occur but can be prevented with petroleum jelly applied to the lower eyelid.

Patient Monitoring/Aftercare

After the animal awakens from sedation/anesthesia, the tubing placement must be monitored, the eye condition being treated must be monitored, and the patency of the tubing must be monitored.

Recommended Reading

Borkowski R, Moore PA, Mumford S, Carastro S. 2007, Sep. Adaptations of subpalpebral lavage systems used for llamas (Lama glama) and a harbor seal (Phoca vitulina). J Zoo Wildl Med; 38(3):453–459.

Giuliano EA, Maggs DJ, Moore CP, Boland LA, Champagne ES, Galle LE. 2000. Inferomedial placement of a single-entry subpalpebral lavage tube for treatment of equine eye disease. Vet Ophthalmol; 3(2–3):153–156.

Sweeney CR, Russell GE. 1997, Nov 15. Complications associated with use of a one-hole subpalpebral lavage system in horses: 150 cases (1977–1996). J Am Vet Med Assoc; 211(10):1271–1274.

72

Conjunctival Pedicle Graft

Tracy Miesner and Matt Miesner

Purpose or Indication for Procedure

This procedure is used for deep corneal ulcers (>50% of corneal thickness), nonhealing ulcers, and corneal stromal abscesses (Figure 72.1).

Equipment Needed

The following equipment is needed: eyelid speculum, Steven's tenotomy scissors, Colibri or tying forceps, ophthalmic needle holders, 6–0 to 8–0 polyglactin 910 suture (smaller is better), and magnifying lens (Gelatt 2007).

Restraint/Position

General anesthesia is used.

Technical Description of Procedure/Method

This technique has been described by multiple people in multiple species. A single case report in published in an alpaca (Rodriquez-Alvaro et al 2005). This technical description was made using Gellat's Veterinary Ophthalmology text as a reference and with personal consultation with Dr. Anne Metzler, DVM, MS, ACVO.

Specific location and size of flap is determined by the corneal defect being covered. The conjunctiva is incised at a position that will allow undermining and transposition to the corneal lesion. The initial incision should be perpendicular to the cornea and undermined parallel to the corneal edge with more width than the abnormal corneal tissue to allow for some contracture (Figure 72.2). Careful dissection is done to remove the conjunctiva from Tenon's capsule without putting holes in the conjunctiva. The pedicle is created by making two long incisions in the undermined conjunctiva at and parallel to the limbus and at a parallel line distal to the limbus creating a flap that is 1–2 mm wider than the defect to be covered and wider at the base than at the tip (Figure 72.2). This creates a pedicle that is roughly rectangular in shape with three sides cut free and one edge attached. Final graft material should be thin enough that the scissors can be seen through it, large enough to more than cover the defect, loose enough to have no tension when sutured in place, and the base should be wider than the tip of the graft.

The conjunctival flap will not adhere to corneal epithelium, necrotic, or collagenolytic corneal stroma. Therefore, preparation of the cornea for graft placement should be done to carefully remove all melting or dead tissue and the corneal epithelium needs to be removed for graft adhesion. The pedicle is rotated to

Veterinary Techniques in Llamas and Alpacas, Second Edition. Edited by David E. Anderson, Matt Miesner, and Meredyth Jones.

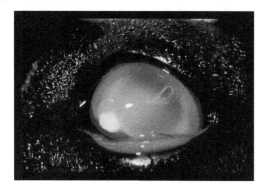

Figure 72.1 Stromal abscess in a llama. (Photo courtesy of Anne Metzler, DVM, MS, ACVO).

the lesion and sutured in place. Other techniques may be used such as bridge flaps that are attached at both short ends of the rectangle and the loosened conjunctiva spans the corneal surface and is sutured at the lesion site. Suturing is done using a simple interrupted pattern with the first suture being at the distal most portion of the flap and then progressing around the lesion at 1–1.5 mm apart until sufficient sutures have been placed to keep the flap secured (Figure 72.3). Some authors described placing an additional holding suture on either side of the base of the pedicle, and some

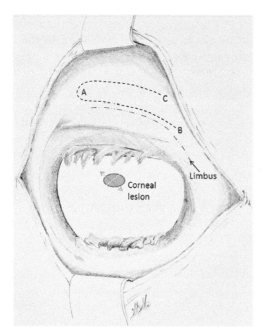

Figure 72.2 Schematic drawing of camelid eye with corneal lesion and conjunctival flap harvest. Initial incision is perpendicular to the cornea at **A** and undermined toward **B** and **C**. The location of **A** is determined by measuring from a location nearest to the lesion, which will be the base of the pedicle at **B** to 1–2 mm beyond the lesions distal edge (*light green dotted line*). The width of the flap is determined by the size of the lesion (*dark green dotted line*). The base of the pedicle must be wider than the tip. After elevation of the conjunctiva, the pedicle is severed from **A** to **B** along the limbus, then from **A** to **C**. (Illustration courtesy of Matt Miesner.)

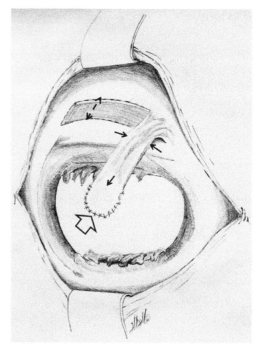

Figure 72.3 After the lesion is cleaned and prepped and a recipient bed of corneal stroma is exposed to accept the graft, then the pedicle is rotated into place and sutured with 6–0 to 7–0 absorbable, monofilament suture in a simple interrupted pattern (*open arrow*). Additional sutures are placed around the lesion 1–1.5 mm apart. Some authors place one additional vertical suture at the apex of the lesion and at the limbus on either side of the pedicle for additional support (*arrows*) (illustration courtesy of Matt Miesner).

describe placing an additional stay suture on the flap at the top edge of the corneal lesion through the center of the flap tissue. This additional suture must be placed vertical to the flap orientation to prevent vascular constriction (Figure 72.3). After the pedicle is sutured to the cornea, the scleral conjunctiva is re-apposed and sutured together. This can be done with either a simple interrupted or a continuous pattern (Figure 72.3). Some authors consider re-suturing to be an optional step. Suture ends should be short.

The corneal lesion should be covered with semitranslucent conjunctival tissue (Figure 72.4). Topical and/or systemic antibiotics and other appropriate medications should be used while the conjunctival flap is supporting the corneal lesion. After the flap has secured to the corneal lesion and when the lesion is stable and the underlying problem has resolved, the graft can be severed from the rest of the conjunctiva using sedation and topical anesthetic. Blunt scissors are slipped under the nonadherent section of the graft and the normal cornea to snip the conjunctival tissue free from the vascular supply of the donor site. The result will be an island of conjunctival tissue. This step is optional, but it leads to a more cosmetic appearance long term. This step must be postponed until the veterinary surgeon is confident

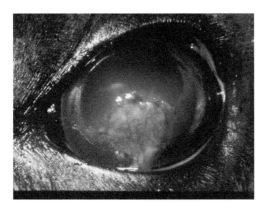

Figure 72.4 Conjunctival flap used to treat stromal abscess in llama (photo courtesy of Anne Metzler, DVM, MS, ACVO).

that the underlying corneal problem has been resolved. This step can be postponed as long as is needed or never performed at all.

Practice Tip to Facilitate Procedure

General anesthesia is used.

Potential Complications

If the flap is sutured in place under tension, the vascular supply will be compromised and the flap will necrose and dehisce. If Tenon's capsule is not adequately removed from the conjunctival flap, the graft will contract and dehisce.

Patient Monitoring/Aftercare

Routine monitoring for recovery from general anesthesia and routine monitoring of corneal lesions should be performed.

Recommended Reading and References

Gelatt K. 2007. *Veterinary Ophthalmology*, 4th Edition. Blackwell, pp. 671–675 and 707–711.

LoPinto AJ, Pirie CG, Bedenice D, et al. 2017. Corneal thickness of eyes of healthy goats, sheep, and alpacas manually measured by use of a protable spectral-domain optical coherence tomography device. *Ajvr*; 78(1):80–84.

Metzler A 2010. The Ohio State University Veterinary Teaching Hospital Ophthalmology Department. *Personal communication.*

Rodriquez-Alvaro A, Gonzalez-Alonso-Alegre EM, Delclaux-real Del Asua M, et al. 2005. Surgical correction of a corneal perforation. *J Zoo Wldlf Med*; 36(2):336–339.

Section XV

Miscellaneous

73

Blood Transfusion

Meredyth L. Jones

Purpose or Indication for Procedure

This procedure is performed to provide volume, protein, and oxygen-carrying support in cases of hypovolemia, hypoproteinemia, or anemia associated with signs of hypoxemia.

Equipment Needed

The following equipment is needed: intravenous (jugular) catheters (16- × or 14-gauge 15-cm catheter) secured in place in donor and recipient animal, acid citrate dextrose (ACD) blood collection bag, filtered administration set, and whole blood and serum from the donor and recipient for crossmatch, if desired (performed at reference laboratories). Where commercial blood bags are not available, sodium citrate (2.5–4%) and a sterile receptacle may be used.

Restraint/Position

Standing, haltered, and chute restraint may be used.

Technical Description of Procedure/Method

The donor is selected based on good general health, a packed cell volume (PCV) and total protein within the reference ranges, and a body weight similar to or greater than the recipient. Both donor and recipient should have jugular intravenous catheters placed aseptically.

Calculations should be made as to the amount of whole blood that will be administered. In the case of anemia, an ideal blood volume to be administered can be calculated when the PCV of the donor and recipient are known.

$$\text{Administration volume}(L) = \frac{\text{PCV}\begin{pmatrix} \text{desired} - \text{PCV}\,(\text{recipient}) \times \\ \text{BW of recipient }(\text{kg}) \times 0.1\,L\,/\,\text{kg} \end{pmatrix}}{\text{PCV}\,(\text{donor})}$$

Donated blood should not exceed 20% of the blood volume of the donor, which equates to about 1.5% of the donor's body weight. It is often encountered that the donor is unable to give the volume of blood that is required to achieve the desired PCV using the above formula. In these cases, if a donor of greater body weight cannot be obtained, the safe donor volume must be administered and a lower PCV achieved.

Veterinary Techniques in Llamas and Alpacas, Second Edition. Edited by David E. Anderson, Matt Miesner, and Meredyth Jones.

In the case of hypoproteinemia caused by hypoalbuminemia, hypoglobulinemia, or pan-hypoproteinemia, whole blood may also be administered where plasma is unavailable using the following formula (using albumin as the target protein):

$$\text{Administration volume}(L) = \frac{\text{Alb}\left(\begin{array}{l} \text{desired} - \text{Alb}(\text{recipient}) \times \text{BW of} \\ \text{recipient}(kg) \times 0.06\,L\,/\,kg \end{array}\right)}{\text{Alb}(\text{donor})}$$

When the collection and administration volumes are calculated, the donor is restrained in the standing position (preferably in a chute) and the catheter connected to the appropriate receptacle containing anticoagulant. The container is lowered to the ground and filled by gravity flow. In the case of commercial blood collection bags (Figure 73.1), they should be filled until turgid and rocked to assure proper mixing of the blood and anticoagulant. Where these bags are not available, any sterile receptacle may be used. Sodium citrate is added to the receptacle at a volume to create a 1:9 ratio of sodium citrate: whole blood.

After the desired volume is collected, the bag is attached to a filtered administration set (Figure 73.2) and administration to the donor initiated. The transfusion should begin at a slow rate of 5 mL/kg/hour for the first 15 to 20 minutes and the recipient monitored for signs of transfusion reaction (see Patient Monitoring below). After this time, if no abnormalities are noted, the rate may be increased to 10 mL/kg/hour for the remainder of the transfusion.

In cases where acute hemorrhage is the cause of anemia, the bleeding must be stopped prior to or during the transfusion, because the volume expansion will worsen the losses. In the case of hemolytic disease, efforts should be made to identify the cause and minimize ongoing hemolysis, as the average lifespan of transfused red blood cells is limited to 3 to 5 days. Severe anemia may be recognized during the physical examination by inspection of the mucous membranes. Extreme anemia causes a pale appearance (Figure 73.3). Assessment of the anemic patient should include examination of peripheral blood. This may allow identification of *Mycoplasma haemolamae* infection of red blood cells (Figure 73.4).

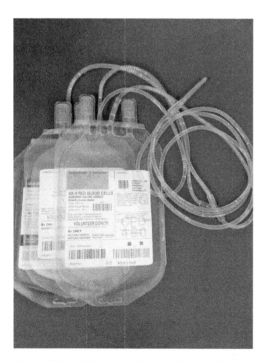

Figure 73.1 Acid citrate dextrose blood collection bags. These commercially available bags come as a set of three for separating blood components, but only one of the bags is used for whole blood collection.

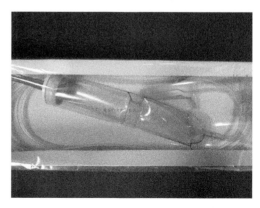

Figure 73.2 Filtered blood transfusion administration set. These should be used to prevent microscopic clots from being transfused.

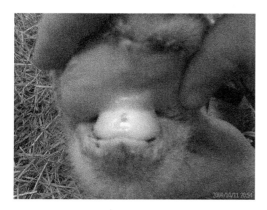

Figure 73.3 The mucous membranes of an alpaca presented for weakness and lethargy. Note the extreme pallor. This animal had a packed cell volume of 9%, was tachycardic, tachypneic, and recumbent.

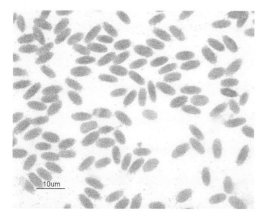

Figure 73.4 Peripheral blood smear (Wright-Giemsa) of an alpaca infected with *Candidatus Mycoplasma haemolamae*, which can result in severe hemolytic episodes. Note the blue organisms in the background of the blood film.

Practice Tip to Facilitate Procedure

It is useful to place the largest gauge catheter possible in the donor animal to facilitate rapid donation of blood.

Where sodium citrate is not readily available, heparin may be used as a substitute anticoagulant at 4.5 to 5 units heparin per 1.0 mL blood, but should be avoided in cases of hemorrhage.

Glass bottles from injectable medications may be cleaned, the mouth covered in aluminum foil or pack wrap sealed with autoclave tape and sterilized in a steam autoclave for blood transfusion. The appropriate amount of anticoagulant is added and a Bell IV (simplex) set attached with the metal injection port removed and the tubing attached to a filtered administration set.

In general, when treating for failure of passive transfer of immunoglobulin, 40 mL/kg of whole blood are administered when plasma is unavailable.

Although crossmatch is desirable in all cases of blood transfusion, it is not performed in most veterinary practices, but it is available through most reference laboratories. The time delay for laboratory testing, as well as the difficulty interpreting the test in camelid species, makes this test impractical in most situations.

Potential Complications

Blood donation is generally a very safe procedure for the donor, and few complications are seen. Hematoma or other catheter complications may occur and, rarely, the donor may show signs of hypovolemia (weakness). This appears to occur in animals that are very stressed during donation. Where there is concern for the vascular volume of the donor, a liter of a balanced intravenous fluid can be administered prior to removal of the catheter.

For the recipient, the primary concern during and after blood transfusion is that of a transfusion reaction. Transfusion reactions can range from minor urticaria to life-threatening anaphylaxis.

Patient Monitoring/Aftercare

The donor should be monitored for 2 to 3 days after blood donation for general health and appetite.

The recipient should be monitored for any evidence of transfusion reaction during and after the transfusion. Prior to initiation of the transfusion, basal temperature, pulse, and respiratory rate findings should be recorded. Signs that should be monitored for include trembling, hives, pruritis, hemoglobinuria, edema, tachypnea, tachycardia, increased rectal temperature, and collapse. If a mild reaction is noted, the transfusion should be stopped and antihistamines administered. If more severe signs occur that indicate anaphylaxis, the transfusion should be stopped and supportive therapy, perhaps including epinephrine, should be initiated.

Recommended Reading

DeWitt SF, Bedenice D, Mazan MR. 2004. Hemolysis and Heinz body formation associated with ingestion of red maple leaves in two alpacas. *J Am Vet Med Assoc*; 225(4):578–583.

Divers TJ. 2005. Blood component transfusions. *Vet Clin N Am Food Anim Pract*; 21:615–622.

Miesner MD, Anderson DE. 2006. Factor-VII deficiency in a newborn alpaca. *J Vet Intern Med*; 20:1248–1250.

Tornquist SJ. 2009. Clinical pathology of llamas and alpacas. *Vet Clin N Am Food Anim Pract*; 25(2):311–322.

Tornquist SJ, Boeder LJ, Cebra CK, et al. 2009. Use of a polymerase chain reaction assay to study response to oxytetracycline treatment in experimental *Candidatus* Mycoplasma haemolamae infection in alpacas. *Am J Vet Res*; 70:1102–1107.

74

Plasma Transfusion
Meredyth L. Jones

Purpose or Indication for Procedure

This procedure is to provide intravascular volume and protein in cases of hypovolemia, hypoalbuminemia, hypoglobulinemia, or panhypoproteinemia.

Equipment Needed

Intravenous (jugular) catheter in place in the recipient, commercial frozen plasma, and filtered administration set are needed.

Restraint/Position

Standing (chute) or cushed positions may be used.

Technical Description of Procedure/Method

Commercial llama plasma is available for use in transfusions (Figure 74.1). Volume to be thawed may be calculated by providing 20–40 mL plasma per kg of body weight. The plasma should be thawed slowly by immersion in warm water. Active heating by microwave or other means must be avoided to prevent denaturing of proteins.

The recipient should have a jugular intravenous catheter placed aseptically. The thawed plasma should be attached to a filtered administration set (Figure 74.2) and administration to the recipient initiated. The transfusion should begin at a slow rate of 5 mL/kg/hour for the first 15 to 20 minutes and the recipient monitored for signs of transfusion reaction. After this time, if no abnormalities are noted, the rate may be increased to 10 mL/kg/hour for the remainder of the transfusion.

Practice Tip to Facilitate Procedure

In sick crias, it has been shown that 2 or more units of plasma may be needed to achieve IgG levels over 1,000 mg/dL (Gerspach et al. 2007).

Potential Complications

The primary concern during and after plasma transfusion is a transfusion reaction. Transfusion reactions can range from minor urticaria to life-threatening anaphylaxis.

Plasma components may be absorbed across the peritoneum, leading many to administer plasma via abdominal catheter rather than intravenously. This technique may result in

Veterinary Techniques in Llamas and Alpacas, Second Edition. Edited by David E. Anderson, Matt Miesner, and Meredyth Jones.

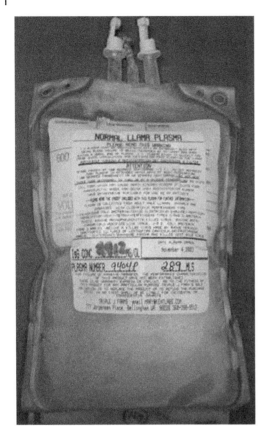

Figure 74.1 Commercially available frozen llama plasma. The total volume of plasma in each bag varies but is generally around 250–300 mL. The IgG concentration is recorded on each bag.

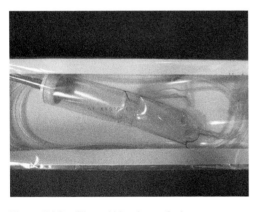

Figure 74.2 Filtered blood transfusion administration set. These should be used to prevent microscopic clots and fibrin from being transfused.

signs of colic in crias and provides a ready media for bacterial growth. The author elects to avoid this method of administration and if it is chosen, strict asepsis must be practiced.

Patient Monitoring/Aftercare

The recipient should be monitored for any evidence of transfusion reaction during and after the transfusion. Prior to initiation of the transfusion, basal temperature, pulse, and respiratory rate findings should be recorded. Signs that should be monitored for include trembling, hives, pruritis, hemoglobinuria, edema, tachypnea, tachycardia, increased rectal temperature, and collapse. If a mild reaction is noted, the transfusion should be stopped and antihistamines administered. If more severe signs occur that indicate anaphylaxis, the transfusion should be stopped and supportive therapy, perhaps including epinephrine, should be initiated.

Recommended Reading

Divers TJ. 2005. Blood component transfusions. *Vet Clin N Am Food Anim Pract*; 21:615–622.

Dolente BA, Lindborg S, Palmer JE, et al. 2007. Culturepositive sepsis in neonatal camelids: 21 cases. *J Vet Intern Med*; 21:519–525.

Gerspach C, Varga A, Niehaus A, et al. 2007. Serum IgG Concentrations in crias: how much is enough? *In: Proceedings of the American College of Veterinary Internal Medicine Forum*, Seattle, WA.

Sharpe MS, Lord LK, Wittum TE, et al. 2009. Pre-weaning morbidity and mortality of llamas and alpacas. *Aust Vet J*; 87:56–60.

Tornquist SJ. 2009. Clinical pathology of llamas and alpacas. *Vet Clin N Am Food Anim Pract*; 25(2):311–322.

Whitehead CE. 2009a. Management of neonatal llamas and alpacas. *Vet Clin N Am Food Anim Pract*; 25(2):353–356.

Whitehead CE. 2009b. Neonatal diseases in llamas and alpacas. *Vet Clin N Am Food Anim Pract*; 25(2):367–384.

Index

Note: Page numbers followed by "*f*" refer to figures and "*t*" refer to tables.

Veterinary Techniques in Llamas and Alpacas, Second Edition. Edited by David E. Anderson, Matt Miesner, and Meredyth Jones.
© 2023 John Wiley & Sons, Inc. Published 2023 by John Wiley & Sons, Inc.